Diffuse

Diseases

of

the

Lung

W.M. Thurlbeck, M.B., FRCPC
Professor of Pathology, University of British Columbia
Pathologist, British Columbia's Children's Hospital
Consultant Pathologist, University Hospital, Vancouver, British Columbia

Roberta R. Miller, M.D., FRCPC
Consultant Pathologist, Vancouver General Hospital
Clinical Associate Professor of Pathology and Associate Member
Division of Respiratory Medicine
University of British Columbia, Vancouver, British Columbia

Nestor L. Müller, M.D., FRCPC
Associate Professor of Radiology, University of British Columbia
Director of Chest Radiology, Vancouver General Hospital
Vancouver, British Columbia

Edward C. Rosenow III, M.D.
Arthur M. and Gladys D. Gray Professor of Medicine
and Chairman, Thoracic Division,
Mayo Medical School, Rochester, Minnesota

Diffuse Diseases of the Lung

A Team Approach

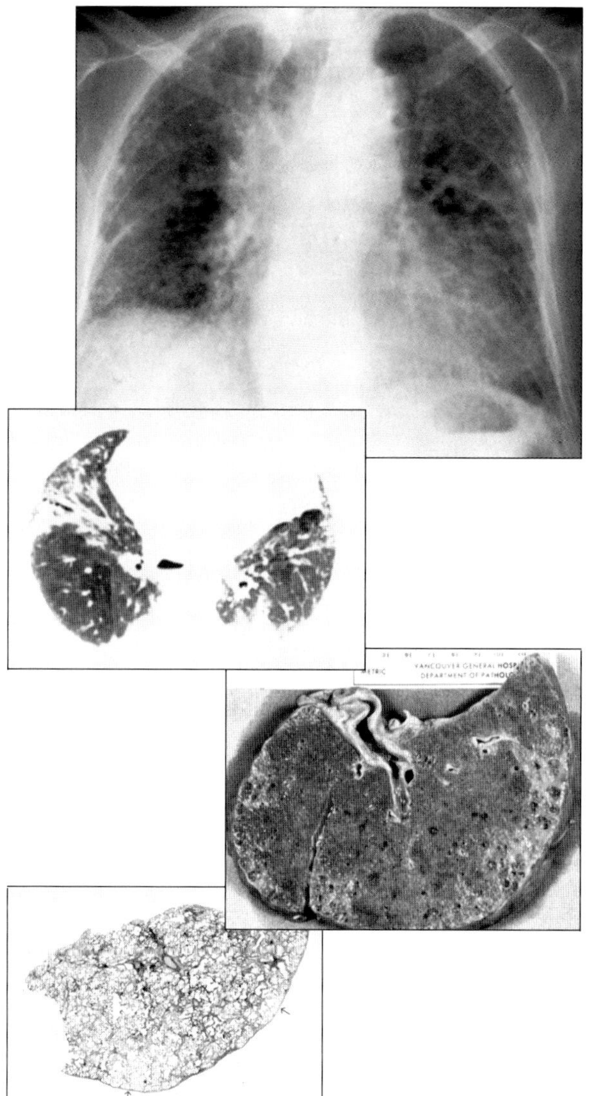

B.C. Decker

Philadelphia

Publisher

B.C. Decker
320 Walnut Street
Suite 400
Philadelphia, Pennsylvania 19106

Sales and Distribution

United States and Puerto Rico
Mosby–Year Book Inc.
11830 Westline Industrial Drive
Saint Louis, Missouri 63146

Canada
Mosby–Year Book Limited
5240 Finch Avenue E., Unit 1
Scarborough, Ontario M1S 5A2

Australia
**McGraw-Hill Book Company Australia
Pty. Ltd.**
4 Barcoo Street
Roseville East 2069
New South Wales, Australia

Brazil
Editora McGraw-Hill do Brasil, Ltda.
rua Tabapua, 1.105, Itaim-Bibi
Sao Paulo, S.P. Brasil

Colombia
**Interamericana/McGraw-Hill de
Colombia, S.A.**
Carrera 17, No. 33-71
(Apartado Postal, A.A., 6131)
Bogota, D.E., Colombia

*Europe, United Kingdom, Middle East
and Africa*
Wolfe Publishing Limited
Brook House
2-16 Torrington Place
London WC1E 7LT England

Hong Kong and China
McGraw-Hill Book Company
Suite 618, Ocean Centre
5 Canton Road
Tsimshatsui, Kowloon
Hong Kong

India
Tata McGraw-Hill Publishing Company, Ltd.
12/4 Asaf Ali Road, 3rd Floor
New Delhi 110002, India

Indonesia
Mr. Wong Fin Fah
P.O. Box 122/JAT
Jakarta, 1300 Indonesia

Japan
Igaku-Shoin Ltd.
Tokyo International P.O. Box 5063
1-28-36 Hongo, Bunkyo-ku,
Tokyo 113, Japan

Korea
Mr. Don-Gap Choi
C.P.O. Box 10583
Seoul, Korea

Malaysia
Mr. Lim Tao Slong
No. 8 Jalan SS 7/6B
Kelana Jaya
47301 Petaling Jaya
Selangor, Malaysia

Mexico
**Interamericana/McGraw-Hill de Mexico, S.A.
de C.V.**
Cedro 512, Colonia Atlampa
(Apartado Postal 26370)
06450 Mexico, D.F., Mexico

New Zealand
McGraw-Hill Book Co. New Zealand Ltd.
5 Joval Place, Wiri
Manukau City, New Zealand

Portugal
Editora McGraw-Hill de Portugal, Ltda.
Rua Rosa Damasceno 11A-B
1900 Lisboa, Portugal

Singapore and Southeast Asia
McGraw-Hill Book Co.
21 Neythal Road
Jurong, Singapore 2262

South Africa
Libriger Book Distributors
Warehouse Number 8
"Die Ou Looiery"
Tannery Road
Hamilton, Bloemfontein 9300

Spain
McGraw-Hill/Interamericana de Espana, S.A.
Manuel Ferrero, 13
28020 Madrid, Spain

Taiwan
Mr. George Lim
P.O. Box 87-601
Taipei, Taiwan

Thailand
Mr. Vitit Lim
632/5 Phaholyothin Road
Sapan Kwai
Bangkok 10400
Thailand

Venezuela
Editorial Interamerica de Venezuela, C.A.
2da. calle Bello Monte
Local G-2
Caracas, Venezuela

NOTICE

The authors and publisher have made every effort to ensure that the patient care recommended herein, including choice of drugs and drug dosages, is in accord with the accepted standards and practice at the time of publication. However, since research and regulation constantly change clinical standards, the reader is urged to check the product information sheet included in the package of each drug, which includes recommended doses, warnings, and contraindications. This is particularly important with new or infrequently used drugs.

Diffuse Diseases of the Lung: A Team Approach

ISBN 1-55664-197-4

Library of Congress catalog card number: 90-83571

10 9 8 7 6 5 4 3 2 1

Preface

This book is the product of two unlikely parents. Two of us (RRM, WMT) contributed a chapter entitled "Diffuse Diseases of the Lungs" in Steve Silverberg's *Principles and Practice of Surgical Pathology* (2nd Ed, Churchill Livingstone 1990). While we were pleased with our product, it had a number of defects; it was written with only practicing surgical pathologists in mind and had no radiologic and little clinical information, and it also suffered from understandable space and illustration constraints. The other parent is the weekly Chest Rounds at the Vancouver General Hospital, where two of the authors (RRM, NLM) are active participants and another (WMT) is an enthusiastic observer. The observer's enthusiasm is derived from the fact that actual active cases are discussed. These are chosen with no preparation ahead of time, and they represent spontaneous presentation of cases. What was apparent to the observer was the high degree of interaction between internist, surgeon, radiologist, and pathologist and that each member of the team knew the details of all the aspects of the case, not merely from his or her particular discipline.

Both surgical and medical cases are discussed in this book, but the need for intermember team cooperation is most apparent in the case of biopsy for diffuse lung disease. We had difficulty selecting the title because, for example, emphysema and pulmonary edema are diffuse lung diseases, as are some pleural diseases. We did not wish to limit the content to infiltrative or interstitial lung disease. Further, neither of these terms is suitably precise. What the conditions presented here have in common is that they frequently come to biopsy for diagnostic purposes.

The outcome and the diagnosis depend very much on interdepartmental cooperation. Because the site of the lung biopsy is usually dictated by computed tomography, the surgeon must be aware of the findings so that he or she can take a representative and adequate biopsy or biopsies. The pathologist in the final analysis needs to know the clinical data. For example, a previously known lymphoma or malignant tumor (and its site) may be important information. The internist must be able to understand the limitations of biopsy diagnosis in general and, in that case, in particular. Hence the subtitle "A Team Approach." In this monograph all authors have contributed to and edited all chapters and have worked interactively on many occasions.

It became apparent that there was a danger of parochialism because of the close communication among authors associated with the same institution. Therefore, we believe that the contributions of a distinguished chest physician (ECR, III) from another institution with a somewhat different attitude and type of practice would be welcome. The difference is best illustrated in the handling of open lung biopsies in the immunocompromised host, where the Mayo Clinic approach is to follow a specific protocol. In contrast, the approach at Vancouver General Hospital is more individualistic depending on the pathologist's knowledge of the clinical, radiologic, and gross findings in the case. Also, all the biopsies are handled by one pathologist.

The monograph starts with a series of chapters on normal structure, function, and imaging, followed by sections on "how to" or practical background information. Then the topics are presented in chapters based primarily on clinical groupings. As indicated in the various chapters, it is not possible to impose a rigid division of all diseases into special chapters and within this caveat we have done our best.

William M. Thurlbeck, M.B., FRCP(C)

Contents

CHAPTER 1

NORMAL STRUCTURE AND FUNCTION OF THE LUNG

This chapter describes the normal histology relevant to the subject of this book, arbitrarily considered to be that of bronchioles, the gas-exchanging units of the lung, and the pulmonary vessels. The review is brief; excellent, more extensive reviews of lung structure are available (Breeze and Wheeldon, 1976; Kuhn, 1976, 1978, 1988; Reid, 1979).

Bronchi are defined as airways that have cartilage in their walls; the airways distal to them, without alveoli in their walls, are referred to as membranous bronchioles or, simply, bronchioles. Bronchioles have an irregular dichotomous branching pattern, except for their distal three orders, which show regular dichotomy (Horsfield and Cumming, 1968). An important feature is that while each succeeding generation has a smaller diameter than the preceding one, the total cross-sectional area increases with succeeding generations (Weibel, 1963), since the daughter bronchioles are more than half the diameter of the parent one (Fig. 1-1). It is this increase in total cross-sectional area, which becomes rapid distally, that accounts for the fact that there is little resistance to flow in the peripheral airways (see "Chronic Airflow Obstruction," chapter 12). Bronchiolar mucosa lacks the compound mucus-secreting subepithelial glands so characteristic of bronchi. The lining epithelium of the largest bronchioles when fully distended loses some of the pseudostratified appearance of bronchi (Fig. 1-2). The great majority of the cells lining the bronchioles are ciliated cells (see Fig. 1-2). Their nuclei are basal, rather square in shape, and are arranged in a single row in the smaller bronchioles and mostly pseudostratified in larger bronchioles. Scattered basal cells with elongated nuclei lie deep to the nuclei of the ciliated cells (see Fig. 1-2). Mucus-secreting cells are extremely scanty in nonsmokers. When these cells are distended with mucus they are referred to as goblet cells (Fig. 1-3).

Neuroendocrine cells ("K cells," Kulchitsky cells) of the lung occur either singly or in clusters, the latter generally referred to as neuroepithelial bodies. With hematoxylin and eosin (H&E) staining, these cells have a clear or slightly eosinophilic cytoplasm; with appropriate silver stains, they may be argyrophilic. They are considerably more numerous in fetal lungs than adult lungs and are distributed mostly in the epithelium of subsegmental bronchi. They are a part of the APUD (*Amine Precursor Uptake and Decarboxylation*) cell system throughout the body and ultrastructurally contain characteristic dense core cytoplasmic granules. Normally they may be shown to contain gastrin-releasing peptide (bombesin), leu-enkephalin, calcitonin, serotonin, and neuron-specific enolase, although the precise role of these substances in the regulation of growth,

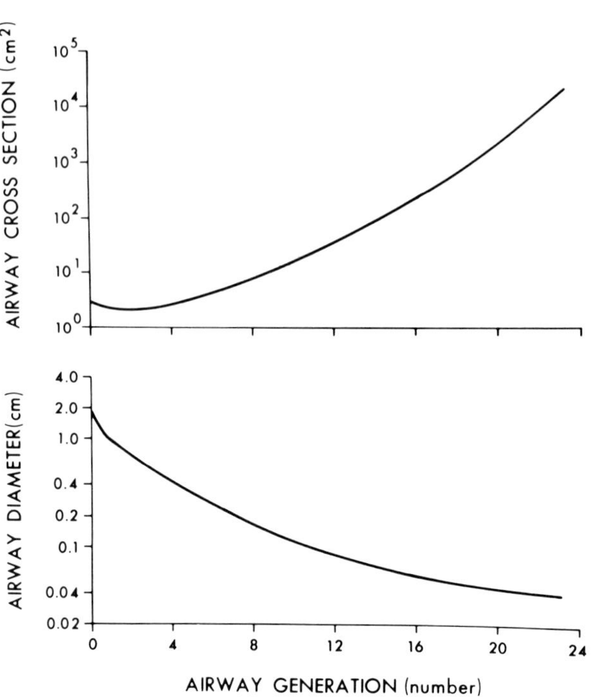

Figure 1–1   The cross-sectional area of individual generations (*bottom*) and the summed cross-sectional area of generations (*top*) are shown. In this model generation 0 is the trachea, and symmetric dichotomy is assumed. Proceeding peripherally, the total cross-sectional area increases dramatically (note that the cross-sectional area is expressed on a logarithmic scale). The end of the bronchial tree corresponds approximately to generation 7 and terminal bronchioles are generation 16. (Reprinted with permission from Weibel ER. Morphometry of the human lung. Berlin: Springer Verlag, 1963.)

development, and gas exchange is still uncertain. Carcinoid tumors and small-cell carcinomas show differentiation toward neuroendocrine cells. In addition to bombesin and other indigenous peptides, hormones, such as ACTH and antidiuretic hormone (ADH), which are not demonstrable in normal lung epithelium may also be produced by these tumors. (Gail and Lenfant, 1983; Gould et al, 1983).

The columnar, nonciliated secretory cell (Clara cell) is inconspicuous in humans compared with small laboratory animals. Characteristically, the cells are taller than other epithelial cells, projecting into the lumen of the bronchioles. The function of these cells is not known with certainty. Some consider them to be the major source of pulmonary surfactant. Others consider them to secrete the hypophase of protein and liquid on which surfactant lies. In laboratory animals, Clara cells are the progenitor cells of the

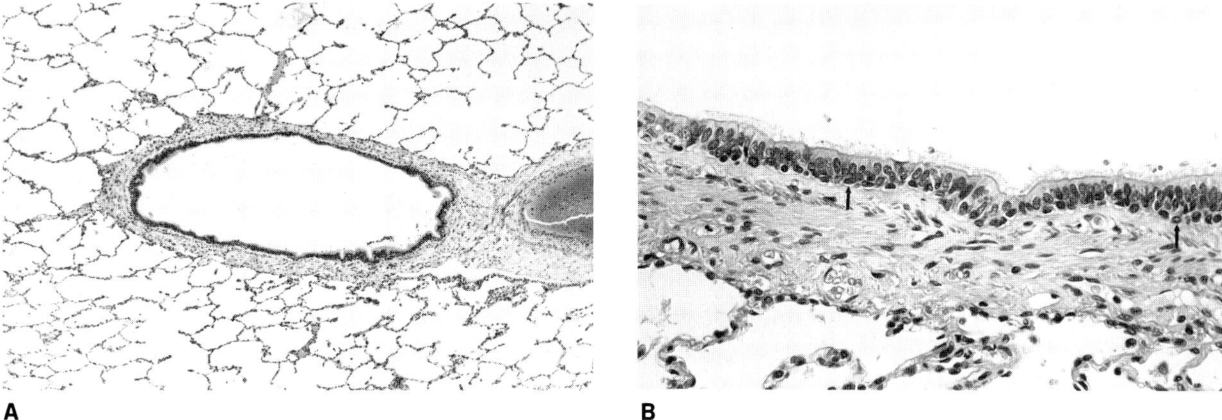

A   **B**

Figure 1–2   Large (membranous) bronchiole, approximately 2 mm in diameter. *A*, Cartilage and compound mucus-secreting glands are not present in the walls of the bronchiole (H&E, × 63). *B*, Most of the cells of the epithelium are ciliated. Flattened basal cell nuclei are also seen (*arrows*). Mucus-secreting (goblet) and nonciliated columnar (Clara) cells are not apparent. The basal lamina is thin (H&E, × 400).

bronchioles and may differentiate into other Clara cells, ciliated cells, or mucus-secreting cells. The epithelial basal lamina is very thin (see Fig. 1-2), and it is the collagen associated with the basal lamina that makes the basement membrane visible by light microscopy. An elastic tissue net is closely applied to the basal lamina (Fig. 1-4). The muscle of the bronchioles is arranged in a geodesic pattern, which in smaller bronchioles leads to an appearance of an incomplete muscular layer (see Fig. 1-4). A few mononuclear inflammatory cells are present in most bronchioles, but even a modest collection of cells and any neutrophils should be regarded as abnormal. Outside of the muscular layer the arteries and bronchioles share a common adventitia. There is loose

connective tissue outside this, forming part of the lung interstitium. The surrounding connective tissue becomes progressively more scanty in the smallest bronchioles.

The last purely conducting bronchiole, without alveoli in its walls, is the terminal bronchiole. Distal to it is the gas-exchanging unit of the lung, known as the acinus. In order, it comprises respiratory bronchioles, alveolar ducts, and sacs. Respiratory bronchioles have both alveolated and nonalveolated walls (Fig. 1-5). Nonalveolated walls have epithelium like that of bronchioles, except that the cells are flatter. The majority of the cells are still ciliated. There is a relatively abrupt transition between the ciliated cells and flattened epithelium, resembling that of the

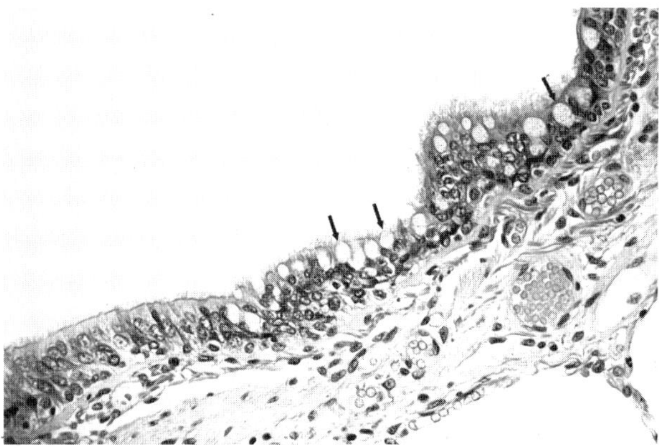

Figure 1–3   Bronchiole comparable in size to Figure 1–2 from a cigarette smoker. Note goblet cells (*arrows*) (H&E, × 400).

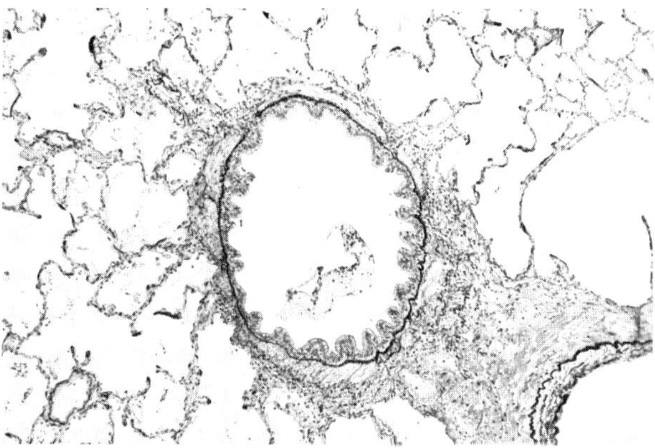

Figure 1–4   Subepithelial elastic layer is closely adherent to the epithelium, with underlying interrupted smooth muscle (VVG, × 100).

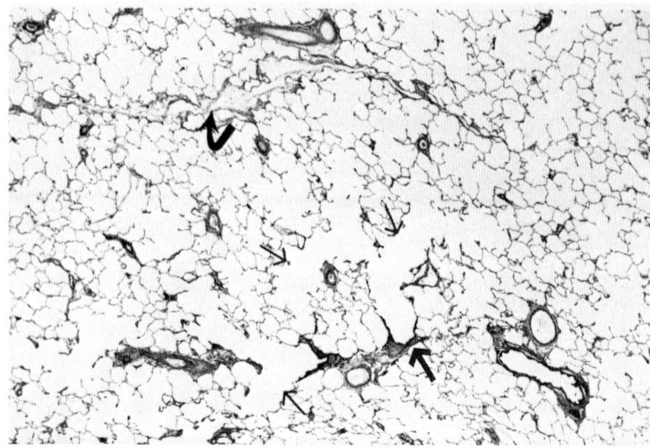

Figure 1–5 Acinus, showing respiratory bronchioles (*large arrow*), alveolar ducts (*small arrows*), and lobular septum (*curved arrow*) (H&E, × 25).

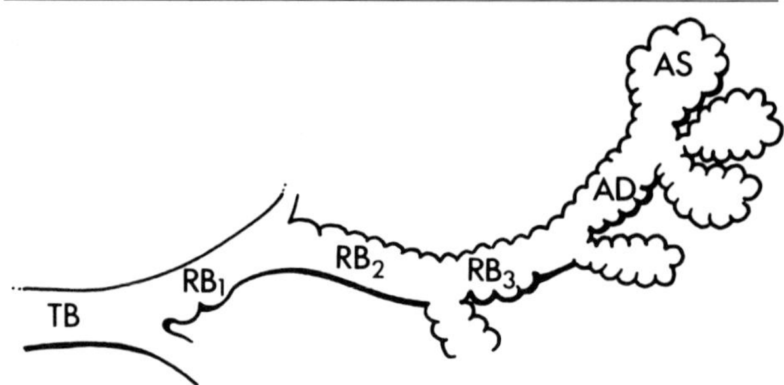

Figure 1–6 Diagrammatic representation of the acinus shows the terminal bronchiole (TB); three orders of respiratory bronchioles (RB) with increasing numbers of alveoli in their walls; a single order of alveolar duct (AD), whose wall is entirely alveolated; and the terminal structure, the alveolar sac (AS).

alveoli. A simplified model of the acinus is shown in Figure 1-6. Respiratory bronchioles have more alveoli in their walls in succeeding generations and are succeeded by alveolar ducts, entirely alveolated conducting structures. The terminal unit of the acinus is the alveolar sac, which is likewise entirely alveolated. The acinus is important as the gas-exchanging unit of the lung, and it is this structure that is enlarged and its walls destroyed in emphysema.

A traditional structural unit of the lung is the lobule. Sheets of connective tissue containing veins and lymphatics subdivide the lung into macroscopic units, and the smallest units surrounded by (lobular) septa are referred to as lobules. The problem is that lobular septa are quite variable in extent, being more obvious in the upper lobe than the lower lobe and more obvious in infants than adults (Fig. 1-7). Also there are quite considerable differences between individuals. Thus the size of lobules is variable and different lobules contain different numbers of acini. While the boundaries of lobules are easier to identify morphologically (i.e., interlobular septa), the acinus is a more useful unit.

The surface of human alveoli is lined by type-I and type-II epithelial cells. The majority of the surface is covered by the thin, greatly extended cytoplasm of type-I epithelial cells, which contain few organelles. There are actually more type-II epithelial cells but, because they are columnar, they cover only about 5 percent of the surface of the alveoli. They are characteristically situated in the angles of the alveoli and are thus sometimes called corner cells or niche cells. They contain large numbers of organelles and the characteristic osmiophilic lamellar bodies (Fig. 1-8), which, when secreted into the alveolus, constitute the surface-active material essential for alveolar stability. Type-II cells have another vital function, that of being the progenitor cell of alveolar epithelium. They have the ability to divide and produce two type-II cells; this happens during lung development and following injury. Alternatively they can divide to form one type-II cell and one type-I cell; this is a normal process in mature lungs and in the recovery phase of lung injury. Type-I and type-II cells are joined by tight junctions and thus represent the major barrier to passage of large molecules from the capillary lumen to the airspace.

Alveolar macrophages play a major role in the lung's defense mechanism, but the source of these cells is controversial. Some consider that they are mainly derived from the monocytes of the bone marrow and undergo a maturation division in the alveolar interstitium before passing into the airspaces.

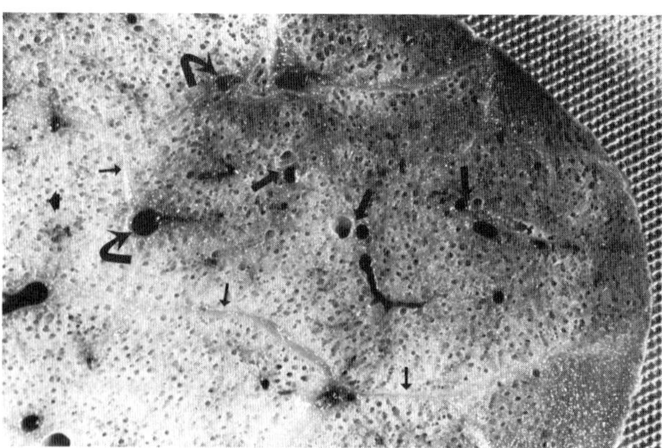

Figure 1–7 Gross view of lobules, showing centrilobular bronchovascular structures (*large arrows*), septa (*small arrows*) and veins within septa (*curved arrows*).

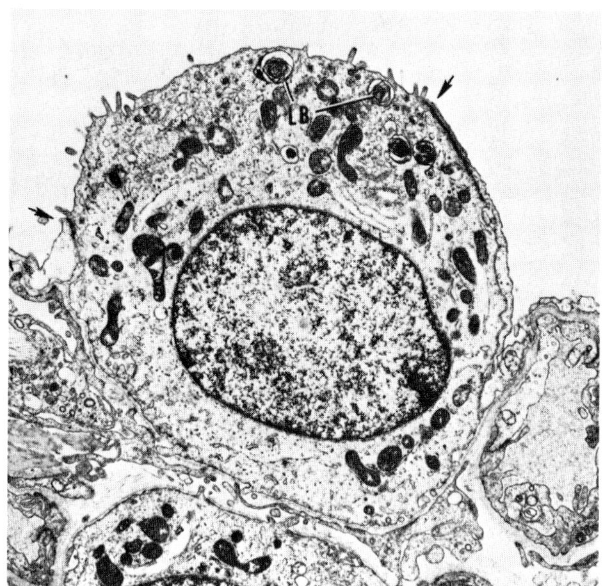

Figure 1–8 A type-II cell contains many lamellar bodies (LB). The type-II cell is partially covered by extensions of type-I cells, extending up to the intercellular junctions (*arrows*). Microvilli are present on the exposed apical surface. (Reprinted with permission from Kuhn C III. Normal anatomy and histology. In Thurlbeck WM, ed. Pathology of the lung. New York: Thieme, 1988.)

Considerable multiplication of alveolar macrophages also may occur within airspaces especially in the neonatal period (Evans et al, 1987). They differ from peritoneal macrophages in that alveolar macrophages are more dependent on aerobic metabolism.

The alveolar wall contains capillaries, collagen fibers, elastic fibers, glycosaminoglycans, and interstitial cells. The latter include mast cells, smooth muscle cells, occasional lymphocytes, pericytes, and connective tissue cells. The last type of cells are usually referred to as fibroblasts, but they appear quiescent and have few organelles. Bundles of filaments identified as actin and myosin have been noted in these cells, and it has been suggested that they may have a contractile role and may control perfusion in the lung. Capillary endothelial cells are joined by tight or "semitight" junctions. The latter are relatively sparse but permit the passage of large molecules. Endothelial cells are metabolically active and metabolize serotonin, norepinephrine, acetylcholine, adenine monophosphate, adenine triphosphate, bradykinin, angiotensin I, very low density lipoproteins, and prostaglandins E_1, E_2, and F_2. Cells of the alveoli differ in their susceptibility to injury. The type-I cell is the most sensitive, with damage leading to increased permeability and alveolar edema. The capillary endothelial cells are the next most sensi-

tive, followed by the type-II cell. The alveolar wall has a "thin" and a "thick" side (Fig. 1–9). On the thin side the basal lamina of epithelial cells and that of endothelial cells fuse, and gas exchange is most easily accomplished here. On the thick side the basal laminae are separate, and in this space lies another part of the interstitium of the lung with the components noted above. There is a single capillary layer in the alveolar wall, with capillaries winding from one side of the alveolar wall to the other.

The pulmonary arterial tree is a high-capacitance system, with the resistance vessels being the muscular pulmonary arteries. These arteries accompany the airways, and it is usual to refer to this arrangement together with the common adventitia as the bronchovascular bundle. Age-dependent structural differences exist in the pulmonary arterial system, with increased intimal thickening occurring with age. In the adult, the elastic arteries (Fig. 1–10A), which have more than two elastic laminae, are larger than 1000 μm in diameter, whereas arteries between 100 and 200 μm are muscular, in which the muscle is enclosed by an internal and an external elastic lamina (Fig. 1–10B). Smaller vessels may be muscular, partially muscular (when the muscle is spirally arranged around the vessel so that parts of the wall appear muscular and parts nonmuscular), and nonmuscular. The two elastic laminae fuse where muscle is absent, and a single fragmented elastic lamina separates the intima from the adventitia (Fig. 1–10C). The term "pulmonary arteriole" (arterial vessels less

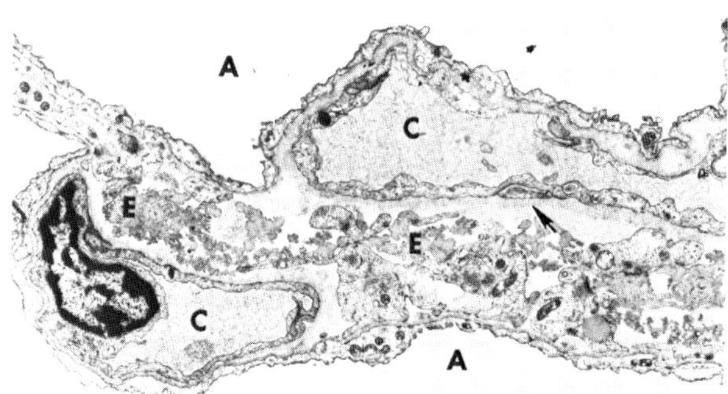

Figure 1–9 Electron micrograph of alveolar wall showing alveolar space (A), capillary (C), and elastic tissue (E). Note that the basal lamina of endothelium and epithelium are joined on the thin side of the alveolar wall (*top right*). On the thick side of the alveolar wall the basal lamina of the capillary (*arrow*) is separated from the basal lamina of a type-I epithelial cell (*lower right*). In the space, elastic tissue can be seen as well as cytoplasm of an interstitial cell. (Reprinted with permission from Kuhn C III. Normal anatomy and histology. In Thurlbeck WM, ed. Pathology of the lung. New York: Thieme, 1988.)

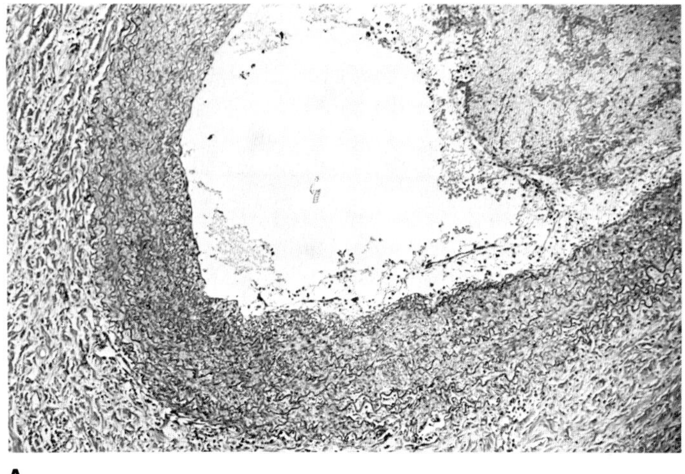

A

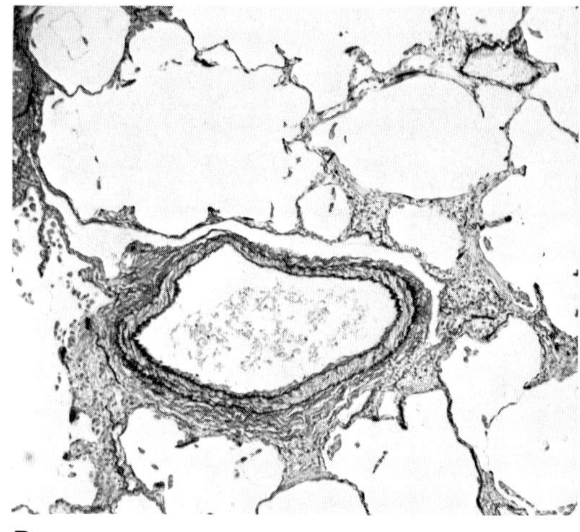

B

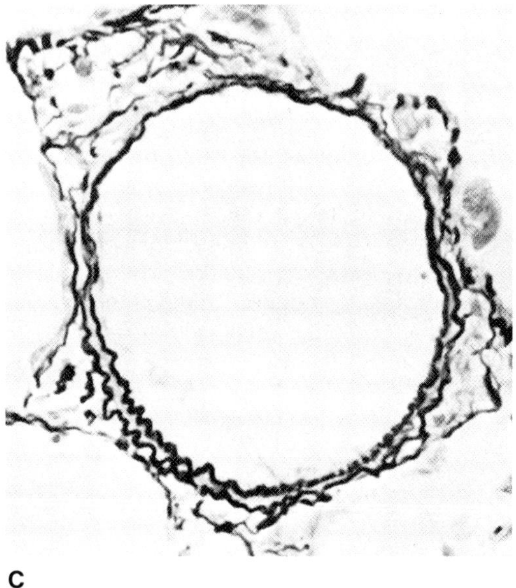

C

Figure 1–10   Varieties of pulmonary arteries. *A*, Large elastic artery with multiple elastic laminae (H&E, × 100). *B*, Large muscular pulmonary artery (VVG, × 100). *C*, Transverse section of a small pulmonary artery. The lower half of the circumference has a muscular media, but the rest has a single elastic lamina. (Elastic Van Gieson, × 420). (Reprinted with permission from Kuhn C III. Normal anatomy and histology. In Thurlbeck WM, ed. Pathology of the lung. New York: Thieme, 1988.)

than 100 μm in diameter) has become obsolete. The appearance, in terms of vessel size, is surprisingly similar in adults, children, and fetuses (Reid, 1979), but this is because vessels of similar size represent different generations of artery in infants compared with adults. When compared by position in the lung, the structure of vessels is quite different at different ages. In the fetus and soon after birth, the intra-acinar arteries are all nonmuscular. There is increasing muscularity of the intra-acinar arteries during childhood, but even at age 11 this process is not complete, with muscle extending only to the level of the alveolar ducts. In the adult, arterial muscle reaches as far as the alveoli. The ratio of arterial wall thickness to external arterial diameter is a useful parameter to assess abnormality, but it should be noted that the values for arteries distended with contrast medium are lower when high pressures are used to distend the vessel. In undistended muscular arteries, the ratio of medial thickness to external arterial diameter is about 5 percent (3 to 7 percent).

Pulmonary veins commence at the distal end of alveolar capillaries and proceed in the interstitium of the lung toward the lobular septa. Small pulmonary veins are indistinguishable from nonmuscular pulmonary arteries by histology, but the distinction can be made by the juxta-airway position of pulmonary arteries. The veins drain centrally in the septa and then form larger structures that lie separate from arteries and airways. The walls of veins are much thinner than arteries and, in general, have a single, poorly formed external elastic lamina and no muscle

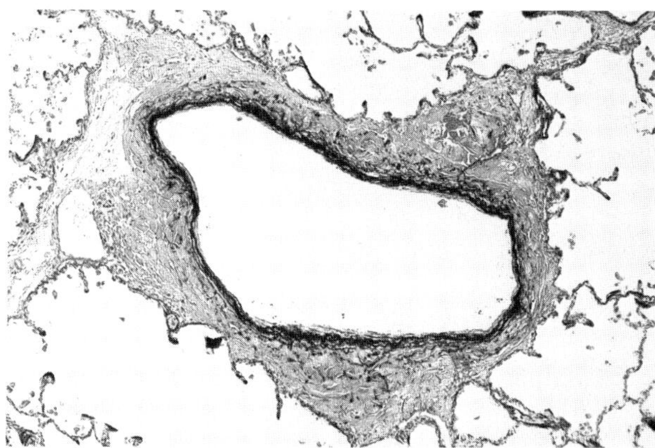

Figure 1–11   Medium-sized pulmonary vein with several incomplete elastic laminae, and virtually no muscle (VVG, × 100).

(Fig. 1–11). Larger veins may contain more than one elastic lamina, also poorly formed; muscle is scanty.

Bronchial arteries arise from the aorta or the intercostobrachial trunk, and course with the airways and pulmonary arteries in the bronchovascular tree. They are usually two to four in number. The bronchial arteries have the structure of systemic arteries, i.e., have a relatively thick media and supply the structures in the interstitium. The bronchial arteries extend as far as the terminal bronchiole and then anastomose with branches of the pulmonary artery at this point and beyond. Bronchial veins arise from the bronchial capillaries and drain into the bronchovascular bundle to join the azygos and hemiazygos veins. The bronchial vessels that have precapillary, capillary and postcapillary anastomoses with the pulmonary arteries drain into the pulmonary vein. The bronchial arteries also supply the medial and diaphragmatic visceral pleura and the tracheal, carinal, hilar, and intrapulmonary lymph nodes.

Pulmonary lymphatics are not present between alveolar walls but start where alveoli are juxtaposed to lobular septa and the bronchovascular bundles. These vessels have walls that are quite thin with a lining of endothelial cells lying on a basal lamina, embedded in a loose connective-tissue matrix. They contain valves that direct the flow of lymph. Lymphatics proceed centrally with the bronchovascular tree, in lobular septa and with veins, and also to the pleural surface. Pleural lymphatics course in the visceral pleura and send numerous connections into the interior of the lung to anastomose with perivenous lymphatics.

The interstitium of the lung is an important concept (Fig. 1–12). It has never been officially defined, but our understanding is that it is tissue between structures concerned with gas exchange. It is thus the loose connective tissue outside airways and arter-

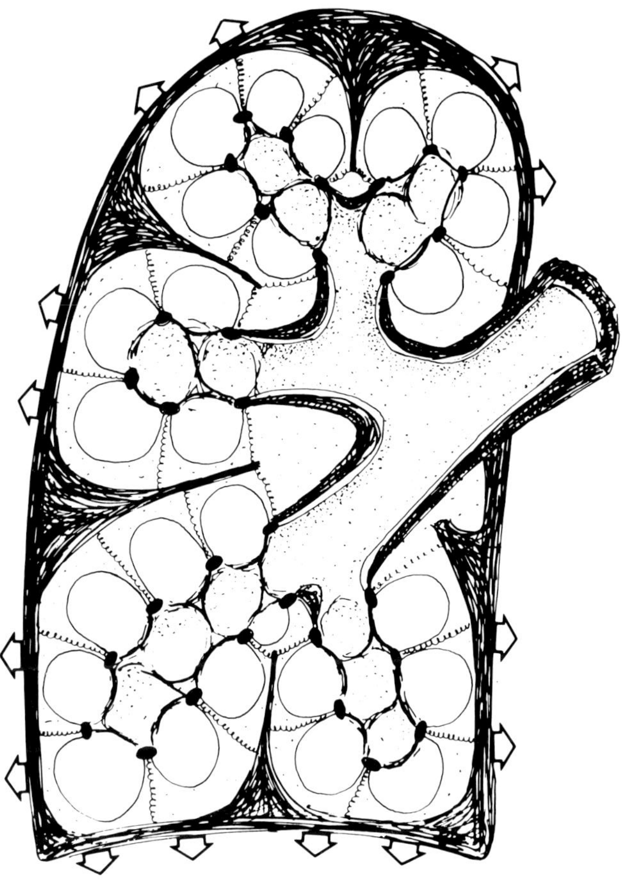

Figure 1–12   The interstitium of the lung represents a continuum of connective tissue. It extends around airways (and arteries) to the walls of alveoli, represented as circles. In addition, the interstitium extends from alveolar walls to lobular septa (deep indentations from pleura), in which veins are found in the pleura. Lymphatics are also found in the interstitium which has its blood supply from the bronchial arteries. (Reprinted with permission from Weibel ER, Gil J. Structure-function relationships at the alveolar level. In West JB, ed. Bioengineering aspects of the lung. New York: Marcel Dekker, 1977.)

ies, outside veins and lymphatics, and the tissue between the capillary and epithelium on the thick side of the alveolar wall.

RADIOLOGY

Chest Radiograph

A properly exposed chest radiograph allows visualization of small blood vessels in the lung periphery, and faint visualization of the intervertebral disk spaces, ribs, and blood vessels behind the heart. As any degree of rotation will result in changes in density of one lung as compared with the other, the position of the patient should be assessed. On a well-centered radiograph, the medial aspect of the clavicles is equidistant to the spinous processes. Provided that the individual is not rotated, normally the density of the right lung is similar to that of the left.

Analysis of the chest radiograph may be made by a free global search, a directed search, or preferably a combination of both methods (Fraser et al, 1988). Up to 70 percent of abnormalities can be detected within 0.2 second by a global overview, or gestalt, of the radiograph (Kundel and Nodine, 1975). However, detection of more subtle abnormalities requires an orderly, directed search that includes analysis of the extrathoracic soft tissues, bony thorax, diaphragm, pleura, mediastinum, as well as the lungs. The lungs are inspected most easily by comparing right and left lungs from apex to base. Approximately 15 percent of the lung is hidden behind the diaphragm and the cardiothoracic structures.

On the normal radiograph, the visualized shadows in the lung parenchyma are made up almost exclusively by the pulmonary vessels. The right hilar vessels are 1 to 3 cm lower than the left hilum in 97 percent of individuals and seem to extend farther out than the left because a portion of the left hilum is obscured by the heart. The vessels branch and taper, and on high-quality radiographs may be seen to extend to the periphery of the lungs. The pulmonary circulation is a low-pressure system, the vessel walls being thin and readily distensible. Because the pulmonary arterial pressure is low, blood flow to the different lung regions is markedly influenced by changes in posture. In the upright individual, there is a gradient in hydrostatic pressure of approximately 30 cm H_2O from the lung apices to the lung bases. As a consequence, the blood flow to the bases is normally severalfold greater than that to the apices. On the radiograph, the increased hydrostatic pressure is reflected by the greater caliber of the lower-lobe vessels as compared with that of the upper-lobe vessels. In the supine individual, although flow to the upper lobe increases, because of the larger anteroposterior diameter in the lung bases, blood flow and blood-vessel diameter are still greater in the lower lobes.

Apart from the interlobar pulmonary arteries, the superior and inferior pulmonary veins, and perhaps their major branches, it is usually not possible to determine which of these vessels are arteries and which are veins. This, however, is not of much consequence, as arteries and veins usually change in caliber equally (Trapnell, 1983). Thus, in left-sided heart failure, the prominent upper-lobe vessels do not represent "engorged veins" but rather redistribution of blood flow to the upper lobes.

Apart from the vessels, the only normal structures seen are the major bronchi and interlobar fissures. The walls of the segmental bronchi are often seen end-on and are normally about 1 mm thick.

The normal interstitium, including the interlobular septa, is not visualized.

Computed Tomography

Computed tomography (CT) scan images should be analyzed systematically, taking into consideration the findings on the images immediately above and below. As on the radiograph, the main structures seen on CT are the pulmonary vessels (Fig. 1–13). Vessels equal to or greater than 0.8 mm in diameter can be clearly visualized (Zerhouni et al, 1985). Bronchi are much better seen on CT than on the radiograph. The lobar and segmental bronchi coursing vertically or horizontally are clearly identified. Their walls normally measure approximately 1 mm in thickness. Subsegmental bronchi can often be seen as small lucencies adjacent to pulmonary arteries. The middle lobe and lingular bronchi course obliquely and are well seen on routine 1-cm collimation scans in about 75 percent of patients, but can be visualized in almost all individuals with 1.5-mm collimation scans.

The major fissures appear on 10-mm collimation scans as white lines or as ill-defined bands of increased or decreased density (Frija et al, 1982). On 1.5-mm collimation scans, they are almost always seen as thin white lines. The minor fissure is seen as

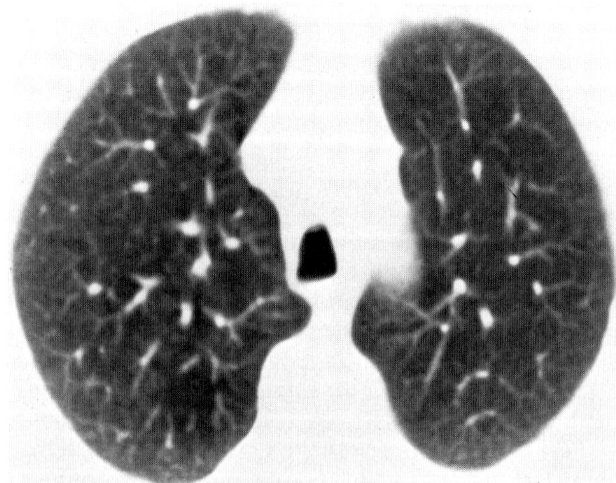

Figure 1–13   Normal 10-mm collimation CT scan through the upper lobes. The vessels can be seen as branching structures.

a hypovascular triangle, circle, or oval on 10-mm collimation scans and as a white line on 1.5-mm scans.

There is normally a density (attenuation) gradient between lung apex and base, and between dependent and nondependent portions of lung related to the influence of gravity on blood flow. Often a localized band of increased density is seen in the dependent lung. The nature of this is not clear, but presumably it is related to airway closure. These gravity-dependent changes can hinder the assessment of subtle parenchymal abnormalities. The problem can be solved, however, by rescanning the area of interest with the patient prone.

CT scans are routinely done using 10-mm collimation. This leads to volume averaging of the structures within that thickness and allows for clear identification of vessels as they course through the thickness of the slice and thus, usually, easy distinction of vessels from nodules (see Fig. 1–13). However, volume averaging also results in lower spatial resolution. Therefore, in the assessment of diffuse lung disease, the conventional CT should be supplemented with 1.5-mm collimation scans (thin-section CT). These images may be further optimized by using a high-spatial-frequency reconstruction algorithm ("bone algorithm" on the GE 9800 scanner) and a smaller field of view. The bone algorithm and the smaller field of view improve the spatial resolution and give a sharper image (Fig. 1–14). These high-resolution images, known as high-resolution CT scans, allow identification of smaller parenchymal

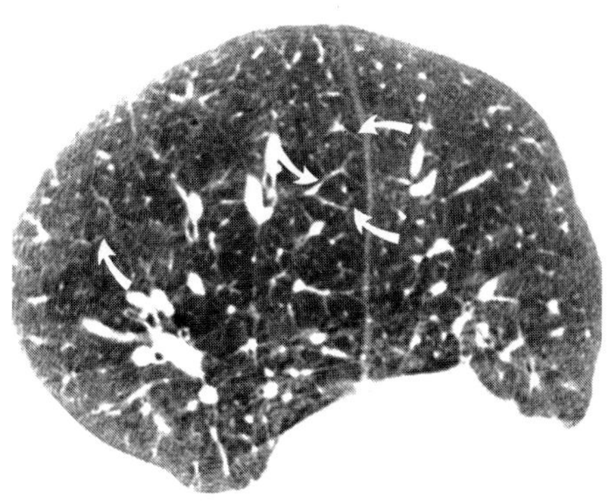

Figure 1–15   Normal high-resolution CT through the right lower lung zone allows identification of secondary pulmonary lobules. The pulmonary veins in the septa appear as polygonal lines (*curved arrows*), and the artery and the accompanying bronchiole are seen as dots near the center of the lobule.

structures including secondary pulmonary lobules. These lobules are identified by the centrally situated artery and accompanying bronchus and by the surrounding interlobular septa (Fig. 1–15). The septa can also often be identified in the lung periphery as thin lines extending to the pleural surface.

Other modalities of lung imaging and their application are discussed in Chapter 3.

PULMONARY FUNCTION TESTS

Standard tests of pulmonary function often play an important role in the diagnosis of lung disease. Even a moderately brief review of pulmonary physiology is inappropriate for this book, but an outline of standard tests of pulmonary function may be useful, as they will be referred to repeatedly.

Subdivisions of Lung Volumes

During quiet breathing the diaphragm and intercostal muscles contract to produce inspiration. The amount of air breathed in is referred to as the tidal volume or V_T (Fig. 1–16). Expiration results from the elastic recoil of the lungs and occurs passively. Expiration ceases when the elastic recoil of the lungs inward is equal to the outward elastic recoil of the chest wall. This is the functional residual capacity (FRC) and is the amount of air in the lung at the end of a normal quiet expiration. Residual volume (RV) is the amount of air left in the lung at the end of the

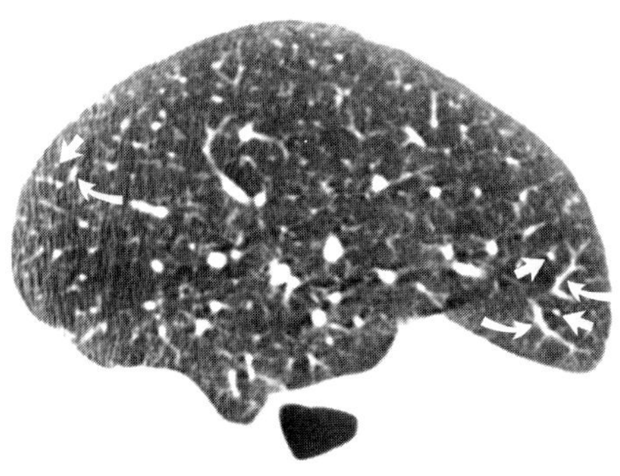

Figure 1–14   A 1.5-mm collimation scan targeted to the right lung at the same level as Figure 1–13 and reconstructed using a high-spatial-frequency algorithm (high-resolution CT) allows much better assessment of parenchymal detail. However, as most vessels appear as nodular densities, it would be easy to miss small nodules. In some areas, veins in the interlobular septa (*curved arrows*) can be seen as well as the centrilobular artery and bronchiole (*straight arrows*).

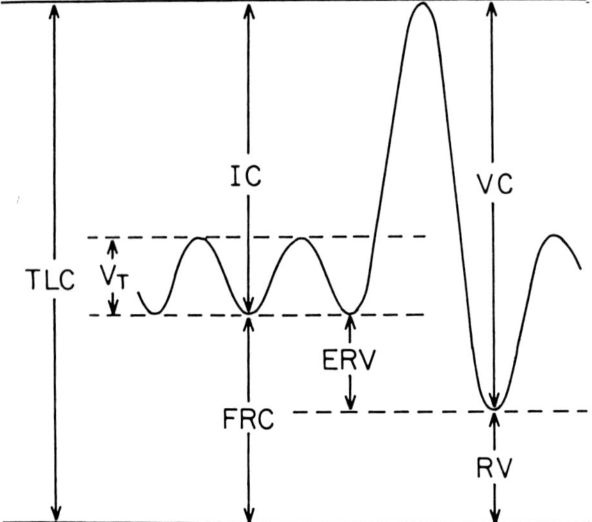

Figure 1–16 Subdivisions of lung volume: total lung capacity (TLC), vital capacity (VC), residual volume (RV), tidal volume (V_T), expiratory reserve volume (ERV), functional residual capacity (FRC), and inspiratory reserve capacity (IC). (From Bates DV, Christie TRV. Respiratory function in disease. 3rd ed. Philadelphia: WB Saunders, 1989.)

deepest possible expiration. If the lungs are normal, this point is determined by the chest wall because at low lung volumes the chest wall becomes very stiff and can move no further inward. Residual volume is also in part determined by airway closure. In young subjects airway closure plays a very small part, but in middle-aged or older subjects airways close before maximum chest wall stiffness is reached, so that RV increases with age. The amount of air in the lung at the end of a maximum inspiration is called total lung capacity (TLC). It represents the dissipation of forces applied to the chest wall on the lungs and is limited primarily by the lungs because they become very noncompliant as they approach full inspiration. Vital capacity (VC) is the maximum amount of air that can be exhaled following full inspiration and thus represents the volume of air between TLC and RV. Two subdivisions of lung volume are seldom used clinically: expiratory reserve volume (ERV), which is the difference between FRC and RV, and inspiratory capacity (IC), the difference between FRC and TLC. By convention, the term "capacity" means a sum of two or more volumes: e.g.,

$$VC = IC + V_T + ERV.$$

Lung volume and its subdivisions are determined by stature, sex, and age, with stature being the most important. Even prediction data using these variables

have a wide range of normal, usually considered ± 20 percent of predicted normal.

Expiratory Flow

Tests of expiratory flow are mainly related to airflow resistance within the airways. However, this measurement is not easily made and thus airway resistance is usually measured indirectly. The most common and most popular test is the forced expiratory volume in one second (FEV_1). This is the amount of air that is expired in the first second of forced expiration from TLC and is decreased when expiratory flow resistance is increased. It is volume differentiated by time, and therefore represents a measurement of flow. One of the difficulties is that like lung volumes, the FEV_1 is stature, sex, age, and effort dependent. One way of correcting for this is to express it as a percentage of the forced vital capacity (FVC), which is likewise stature, age, sex, and effort dependent. Thus the FEV_1/FVC ratio is body size independent and reduction indicates airflow obstruction.

Formerly it was believed that the peripheral ("small") airways contributed very little to total flow resistance, and it has been argued that considerable disease could occur in these airways without the FEV_1 being abnormal. Thus a large number of tests had a great vogue 10 to 15 years ago. These included measurements of flow at low lung volumes (which reflect flow in the peripheral airways). Another popular test is the single-breath nitrogen test (SBNT), which is largely a reflection of airway narrowing at low lung volumes and airway closure. The slope of phase III of the SBNT reflects irregular airway closure, and closing volume (CV) represents a volume at which airways close.

Gas Exchange

The transfer of gas from alveolar air to blood is referred to as the transfer factor or diffusing capacity. This is measured by assessing the ability of very dilute carbon monoxide inspired into the airspaces to transfer itself into the blood (diffusing capacity for carbon monoxide [D_LCO]). It has two components: the membrane component, which reflects the transfer of gas from alveolar air to the intravascular space, and the capillary component, which reflects the amount of available blood. Most commonly these are expressed together as the D_LCO. The most important, but relatively insensitive, measurements of gas exchange are the partial pressure of oxygen in the arterial blood (PaO_2) and the partial pressure of carbon dioxide in the arterial blood ($PaCO_2$).

Lung Mechanics

Like the volume of any distensible structure, that of the lung will vary with the pressure used to distend it. When the amount of air is related to the transpulmonary pressure, or to the distending force applied to the lung, this is expressed as the volume-pressure curve. This curve is best thought of as an exponential with small changes in volume occurring at high pressures. (As explained previously, at high lung volumes the lungs become very stiff, and thus changing pressures have very little effect.) At lower lung volumes, pressures result in much larger changes in volume (Fig. 1-17). Volume-pressure volume curves are tedious to measure and uncomfortable for the patient. Much argument exists as to the correct way of expressing the volume-pressure curve. These include compliance or change in volume per unit of pressure on the relatively linear part of the pressure volume curve. Because lung volumes are related to body size, correction can be made by expressing the volume change as percentiles of TLC. Other methods of expressing the data include the recoil pressure of the lung either at TLC or at 90 percent of TLC (P_L90). A method that has become popular in the last decade is fitting the volume-pressure curve above FRC to a single exponential of the form

$$V = A - Be^{-KP}$$

where V is volume at pressure P, A is the theoretical volume at infinite pressure, B the volume intercept at 0 pressure, and K the shape of the curve. When elasticity of the lung is reduced, lung volumes are increased for given pressures. The curve is then described as being shifted upward and to the left (traditionally, volume is the ordinate, and pressure, the abscissa). The shape constant is increased, and P_L90 and recoil pressures at TLC are decreased. Loss of elasticity is thought to be characteristic of emphysema, and increased "elasticity" is typical of many examples of infiltrative lung disease. However, it is not an increase in elasticity but more an increase of stiffness or loss of compliance.

REFERENCES

Bates DV. Respiratory function in disease. 3rd ed. Philadelphia: WB Saunders, 1989.

Breeze RG, Wheeldon EB. The cells in the pulmonary airways. In Murray JF, ed. Lung disease: state of the art. New York: American Lung Association, 1976–1977:111–183.

Evans MJ, Sherman MP, Campbell LA, Shami SG. Proliferation of pulmonary alveolar macrophages during postnatal development of rabbit lungs. Am Rev Respir Dis 1987; 136:384–387.

Fraser RG, Paré JAP, Paré PD, et al. Diagnosis of diseases of the chest. WB Saunders, 1988:1–314.

Frija J, Schmit P, Katz M, et al. Computed tomography of the pulmonary fissures: normal anatomy. J Comput Assist Tomogr 1982; 6:1069–1074.

Gail DB, Lenfant CJM. Cells of the Lung: biology and clinical implications. Am Rev Respir Dis 1983; 128:366–387.

Gould VE, Linnoila RI, Memoli VA, Warren WH. Neuroendocrine components of the bronchopulmonary tract: hyperplasias, dysplasias and neoplasms. Lab Invest 1983; 49:519–537.

Horsfield K, Cumming G. Morphology of the bronchial tree in man. J Appl Physiol 1968; 24:373–383.

Kuhn C III. Ciliated and Clara cells. In Bouhuys A, ed. Lung cells in disease. Amsterdam: North-Holland, 1976:91

Kuhn C III. Ultrastructure and cellular function in the distal lung. In Thurlbeck WM, Abel MR, eds. The lung: structure, function and disease. Baltimore: Williams & Wilkins, 1978:1.

Kuhn C III. Normal anatomy and histology. In Thurlbeck WM, ed. Pathology of the Lung. New York: Thieme, 1988:11–50.

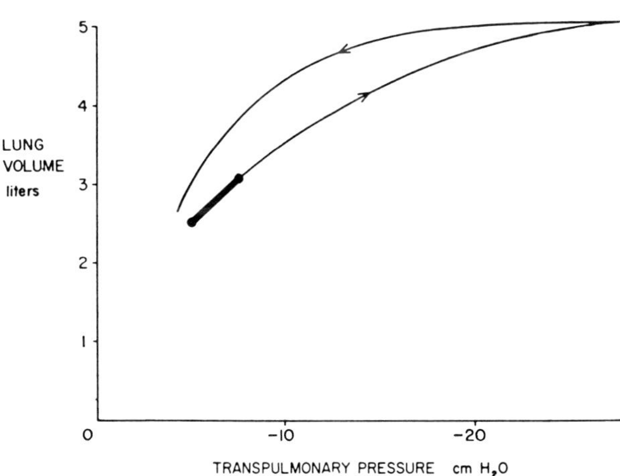

Figure 1–17   A volume-pressure curve. Note that the inspiratory curve (*arrow going to right*) is different from the expiratory curve (*arrow going to the left*), a phenomenon known as hysteresis. At high lung volumes the change in volume with changing pressure is small. The *solid line* represents the tidal volume range at which compliance (change in volume per cm H₂O pressure) is usually measured (From Bates DV, Christie TRV. Respiratory function in disease. 1st ed. Philadelphia: WB Saunders, 1964).

Kundel HL, Nodine CF. Interpreting chest radiographs without visual search. Radiology 1975; 116:527–532.

Milne ENC, Pistolesi M, Miniati M, Giuntini C. The radiologic distinction of cardiogenic and noncardiogenic edema. AJR 1985; 144:879–894.

Reid LM. The pulmonary circulation: remodeling in growth and disease. Am Rev Respir Dis 1979; 119:531–546.

Trapnell DH. Design, dynamics and deduction: a radiologist looks at the human lung. Clin Radiol 1983; 34:479–490.

Weibel ER. Morphometry of the human lung. Berlin: Springer Verlag, 1963.

Weibel ER, Gil J. Structure-function relationships at the alveolar level. In West JB, ed. Bioengineering aspects of the lung. New York: Marcel Dekker, 1977.

Zerhouni EA, Naidich DP, Stitik FP, et al. Computed tomography of the pulmonary parenchyma. Part 2: interstitial disease. J Thorac Imag 1985; 1:54–64.

CHAPTER 2

ABNORMAL STRUCTURE AND FUNCTION OF THE LUNG

TERMINOLOGY AND CONCEPTS

Diffuse Infiltrative Lung Disease and Diffuse Interstitial Lung Disease

The term "diffuse interstitial lung disease" implies a diffuse increase in tissue in the interstitium of the lung, i.e., the supporting tissue around airways, vessels, lobular septa, and the thick side of the alveolar wall. However, certain conditions such as cryptogenic organizing pneumonia (also known as bronchiolitis obliterans and organizing pneumonia), diffuse pulmonary hemorrhage, pulmonary edema, alveolar microlithiasis, and pulmonary alveolar proteinosis are primarily intra-alveolar processes, with only a slight or no interstitial component. Thus, to be all-inclusive, we prefer the term "diffuse infiltrative lung disease," meaning an increase in tissue within the lung, usually within the interstitium, but possibly also in the airspaces. A rigid definition cannot be applied—e.g., widespread bronchopneumonia might fall under this definition. The increased amount of tissue produces radiologically observable opacities that are generally diffuse and bilateral.

End-stage or Honeycomb Lung

When alveolar walls are damaged in infiltrative lung disease, fibrosis may ensue. This has best been described in what is usually termed "usual interstitial pneumonia" (UIP) or fibrosing alveolitis (Basset et al, 1986). It is thought that damage and disruption of alveolar basal lamina is an essential part of this process. Granulation tissue forms either within alveolar walls or as polypoid masses protruding into alveolar lumina from alveolar walls. This is accompanied by proliferation of fibroblasts and deposition of collagen within the interstitium. The newly formed granulation tissue is re-epithelialized by proliferation of alveolar type-II cells, with the end result being gradual obliteration of alveoli. As this happens, more and more gas-exchanging tissue is lost and becomes incorporated into scars. The respiratory bronchioles and alveolar ducts proximal to the scar dilate, and their normal epithelium is replaced to a varying extent by other types of epithelium. The epithelium lining the spaces is highly variable. It may consist of alveolar type-I epithelium, alveolar type-II epithelium, bronchiolar cells, squamous cells, or a mixture of cells. The spaces are dilated airways, rather than true cysts (Pimentel, 1967), but their shapes are greatly distorted. The resultant appearance is one of multiple cysts usually 0.5 to 2 cm in diameter, lined by various types of epithelium and containing accumulated secretions. The "cysts" are separated from each other by connective tissue of varying thickness and cellularity, in which there may be smooth muscle and even fat (Fig. 2–1). This appearance is referred to as end-stage lung (Genereux, 1975) or "honeycomb lung." The former term is preferred since the resemblance to the appearance of a honeycomb is not actually very great.

The concept of end-stage lung is critical. A variety of diseases such as usual interstitial pneumonia, rheumatoid lung, scleroderma, desquamative interstitial pneumonia, extrinsic allergic alveolitis, sarcoidosis, and asbestosis may result in this appearance. Similarly, focal areas of scarring resembling end-stage lung may occur in otherwise normal lungs. End-stage lung is nonspecific and should be thought of in the same way as end-stage renal disease. A common error is to confuse end-stage lung with UIP. This is discussed further in Chapter 7, where the relationship between desquamative interstitial pneumonia (DIP) and UIP is examined (see p. 105).

Restrictive Lung Disease

There is no universally accepted definition of restrictive lung disease. Most often the term is applied to patients who also have extensive bilateral pulmonary radiopacities. Under these circumstances, a relatively uniform clinical picture emerges in terms of symptoms, signs, radiologic findings, and pulmonary function. These patients correspond closely to patients who have infiltrative lung disease, and on that account the lungs may be stiff. However, the picture is incomplete and a wider concept is sometimes useful.

In the broadest sense, restrictive lung disease implies impaired maximal filling of the lung with air, i.e., diminished total lung capacity (TLC). The amount of air that the lung can contain depends on the force applied to the respiratory system, the degree to which the respiratory system can respond to the force applied to it, and whether or not the airspaces in the lung can be filled with air. Thus, in simplistic terms, restrictive lung disease can be classified by both the mechanism and the site of limitation (Table 2–1).

By far the most common cause of restrictive lung disease is diffuse infiltrative lung disease, and this may be the consequence of nearly 200 different conditions. Because they have lung stiffness in common, these conditions show fairly uniform alterations of tests of pulmonary function. Compliance—an expression of lung distensibility in terms of the change in volume of the lung per cm H_2O transpulmonary pressure—is decreased because the lung is "stiff," requiring greater pressures to distend the

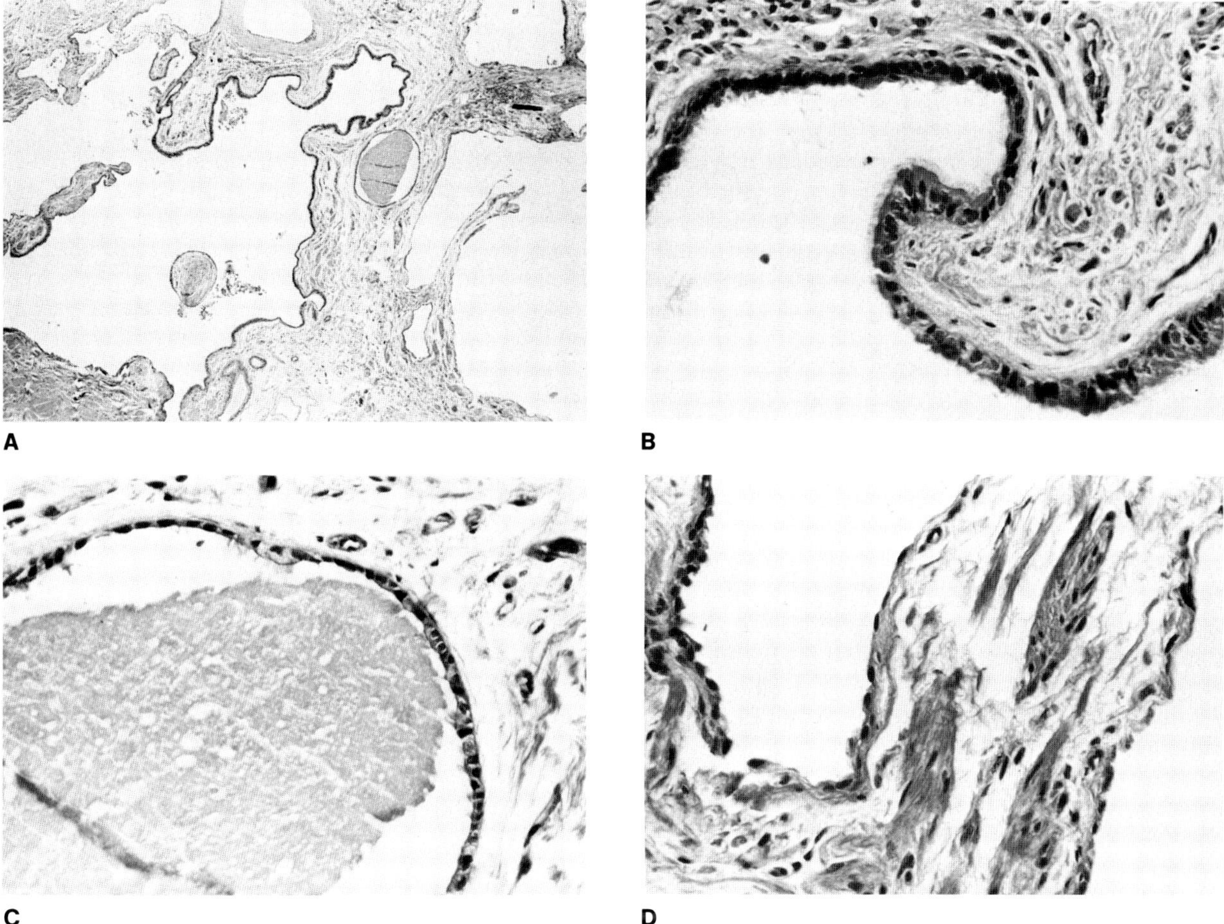

Figure 2–1   *A*, "Cyst" formation, in reality bronchiolectasis. The dilated airspaces are separated from each other by dense fibrosis (H&E, $\times$ 25). *B*, Lining of spaces may be ciliated, columnar, cuboidal or squamous epithelium (H&E, $\times$ 400). *C*, Debris with bronchiolectasis. *D*, Prominent smooth muscle in the fibrotic areas (H&E, $\times$ 400). These changes are not specific and may be seen in the end stage of UIP, DIP, extrinsic allergic alveolitis, sarcoidosis, asbestosis, or other forms of infiltrative lung disease. Focal areas of honeycombing are also occasionally found in otherwise normal lungs.

TABLE 2–1

PATHOGENESIS OF RESTRICTIVE LUNG DISEASE

MECHANISM OF LIMITATION	SITE OF LIMITATION		
	Chest wall	Pleura	Lungs
Increased stiffness of respiratory system	Kyphoscoliosis, chest wall scarring	Pleuritis	—
Decreased compliance of lungs	Normal	Usually normal	Infiltrative lung disease (e.g., usual interstitial pneumonia)
Normal compliance of the respiratory system	Paralysis of muscles, obesity	Pleural effusion	Tumors, alveolar edema

lungs. The effects on lung volumes are predictable. TLC is decreased because at high lung volumes the respiratory muscles are relatively weak and cannot stretch the stiffened lung to reach maximal volume. Functional residual capacity (FRC), i.e., the resting volume of the lungs, is also decreased, as it is determined by the balance between the force of the lungs, which tend to collapse inward, and the force of the chest wall, which tends to spring outward at low lung volumes. In fibrotic lung disease, this balance of forces occurs at a lower lung volume because the lung has increased recoil and overcomes the outward recoil force of the chest wall at a lower lung volume. Other than in young subjects, residual volume (RV) is mainly determined by airway closure. Because of increased recoil pressure, airways will be kept open at lower lung volumes in patients with infiltrative lung disease, and RV will decrease. TLC is affected to a greater extent than RV, and vital capacity (VC) is therefore reduced. Thus, characteristically, all the major subdivisions of the lung—RV, FRC, TLC, and VC—will be decreased in restrictive lung disease due to infiltrative lung disease.

The results of standard tests of expiratory function may appear anomalous. Because VC is decreased, expiratory volumes will be reduced; therefore, tests of expiratory flow, such as the forced expiratory volume in one second (FEV_1) and the maximal midexpiratory flow rate, will be reduced when expressed as a percentage of predicted values. However, because the recoil pressure of the lung is increased, the driving force applied to expiratory flow in the lung (which is recoil pressure) is increased and the airways are held open more widely at corresponding lung volumes. Thus, the flows may be greater than predicted when corrected for the reduction in lung volume unless the disease also affects airways or there is concomitant disease. For example, the ratio of FEV_1 to forced vital capacity or to VC is characteristically abnormally high in pulmonary fibrosis. Total airway resistance is primarily dependent on large airway size and is unchanged. However, peripheral airway resistance is increased because of distortion and narrowing of the airways. Since peripheral resistance contributes little to total airway resistance, the increase in peripheral airway resistance has little effect on total airway resistance, but tests of peripheral airway function may be abnormal.

Most characteristically of all, the diffusing capacity (transfer factor) for carbon monoxide ($D_L CO$) is reduced in patients with infiltrative lung disease. The main reason for this reduction is an abnormality in ventilation-to-perfusion matching, rather than an alteration in diffusion, although the latter abnormality is now regarded as contributing about 20 percent of the abnormality in gas exchange, as a result of thickening of the air-blood barrier. Ventilation-perfusion abnormalities are brought about by varying degrees of alteration or unevenness of lung compliance within small units of the lung and by varying degrees of small airway resistance. In addition, increased pulmonary artery pressure (because of obliteration of the capillary bed and increased cardiac output) shifts blood flow to the upper part of the lung, which is relatively poorly ventilated.

Diffusion limitation may be an important factor in the increased hypoxemia that patients with infiltrative lung disease develop with exercise. The obliteration of pulmonary capillaries that occurs in many interstitial lung diseases results in reduction of capillary blood volume, one of the principal determinants of the diffusing capacity. Blood gas abnormalities are also characteristic. For an unknown reason, patients with restrictive lung disease due to infiltrative lung disease tend to ventilate much more than patients with equivalent hypoxemia due to other causes. Overventilation does little to increase oxygen content of the blood since patients are generally breathing on the "flat" part of the oxygen dissociation curve (Fig. 2-2). This means that pulmonary venous blood from overventilated parts of the lung does not contain much more oxygen than normal. When mixed with poorly oxygenated pulmonary venous blood from the underventilated parts of the lung, the oxygen content of the blood of the whole lung is in the low to low-normal range. By contrast, overventilation has a marked effect on the carbon dioxide content of the blood since patients are on the "steep" slope of the carbon dioxide dissociation curve (see Fig. 2-2). The carbon dioxide content of blood from overventilated parts of the lung is greatly decreased and when mixed with blood from the underventilated areas, the carbon dioxide content of the blood is generally in the low-normal or normal range until advanced states of the disease. Classically, the ratio of the dead space to tidal volume is increased.

As pointed out earlier, not all patients with restrictive lung disease have infiltrative lung disease. Also, not all patients with infiltrative lung disease have restrictive lung disease; for example, lung volumes are often normal in desquamative interstitial pneumonia and increased in lymphangiomyomatosis. In general terms, although it is useful to equate restrictive lung disease with infiltrative lung disease, it should be remembered that one is a functional concept and the other is a morphologic one. Thus it is not surprising that the congruence of the two is incomplete.

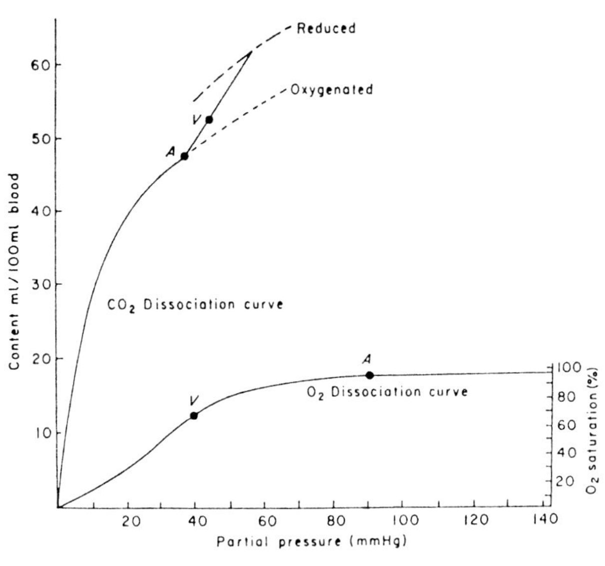

Figure 2–2   Carbon dioxide and oxygen dissociation curves of blood. A and V represent values in arterial (A) and venous (V) blood in normal subjects. Alterations in blood gas abnormalities in diffuse pulmonary fibrosis, such as UIP, can be explained by considering the carbon dioxide and oxygen dissociation curves. Normally, ventilation oxygenates blood on the flat part of the oxygen dissociation curve and thus overventilation produces little change in oxygen content. However, the carbon dioxide dissociation curve is steep and overventilation lowers the PCO_2 markedly. Underventilated areas have a low oxygen and high carbon dioxide content, but the arteriovenous difference is much greater for oxygen than for carbon dioxide. A combination of overventilated and underventilated areas relative to perfusion thus produces hypoxemia associated with normocapnea or hypocapnea. (From Forster RE II, Dubois AB, Brisco WA, Fisher AB. Lung physiological basis of pulmonary tests. 3rd ed. Chicago: Year Book, 1986.)

Diffuse Alveolar Damage

Many injurious agents may produce a similar, if not identical, acute reaction pattern in the lung. The morphologic reaction pattern of many types of acute interstitial injury is diffuse alveolar damage. In experimental animals, the initial lesion after injury may be characteristic for a particular substance as assessed by electron microscopic evidence of damage. For example, capillary endothelium is primarily affected in oxygen toxicity (Kapanci et al, 1969), type-I epithelial cells are affected in paraquat poisoning (Smith and Heath, 1974), type-II cells in N-nitrosamine-thiourea administration (Ryan et al, 1976), and the vascular endothelium of small vessels in bleomycin toxicity (Adamson and Bowden, 1974). However, other cells also become damaged, and the initial specific lesions become obscured in a matter of days. The most common clinical cause of diffuse alveolar damage is the adult respiratory distress syndrome

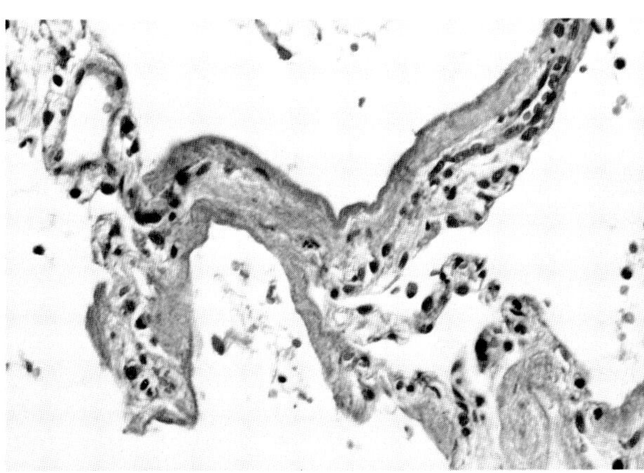

A

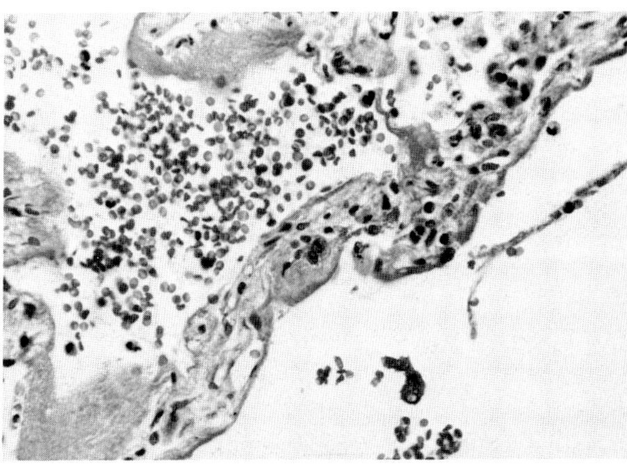

B

Figure 2–3   *A*, Hyaline membranes are closely adherent to alveolar walls (H&E, × 400). *B*, The interstitium is thickened with an excess of mononuclear cells (H&E, × 400). The patient was a 75-year-old man who developed ARDS due to influenza A Victoria. The biopsy was performed 3 days after the onset of his illness, and he died the following day.

(ARDS), which may be due to multiple causes. These are discussed further in Chapter 4.

After the initial injury, extensive lesions occur in other cell types (Katzenstein et al, 1976). When type-I cells are damaged, the integrity of the alveolar wall to fluid is lost, leading to increased permeability and alveolar edema. Passage of proteins, and probably fibrinogen in particular, together with tissue debris, lead to the formation of hyaline membranes in the alveolar spaces (Fig. 2–3). If the basement membrane remains intact and the damage limited, there is a proliferation of type-II cells to line the alveolar walls. The degree and nature of the cellular infiltration depend on the nature of the insult, but an accumulation of mononuclear cells, mostly macrophages, usually occurs, and in large part this represents the attempt by the host to clear the airspaces of debris. This represents the exudative phase and is succeeded by the proliferative phase, in which there is proliferation of interstitial fibroblasts that lay down collagen in the interstitium (Fig. 2–4). Collagen is formed first, whereas elastic tissue is not synthesized until after a period of weeks.

If the basement membrane remains intact and the insult is limited, the amount of fibrous tissue laid down is minimal, consistent with lung structure that has returned to normal, or almost normal. (Kapanci et al, 1969). Clinically, most patients who recover from the ARDS have no, or trivial, deficits in lung function (Lakshminarayan et al, 1976). Similarly, most infants who recover from the infantile respiratory distress syndrome (hyaline membrane disease)

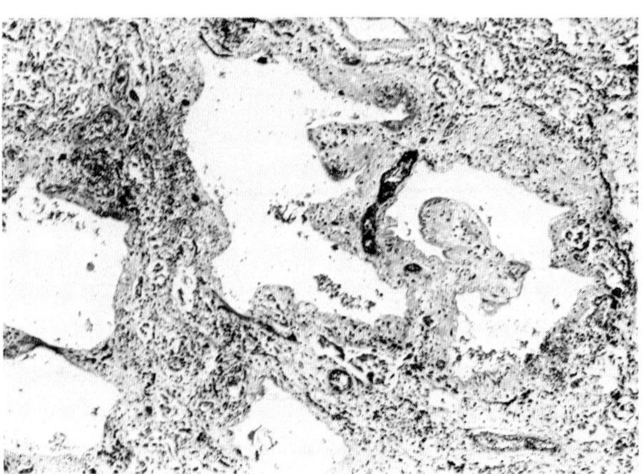

Figure 2–5 This is the same patient as in Figure 2–4. The lung is now restructured, and numerous cyst-like spaces are present, which represent dilated alveolar ducts with thick walls. The patient died 12 days after the lung biopsy, on the nineteenth day of his illness (H&E, × 250).

have relatively slight evidence of pulmonary dysfunction (Bertrand et al, 1985). However, some of these infants proceed to develop bronchopulmonary dysplasia (BPD), characterized by diffuse pulmonary fibrosis, airspace enlargement, and varying degrees of bronchiolar inflammation and obliteration (Anderson and Engel, 1983). Occasionally, an appearance very similar to BPD is found in patients consequent upon ARDS (Churg et al, 1983) (Fig. 2–5). These patients had a long period of survival (19 to 46 days) following the onset of ARDS.

CLINICAL APPROACH TO DIFFUSE INFILTRATIVE LUNG DISEASE

The clinician must recognize that diffuse infiltrative lung disease by definition can be limited to one lobe radiologically but involves all five lobes histologically. It is also not uncommon for the process to be very asymmetric, either involving predominantly one whole lung or selectively involving the upper half. With nearly 200 causes of diffuse infiltrative lung disease, the clinician must have some working knowledge of the various presentations of every one of these diseases in order to narrow down the differential diagnosis. The clinician must also keep in mind that a number of diffuse infiltrative diseases can be diagnosed without an invasive procedure, including even bronchoscopy, transbronchoscopic lung biopsy, and bronchoalveolar lavage. It behooves the clinician to do everything he or she can to avoid an open lung biopsy if the diagnosis can be made by other means. There are a number of entities that will

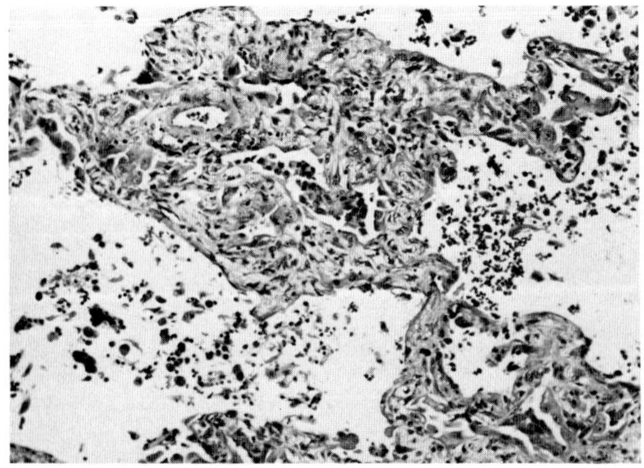

Figure 2–4 The interstitium is markedly thickened, there is type-II cell metaplasia, and numerous macrophages are present in the airspaces (H&E, × 400). The patient was a 66-year-old man with lymphoma diagnosed 2 months before he presented with ARDS. Lung biopsy was performed 7 days after the onset of illness. The cause of ARDS was never established.

TABLE 2–2

DIFFUSE LUNG DISEASE

KNOWN CAUSES

Infection
Neoplasm
Drug/radiation/oxygen
Pulmonary emboli
Organic and inorganic dust/gases
Some causes of ARDS

The rest are of *unknown cause.*

be discussed below in which even an open lung biopsy would not be diagnostic, whereas a careful history including a thorough review of systems, a careful physical examination, appropriate laboratory studies, and then a close scrutiny of the chest radiograph must be done to narrow the differential diagnosis and offer a reasonable approach to establishing an exact diagnosis.

There are a number of approaches to categorizing the diffuse infiltrative lung process and then narrowing the differential diagnosis down to a reasonable handful (DeRemee 1987; Fulmer and Crystal, 1979; Crystal et al, 1981; Crystal et al, 1984; Turner-Warwick 1988a, 1988b; Schwarz and King, 1988). Certainly, most pulmonary physicians have their own way of doing this. A "textbook" approach might be to group the diseases under the typical categories that can involve any organ system: e.g., developmental, infectious, immunologic, neoplastic, traumatic, idiopathic. Working through this involves possibly referring to a textbook to make certain you have not overlooked the uncommon one that may indeed be the process you are encountering. This may be the most comfortable approach for the clinician.

Another approach taken by many is to break down causes into those that are known and those unknown, as shown in Table 2-2. It may be appropriate for many clinicians to work in this manner. The point is that you need something to work around, and the best recommendation for the clinician who sees a lot of patients with diffuse infiltrative lung disease would be to develop his or her own approach. One of the authors (ECR, III) has done this and finds it very workable to the point that it includes nearly all 200 causes of diffuse infiltrative lung disease (Table 2-3). Only the category under "Miscellaneous" needs to be memorized and the rest falls into place with a mnemonic that he uses, because he can remember the first three letters sounding like his

TABLE 2–3

"MAONIDPESCHI"

MAONIDPESCHI is a mnemonic for the differential diagnosis of diffuse pulmonary disease. This includes almost all of the over 200 causes of diffuse pulmonary infiltration.

Miscellaneous: allergic bronchopulmonary aspergillosis (ABPA), alveolar microlithiasis, alveolar proteinosis, aspiration, bronchiectasis, bronchiolitis obliterans, cystic fibrosis (CF), lymphangioleiomyomatosis, tuberous sclerosis, veno-occlusive disease

ARDS (more than 30 causes)

Occupational/hypersensitivity (more than 50 causes)

Neoplasm (includes lymphoma and leukemia)

Infection (more than 40 causes)

Drug (more than 25 causes)

Pulmonary emboli
    Protein disorders

Edema: cardiac and noncardiac
    Eosinophilia

Sarcoidosis

Connective tissue disease (10 causes)

Histiocytosis X (eosinophilic granuloma)
    Hemorrhage: Goodpasture's syndrome, idiopathic pulmonary hemosiderosis (IPH)

Idiopathic: Idiopathic pulmonary fibrosis (IPF), desquamative interstitial pneumonitis (DIP), lymphocytic interstitial pneumonitis (LIP)

TABLE 2–4

HEREDITARY FAMILY HISTORY

AUTOSOMAL DOMINANT	AUTOSOMAL RECESSIVE
*Familial interstitial fibrosis	*Cystic fibrosis
*Tuberous sclerosis	*Alveolar microlithiasis
Rendu-Osler-Weber syndrome	*Kartagener's syndrome
Von Recklinghausen's disease	Alpha-1-antitrypsin deficiency
Marfan's syndrome	Familial pulmonary hypertension
	Ataxia-telangectasia syndrome

*Diffuse infiltrative lung disease

own institution. This table lists the mnemonic of MAONIDPESCHI, and for the rest of this discussion on the clinician's approach to diffuse lung disease this mnemonic will be followed. Also listed in this table is an estimate of the number of conditions associated with each entity. As can be seen, the entities of ARDS (more than 30 causes), occupational/hypersensitivity pneumonitis (more than 50), infection (more than 40), and drug (more than 25) add up to over 150 of the 200 causes and can most of the time be clearly eliminated by appropriate history and clinical setting. Thus a much more reasonable number of entities is left to deal with. We will work through all of the categories listed in Table 2–3 during the remainder of this section.

Statistically, the most common causes of diffuse infiltrative lung disease are as follows:

Cardiac pulmonary edema
Sarcoidosis
Usual interstitial pneumonia
Metastatic neoplasm
Pulmonary emboli/infarction
ARDS
Connective tissue disease
Histiocytosis X (eosinophilic granuloma)
Infection

Certainly the clinician does not want to do a lung biopsy on a patient with cardiac pulmonary edema or pulmonary emboli, but it has been known to happen!

History

The approach to any patient with diffuse infiltrative lung disease begins with a history. Important information to obtain is a family history (Table 2–4). Approximately 5 percent of the patients with idiopathic pulmonary fibrosis have a positive history of a family member with this disease (Bitterman et al,

1986). Getting the details of the history and possibly an open lung biopsy or autopsy findings of that member of the family will help to further narrow the differential diagnosis. In the appropriate clinical setting, if all other entities can be reasonably excluded, then an invasive procedure can be avoided. One fourth to one half of the patients with cystic fibrosis have a positive family history, yet the patient may neglect to mention this unless the physican inquires about members of the family with known pulmonary disease.

The taking of a detailed occupational exposure history, going back to the teenage years cannot be stressed strongly enough. It is likely that many exact diagnoses of occupational and/or hypersensitivity lung diseases are missed because of inadequate history-taking. The patient must be carefully asked about medications.

Physical Examination

A thorough review of systems is also essential. Table 2–5 offers examples of symptoms that would

TABLE 2–5

SYMPTOMS AS CLUES TO ETIOLOGY OF DIFFUSE PULMONARY DISEASE

Raynaud's phenomenon (scleroderma)
Dysphagia (scleroderma, dermatomyositis, cancer with metastasis to lung)
Onset of symptoms 4 to 6 hours after exposure to antigen (extrinsic allergic pneumonitis)
Hemoptysis (congestive heart failure, pulmonary embolism, bronchiectasis including cystic fibrosis, diffuse pulmonary hemorrhage)
Erythema nodosum (sarcoidosis, histoplasmosis, coccidioidomycosis)
Systemic manifestations of connective tissue disorders
Hematuria (pulmonary renal syndromes) (see Fig. 6–2)
Less dyspnea than expected from x-ray pattern (sarcoidosis, eosinophilic granuloma, silicosis)

TABLE 2–6

DISEASES TYPICALLY MULTISYSTEM WITH DIFFUSE LUNG DISEASE (IN ORDER BY "MAONIDPESCHI")

ENTITIES

Diabetes Insipidus
    Histiocytosis X
    Neoplasm
    Sarcoidosis
    Connective tissue disorders
    Tuberculosis

Pulmonary-Renal
    Wegener's granulomatosis
    Lymphomatoid granulomatosis
    Goodpasture's syndrome
    Systemic lupus erythematosus
    Polyarteritis
    Scleroderma
    Renal failure-hypervolemia, pulmonary edema
    Metastatic hypernephroma
    Tuberculosis
    Tuberous sclerosis
    Malignant hypertension (left ventricular failure)

Trauma (including nonthoracic)
    Fat embolism
    Aspiration
    Contused lungs
    Hemorrhage into lungs
    Pulmonary emboli
    Shock lungs
    CNS noncardiogenic pulmonary edema

Cystic fibrosis, ARDS (sepsis, shock, pancreatitis, etc.), Neoplasm (extrathoracic primary with metastasis to lung; lymphoma, leukemia), Infection, Protein disorders (all of them), Sarcoidosis, Connective tissue diseases (all of them with rare exception), Histiocytosis X

---

tial to one of several disorders (such as congestive heart failure, sarcoidosis, eosinophilic granuloma, lymphangioleiomyomatosis, and acute nitrofurantoin pneumonitis), provided that there are not two entities present such as bronchial asthma and idiopathic pulmonary fibrosis. Table 2–6 lists the diffuse pulmonary diseases that may be associated with some clinical syndromes.

The approach to the patient with diffuse pulmonary disease can be divided into noninvasive (which includes the history, physical examination, laboratory studies, and bronchoalveolar lavage) and invasive (which includes transbronchoscopic lung biopsy, open lung biopsy, and transthoracic needle aspiration). As mentioned previously, there are a number of conditions in which simple noninvasive tests may make the diagnosis when even an open lung biopsy may not. This is the case of the sweat chloride in cystic fibrosis; the differential blood count in Löffler's

TABLE 2–7

DIAGNOSIS MADE WITH OR WITHOUT LUNG TISSUE

LUNG TISSUE NEEDED*

Alveolar proteinosis
Sarcoidosis
Neoplasm
Chronic interstitial pneumonias
Eosinophilic granuloma
Lymphangioleiomyomatosis
Bronchiolitis obliterans
Veno-occlusive disease
Wegener's granulomatosis limited to lung

LUNG TISSUE GENERALLY NEEDED

Wegener's granulomatosis
Infection
Adult respiratory distress syndrome
Drug
Inorganic pneumoconiosis
Diffuse pulmonary hemorrhage

NO LUNG TISSUE NEEDED†

Connective tissue disease
Cystic fibrosis
Allergic bronchopulmonary aspergillosis
Hypersensitivity pneumonitis
Edema
Pulmonary embolism
Infections

---

*Includes bronchoalveolar lavage, transbronchial biopsy or open lung biopsy
†Diagnosis made by noninvasive means or by biopsying nonpulmonary tissue

---

further narrow the differential diagnosis. A complete physical examination is appropriate also to look for a primary cancer that might point to lymphangitic or hematogenous metastasis to the lungs or clues that might relate to a connective tissue disorder. An S-3 gallop would certainly be a significant finding and probably point to congestive heart failure as a cause of diffuse lung disease. Any cutaneous changes should be pursued, a biopsy of which may disclose an answer consistent with the pulmonary findings. Clubbing essentially excludes sarcoidosis with very rare exceptions and instead points to usual interstitial pneumonia, cystic fibrosis, eosinophilic granuloma (histiocytosis X), bronchogenic carcinoma, and bronchiectasis. The presence of crackling or "Velcro" rales is relatively characteristic of idiopathic pulmonary fibrosis, but moist rales of secretions can be found in many different entities. The presence of prolonged expiratory slowing implies obstructive airways disease and is a clue that narrows the differen-

syndrome and eosinophilic pneumonia; and serum complement, antinuclear antibody, and rheumatoid factor, in connective tissue disorders. Esophageal motility may be of diagnostic value in the patient with scleroderma lung, which can occur in the absence of cutaneous features. It is abnormal in over 80 percent of the cases. An open lung biopsy in the patient with scleroderma lung would show non-specific changes, whereas esophageal motility (a noninvasive test) would be quite specific. Of course, cultures and occasional fungal serologies may be diagnostic in the patient with infection. Table 2–7 lists the entities for which a tissue sample is needed versus those for which it is not needed; this serves as a reminder to attempt to make a diagnosis without resorting to an invasive procedure.

Differential Diagnosis

Using the mnemonic MAONIDPESCHI, each of the categories will be briefly discussed.

Miscellaneous

The *Miscellaneous* category includes some very important entities. *Allergic bronchopulmonary aspergillosis* (ABPA) almost always occurs in the symptomatic asthmatic patient and begins an average of 7 years after the onset of asthma but can occur much sooner (Patterson et al, 1982). These patients are usually steroid-dependent asthmatics with chest radiographs that show migratory pneumonitis almost always in the upper lobes. The chest radiograph may show tramlines, which are widened central bronchi where mucous plugs containing aspergilli can reside. The IgE is characteristically elevated and usually a good bit higher than that seen in the asthmatic without ABPA. A skin-prick test shows an immediate reaction and occasionally a delayed one. A histologic examination of the expectorated brownish mucous plugs will show mycelia within the plug, and bronchograms or chest CT scans characteristically show central bronchiectasis. An open lung biopsy would be of little or no value in this setting. *Alveolar microlithiasis* is a unique diffuse pulmonary disease showing a characteristic, most exclusive alveolar pattern, predominantly in the lower lung zones (Prakash et al, 1983). These concretions are dense and slowly progressive, taking two or more decades before the patient becomes symptomatic. There is a positive family history of this disease in about one-third of the patients.

Alveolar proteinosis or, perhaps a more proper term, alveolar phospholipidosis, is a relatively uncommon diffuse infiltrative disease involving predominantly the lower half of the lungs (Prakash et al,

1987; Wasserman and Mason, 1988). It, too, shows an alveolar pattern, but the alveolar filling is not so dense as in alveolar microlithiasis. The diagnosis can usually be made without an open lung biopsy, either by bronchoalveolar lavage or transbronchoscopic lung biopsy.

Aspiration pneumonitis without ARDS can produce a diffuse infiltrative process. In fact, some clinicians believe that it is a cause of idiopathic pulmonary fibrosis, although this concept is not widely accepted. Widespread *bronchiectasis* is associated with peribronchial fibrosis and eventually honeycombing. *Bronchiolitis obliterans* is associated with an abnormal chest roentgenogram in about one half to three fourths of the patients. It may have an airspace pattern and/or a fibrotic pattern. In bronchiolitis obliterans–organizing pneumonitis, there is a typical ground-glass haze associated with the roentgenologic pattern (Epler et al, 1985).

Cystic fibrosis (CF) is the most common congenital pulmonary disease in the white population (Davis and di Sant'Agnese, 1984). About one third of the patients with CF do not present until their late teen years. An occasional patient is not diagnosed until his or her thirties or early forties. The earliest radiologic pattern is usually limited to the upper lung zones. With more advanced disease, small microabscesses measuring up to 10 mm are seen. These are transient phenomena related to small bronchi obstructed with mucus, resulting in distal microabscesses. Also, hyperinflation on the chest radiograph is present in almost all symptomatic patients with CF.

Cystic fibrosis should always be considered in any individual under 30 years of age with unexplained clubbing, in the young child or adolescent with nasal polyps, and in any individual with *Staphylococcus aureus* and *Pseudomonas aeruginosa* in mucoid sputum without acute pneumonia. Some young adult men with CF will present to infertility clinics.

Lymphangioleiomyomatosis should always be considered in the female patient in the childbearing-age group and is always associated with dyspnea (CPC 24–1988). Many instances are associated with pleural effusions that are frequently chylous and occasionally with spontaneous pneumothorax. It is important to consider this diagnosis, as a significant proportion of these women have partially reversible disease when treated with progesterone and/or oophorectomy. The diagnosis usually requires open lung biopsy but has been made by transbronchial biopsy. The related syndrome *tuberous sclerosis* is a rare congenital disorder frequently associated with involvement of the lungs and other systems.

Pulmonary veno-occlusive disease is sometimes presumed to be a congenital disorder, but this is uncertain (CPC 21–1986). It becomes symptomatic usually in the late teen years or later and presents as progressive dyspnea with radiographic findings that mimic a number of diffuse infiltrative diseases involving the lower lung zones. Kerley's B lines are frequently seen, which can be a clue, and the varying values found on wedge pressure measurements at cardiac catheterization are also useful. The diagnosis, though, must be made with open lung biopsy. There is no treatment for this disorder.

Adult Respiratory Distress Syndrome

Continuing with the mnemonic MAONID-PESCHI, the *adult respiratory distress syndrome* (ARDS) is usually quite obvious, but diagnosing the underlying cause may be difficult (see Chapter 4).

Occupational Lung Disease

With regard to *occupational lung disease*, or, *hypersensitivity pneumonitis*, it has already been stated that thorough probing of previous and current exposures by mentioning specific situations is extremely important in all situations in which the diagnosis of diffuse infiltrative lung disease is not obvious quickly (Salvaggio, 1987; Grammar and Patterson, 1987; Weill and Jones, 1988; Lopez and Salvaggio, 1988). This is particularly true for asbestosis, in which the exposure can be somewhat obscure if it was of limited duration or occurred more than 20 years prior to onset of clinical disease. On the other hand, silicosis, which can produce an upper zonal lung disease, has a more obvious history of exposure. The onset of symptoms 4 to 6 hours after exposure is characteristic of a hypersensitivity pneumonitis but does not occur in every individual with this disorder, especially if the exposure is not very intense or for a long period; in this setting the onset of symptoms may be subacute or insidious.

Neoplasm

Neoplasm in the diffuse setting is usually metastatic and either nodular or interstitial in pattern. A primary lung cancer in the form of diffuse alveolar cell carcinoma must always be considered. When the metastatic disease is from an extrathoracic primary neoplasm, the extrathoracic primary will be known to the clinician in approximately 90 percent of the cases through a history of past illnesses, a change in bowel habits, or hematuria; or through a thorough physical examination and/or routine laboratory studies. Also included in this category are the lymphomas and leukemic infiltrates.

Infection

There are over 40 *infections* that can produce pulmonary disease, usually associated with a history of acute onset of productive cough, fever, sweats, chills, anorexia, and so on; mycobacterial and some fungal diseases can sometimes be more insidious in onset. Ideally, the diagnosis would be made without resorting to an open lung biopsy.

Drugs

Of the more than 25 *drugs* known to induce diffuse infiltrative lung disease (Table 2–8; this topic is discussed in more detail in Chapters 4, 5, and 7), this differential can be quickly eliminated by taking a

---

TABLE 2–8

DRUG-INDUCED DIFFUSE PULMONARY DISEASE

Antibiotics
    Azulfidine
    Nitrofurantoin
    (acute and chronic)

Anti-inflammatory
    ASA
    Gold
    Methotrexate
    Penicillamine

Cardiovascular
    Hydrochlorothiazide
    Amiodarone
    Tocainide

Illicit
    Heroin
    Methadone
    Propoxyphene

Chemotherapeutic
    Azathioprine
    Busulfan
    Cyclophosphamide
    Bleomycin
    Nitrosoureas
    Chlorambucil
    Mitomycin-C
    Melphalan
    Methotrexate
    Procarbazine
    Hydroxyurea
    Ara-C

Miscellaneous
    Blood products
    Bromocriptine
    Dilantin
    Drug-induced systemic lupus erythematosus
    Oxygen
    Tocolytic agents

---

good history and by keeping in mind that patients may not mention a drug that they voluntarily take at their discretion (Cooper et al, 1986a, 1986b; Rosenow 1988a). A good example of this is the chronic use of nitrofurantoin. Patients frequently use this for urinary symptoms but do not include it as a regular medication because they do not take it every day. That drug, more commonly than any other, must be specifically asked for. With the exception of methotrexate (which can produce granulomas) and amiodarone (which is associated with phospholipid-filled macrophages), the histology of drug-induced pulmonary disease is nonspecific and is really a disorder of exclusion. Pulmonary disease induced by chemotherapeutic agents is frequently confused with opportunistic infection because of the usual association with fever.

Pulmonary Emboli; Protein Disorders

Pulmonary emboli can mimic many other diffuse infiltrative processes and should always be considered in the patient with acute to subacute onset of unexplained dyspnea and hypoxemia, especially, for example, in the high-risk setting of the postoperative period. *Protein disorders* include multiple myeloma, Waldenström's macroglobulinemia, amyloidosis, cryoglobulinemia, and a few others that can have pulmonary involvement.

Edema; Eosinophilia

Edema includes both cardiac and noncardiac varieties and occasionally can present in a somewhat insidious variety, especially cardiac edema. Table 2–9 lists the various causes of noncardiac pulmonary edema. *Eosinophilia* can be an important sign, especially in chronic eosinophilic pneumonia and Löffler's syndrome. Chronic eosinophilic pneumonitis is an entity that can be diagnosed without open lung biopsy, specifically with the finding of eosinophils on bronchoalveolar lavage (Jederlinic et al, 1988; Banks et al, 1988). These individuals are usually women, are acutely to subacutely ill, and have fever, asthma, weight loss, mild anemia, and an elevated sedimentation rate. As mentioned in Chapter 7, eosinophilic pneumonia has a characteristic peripheral lung pattern said to be "the x-ray negative of cardiac pulmonary edema." It responds well to corticosteroid therapy.

Sarcoidosis

Sarcoidosis is one of the most common causes of diffuse pulmonary disease in the ambulatory practice of pulmonary medicine (Thomas and Hunninghake, 1987; Johns, 1988; Fanburg and Pitt, 1988). There are three entities that should be considered when a patient has a fairly extensive diffuse infiltrative lung process as seen on the chest radiograph, and is minimally symptomatic or asymptomatic. These are sarcoidosis, pulmonary eosinophilic granuloma and silicosis. Sarcoidosis can have many different radiographic patterns, with one of the more common ones being the predominant involvement of the upper half of the lung (Table 2–10). Stage II of pulmonary sarcoidosis by definition has associated hilar and mediastinal adenopathy. Table 2–11 lists the differential diagnosis of diffuse infiltrative lung diseases with adenopathy; sarcoidosis is the most common one.

Connective Tissue Disease

There are approximately ten *connective tissue diseases*, including Wegener's granulomatosis, and all but a few such as relapsing polychondritis are associated with diffuse infiltrative lung disease (Dickey and Myers, 1988; Stokes and Turner-Warwick, 1988). It is uncommon for symptomatic lung disease to precede systemic disease except in Wegener's granulomatosis. With the exception of Wegener's granulomatosis, the lung histology is nonspecific, and a diagnosis should be made through noninvasive means such as blood tests, nerve or muscle biopsy, or renal biopsy. As previously pointed out, extrapulmonary symptoms cannot be ignored, as in turn they may lead to the obtaining of appropriate tests, such as blood labs or esophageal motility.

Hemorrhage

Hemorrhage is also considered under the connective tissue diseases and is usually associated with

---

TABLE 2–9

NONCARDIAC PULMONARY EDEMA

Direct
    Aspiration: gastric contents, water (near-drowning)
    Inhalation of toxic gases
    Contusion
    Viral pneumonia
    Drug: heroin, methadone, propoxyphene; ASA;
        leukoagglutinin (blood products)
    Post expansion: thoracentesis, chest tube for
        pneumothorax
    Capillary leak (ARDS)

Indirect
    High-altitude pulmonary edema
    Neurogenic

DIFFERENTIAL DIAGNOSIS BASED ON RADIOGRAPHIC PATTERNS

RETICULAR PATTERN
(irregular linear shadows)

Acute	Pulmonary edema
	Viral pneumonia
	Pneumocystis pneumonia
Chronic	
Upper lung zone	Sarcoidosis
	Hypersensitivity pneumonitis
	Eosinophilic granuloma
Lower lung zone	Usual interstitial pneumonia (UIP)
	Rheumatoid lung, scleroderma
	Asbestosis
	Lymphangioleiomyomatosis

SEPTAL LINES (Kerley's A and B lines)

Acute	Pulmonary edema
	Viral pneumonia
	Mycoplasma pneumonia
Chronic	Lymphangitic carcinomatosis
	Lymphoma
	Interstitial fibrosis of any cause (Uncommon)

END-STAGE LUNG (honeycombing)

Upper lung zone predominance	Eosinophilic granuloma
	Sarcoidosis
	Hypersensitivity pneumonitis
Lower lung zone predominance	Usual interstitial pneumonia
	Rheumatoid lung
	Lymphangioleiomyomatosis
Diffuse	Any of the above
	Drug therapy (nitrofurantoin)

NODULES < 5 MM IN DIAMETER

Acute	Viral pneumonia
	Miliary tuberculosis
Chronic	
Upper lung zone	Sarcoidosis
	Coal workers' pneumoconiosis
	Silicosis
	Eosinophilic granuloma
	Hypersensitivity pneumonitis
Diffuse	Any of the above
	Miliary carcinomatosis

NODULES > 5 MM IN DIAMETER

Smooth margins	Metastatic disease
	Rheumatoid nodules
	Wegener's granulomatosis
	Lymphoma
Irregular margins	Septic emboli
	Bronchoalveolar carcinoma
	Tuberculosis
	Lymphoma

AIRSPACE OPACIFICATION

Acute	Pulmonary edema
	Pneumonia (bacterial, viral, e.g., cytomegalovirus, influenza, varicella-zoster)
	Aspiration pneumonia
	Pulmonary hemorrhage
	ARDS
Chronic	Alveolar proteinosis
	Bronchoalveolar carcinoma
	Lymphoma
	Chronic eosinophilic pneumonia
	Cryptogenic organizing pneumonia

TABLE 2–11

DIFFUSE DISEASE WITH MEDIASTINAL ADENOPATHY

Sarcoidosis
Infectious
    Acute disseminated histoplasmosis and
        coccidioidomycosis
    Toxoplasmosis
Occupational
    Asbestosis
    Berylliosis
Neoplastic
    Metastatic carcinoma
    Lymphoma
    Kaposi's sarcoma
Methotrexate
Histiocytosis X

---

hemoptysis, but this is not always the case. It is one of the main symptoms associated with idiopathic pulmonary hemosiderosis. It is quite frequently seen in the immunocompromised host with clotting disorders (CPC 30–1988; Wilson, 1988; Hay and Turner-Warwick, 1988). Most patients with pulmonary hemorrhage syndromes have an iron-deficiency anemia. If the bleeding is at the alveolocapillary level (versus more proximal, as in bronchogenic carcinoma), hemosiderin-laden macrophages should be evident.

Eosinophilic granuloma of the lung appears to be increasing in incidence (Colby and Lombard, 1983; Prophet, 1982; Lacronique et al, 1982; Rosenow, 1988b). It is one of the "sis" diseases that can have predominant upper half lung disease (Table 2–10). It should always be considered in the differential diagnosis of a radiograph with predominant involvement in the upper lung zones. From 80 to 90 percent of adults with the disease are smokers or former smokers, such that the absence of a smoking history makes the disease less likely but, of course, still possible. With few exceptions, the association with pneumothorax, diabetes insipidus, and bone lesions is quite characteristic for a history of eosinophilic granuloma.

Idiopathic Pulmonary Fibrosis

Idiopathic pulmonary fibrosis (usual interstitial pneumonia) is one of the more common diffuse infiltrative lung diseases and is the main criterion for a single lung transplant at this time. Clinically, it is a disease of exclusion (Schraufnagel et al, 1987; Crystal et al, 1981; Crystal et al, 1984; Bitterman et al, 1986; Hay and Turner-Warwick, 1988; Turner-Warwick, 1988b). Approximately half the patients have clubbing and crackling ("Velcro") rales at the bases. Some clinicians accept these two physical findings, the appropriate clinical setting, and the exclusion of other entities as sufficient for a diagnosis to be made without obtaining lung tissue. Most clinicians, however, may not and prefer some confirmation of the disease as well as exclusion of other processes. Also under the "idiopathic" category is desquamative interstitial pneumonia (DIP), which has a somewhat better prognosis than idiopathic pulmonary fibrosis. *Lymphocytic interstitial pneumonia* (LIP) is considered in this category of "idiopathic," and yet many clinicians and pathologists regard this as a pseudolymphoma or "prelymphoma" and categorize it under "Neoplasm."

RADIOLOGIC APPROACH

Chest Radiography

The chest radiograph is a mainstay in the assessment of all patients with diffuse infiltrative disease. It is sensitive in the detection of pulmonary abnormalities and helpful in the diagnosis and management. Radiologically, the differential diagnosis is based on the type and distribution of opacities. Traditionally, diseases have been classified as being "airspace" or "interstitial" (Felson, 1973; Fraser and Paré, 1977). The airspace pattern is characterized by a cloud-like appearance, ill-defined margins, tendency to coalesce, air bronchograms, "butterfly" (perihilar), and segmental or lobar distribution. The interstitial pattern is characterized by the presence of too many lines or small nodules. This classification is useful to some extent but has several limitations:

1. Some diseases classified as airspace on radiographs are predominantly interstitial histologically and vice versa;
2. A number of conditions affect both the interstitium and alveolar airspace;
3. There is often disagreement between observers on whether a particular radiograph shows an interstitial or an airspace pattern, or both;
4. Since the vast majority of chronic infiltrative diseases cause an interstitial pattern, one is still left with a large differential diagnosis (McLoud et al, 1983; Felson, 1979).

Some of these limitations have been overcome by adapting the ILO Classification for Pneumoconioses to the description and assessment of severity of diffuse infiltrative lung disease (McLoud et al, 1983). Comparison with the ILO set of radiographs allows standardization of terminology and description of radiologic patterns without the implication that a particular pattern histologically reflects interstitial disease or airspace disease, or both. Rather than being described with the nondescript and often misleading term "interstitial pattern," the radiograph should be described as showing predominantly nodular opacities (nodules of 1 to 10 mm in diameter), small irregular shadows (reticular pattern), septal lines (Kerley's A and B lines), or end-stage lung (McLoud et al, 1983; Felson, 1979). As stated earlier in this chapter, end-stage lung is characterized radiologically by the presence of extensive abnormalities with numerous cystic spaces ("honeycombing"). "Increased interstitial markings," as a radiologic descriptor, is meaningless. The term "airspace pattern" may be kept or be substituted by "airspace opacification" or "ground-glass appearance," but it must be realized that it does not necessarily reflect histologic airspace disease.

By analysis of the predominant radiologic pattern and its distribution, the differential diagnosis of both acute and chronic infiltrative lung diseases can often be narrowed down considerably. The different patterns and the most common conditions associated with these patterns are summarized in Table 2-10. For example, usual interstitial pneumonia (UIP), interstitial fibrosis in association with rheumatoid arthritis or scleroderma, and asbestosis often present radiologically with a characteristic lower lung zone predominance of small irregular linear opacities (reticular densities). Hypersensitivity pneumonitis, histiocytosis X, and sarcoidosis often present with small nodular or reticulonodular opacities with an upper lung zone predominance. Chronic eosinophilic pneumonia often shows an almost pathognomonic peripheral airspace pattern. Sometimes bronchiolitis obliterans–organizing pneumonia (BOOP) may have a similar appearance. A perihilar distribution of airspace opacification in an acute setting usually implies pulmonary edema; in the chronic situation, it is characteristic for alveolar proteinosis. Diffuse infiltrates with mild or no symptomatology are characteristic of sarcoidosis, histiocytosis X, and silicosis. As described previously, most chronic infiltrative lung diseases are restrictive and thus associated with loss of lung volume; this is perhaps most prominent in UIP. Normal or large lung volumes are characteristic of lymphangioleiomyomatosis and histiocytosis X.

Additional radiologic clues may help to further narrow the differential diagnosis. Pneumothorax may be seen with end-stage lung of any etiology, but it is most common and may be the first finding in lymphangioleiomyomatosis and in histiocytosis X. Recurrent pneumothorax and chylothorax in a young woman are highly suggestive of lymphangioleiomyomatosis. Small nodules in association with eggshell calcification are virtually pathognomonic of silicosis. Nodular or reticulonodular opacities associated with enlarged hilar nodes are most suggestive of sarcoidosis.

Although these radiographic patterns have been shown to correlate statistically with certain disease entities, it must be realized that most infiltrative lung diseases may present with more than one pattern, may be more prominent in one lung zone, or may be diffuse, and that numerous pulmonary diseases may have similar radiologic findings. Adequate assessment of the chest radiograph requires awareness of the clinical history, physical findings and, ideally, comparison with previous radiographs. The differential diagnosis in the immunocompromised host differs markedly from that in the nonimmunocompromised host and will be considered separately in Chapter 5. It is important to note that a normal radiograph does not exclude significant bronchopulmonary disease. It is seen in up to 10 percent of symptomatic patients with diffuse infiltrative lung disease (Epler et al, 1978; Carrington and Gaensler, 1978). The most common conditions presenting with a normal radiograph are sarcoidosis, desquamative interstitial pneumonia (DIP), hypersensitivity pneumonitis, lymphangitic carcinoma, and bronchiolitis obliterans. The radiograph is also of limited value in the evaluation of patients with asthma, chronic bronchitis, and emphysema.

Computed Tomography

CT is useful in the assessment of both acute and chronic infiltrative lung diseases (Naidich et al, 1985; Zerhouni et al, 1985). It closely reflects the macroscopic pathologic appearance, thus giving a better pictorial assessment of disease pattern and extent than the chest radiograph. CT is superior to the conventional radiograph in the differential diagnosis, the decision on whether transbronchial or open lung biopsy is indicated, and the determination of the optimal biopsy site (Bergin and Müller, 1987; Miller et al, 1987; Mathieson et al, 1989).

The pattern of disease on CT may be classified, as on the radiograph, as consisting predominantly of small nodules, irregular linear opacities (reticular pattern), septal lines, honeycombing, or airspace pattern. The distribution of densities can be much better assessed and may be classified into being predominantly peribronchovascular, diffuse, or subpleural. Using this approach, CT allows a specific diagnosis of a number of diffuse infiltrative lung diseases (see Table 2-12).

Small (1 to 5 mm in diameter) nodules in a predominantly peribronchovascular distribution are

TABLE 2–12

COMPUTED TOMOGRAPHY IN THE DIFFERENTIAL DIAGNOSIS OF CHRONIC DIFFUSE INFILTRATIVE LUNG DISEASE

PATTERN	DISTRIBUTION
NODULAR (<5 mm diameter)	
Well defined	Peribronchovascular
	Sarcoid
	Lymphangitic carcinomatosis
	Lymphoma
	Posterior predominance
	Silicosis
	Random
	Eosinophilic granuloma
	Metastatic malignancy
Poorly defined	Random
	Hypersensitivity pneumonitis
IRREGULAR LINEAR DENSITIES	
	Diffuse
	Drug toxicity
	Eosinophilic granuloma
	Neurofibromatosis
	Peribronchovascular
	Sarcoid
	Peripheral
	UIP
	Asbestosis
HONEYCOMBING	
	Diffuse
	Eosinophilic granuloma
	Lymphangioleiomyomatosis
	Peripheral
	UIP
SEPTAL LINES	
Uneven thickening of septal lines, polygonal lines	
	Lymphangitic carcinomatosis
	Lymphoma
AIRSPACE	
	Peripheral
	Chronic eosinophilic pneumonia
	Cryptogenic organizing pneumonia
HAZINESS	
	Patchy, subpleural areas of airspace opacification or haziness
	Active UIP
	Active desquamative interstitial pneumonia

seen in lymphangitic carcinomatosis and in sarcoid (Bergin and Müller, 1987). Although the chest radiograph occasionally has a characteristic appearance in lymphangitic carcinomatosis, in the majority of patients it is normal or shows a nonspecific pattern. On CT, most patients have a virtually pathognomonic appearance consisting of uneven thickening of bronchovascular bundles giving a nodular appearance, and uneven thickening of the interlobular septa (Stein et al, 1987; Munk et al, 1988). In some patients, the abnormality is unilateral or restricted to a localized region of lung. CT may show the characteristic appearance even in patients with normal or non-specific radiologic findings (Stein et al, 1987). In sarcoid, nodules can be seen along the bronchovascular bundles, subpleural region and, to a lesser extent, in the interlobular septa (Müller et al, 1989) (Fig. 2-6). As the process becomes chronic, there is progressive fibrosis which also tends to be predominantly peribronchovascular (Fig. 2-7). Thickening of peripheral septal lines may be seen in sarcoidosis but usually it is not a major feature. The marked involvement of the bronchovascular sheath in sarcoidosis and lymphatic spread of tumor is well known pathologically and corroborated by the ease with which these two conditions, unlike most other chronic lung diseases, can be diagnosed by transbronchial biopsy.

In silicosis, the nodules have a random distribution, but they are more numerous in the upper lung zones, particularly in the posterior aspects of the lungs (Bergin et al, 1986). This posterior distribution cannot be appreciated on the radiograph. Hypersensitivity pneumonitis in the acute or subacute phase may be suspected on CT by the presence of ill-defined nodules and airspace opacification (which is presumably due to bronchiolitis and granulomas)

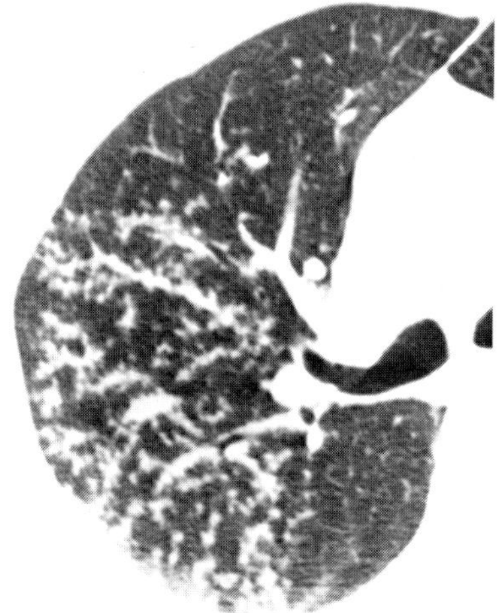

Figure 2–6 High-resolution CT through the right midlung zone in a patient with sarcoidosis shows nodular densities along the bronchovascular bundles, giving a beaded appearance. Nodules are also present in the subpleural regions posteriorly. The distribution of the abnormalities is patchy, with sparing of the anterior and posteromedial regions.

in the sub-acute phase and by edema in the acute phase (Bergin and Müller, 1987).

Irregular linear (reticular) opacities are seen in a variety of chronic lung diseases. Several conditions may cause reticular opacities in a diffuse or random distribution throughout the lung parenchyma. We have seen this distribution in pulmonary fibrosis due to drug toxicity, histiocytosis X, longstanding hypersensitivity pneumonitis, and neurofibromatosis. So far, with few exceptions, we have been unable to distinguish these conditions one from another on CT. On the other hand, we have found CT to be very useful in the diagnosis of UIP (Bergin and Müller, 1987; Müller et al, 1986). On CT, UIP has a virtually pathognomonic appearance consisting of reticular densities and honeycomb cysts in a predominantly subpleural distribution (Fig. 2–8). This peripheral predominance is present in the vast majority of patients on CT, regardless of the stage of the disease (Müller et al, 1986) and is so characteristic as to obviate the need for open lung biopsy for diagnosis. The extent of interstitial changes, as assessed by CT, also correlates much better than the chest radiograph with the clinical and functional impairment in these patients (Staples et al, 1987). CT may also be helpful in the assessment of disease activity in UIP (Müller et al, 1987). This is important because only patients with marked disease activity and little fibrosis respond well to corticosteroid therapy. On CT, disease activity is characterized by the presence of patchy areas of airspace opacification, which, like the reticular densities, are predominantly in a subpleural distribution.

Presently, at the Vancouver General Hospital, CT scans are performed almost routinely in the evaluation of patients with chronic diffuse infiltrative lung disease. Particularly in patients with UIP, the characteristic findings on CT often establish the

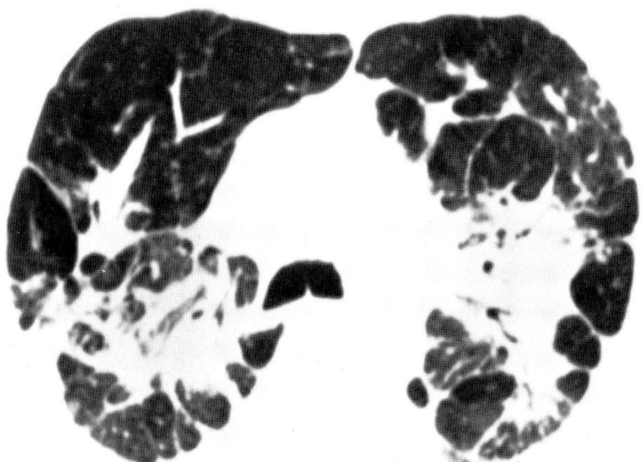

Figure 2–7 CT scan at the level of the tracheal carina in a patient with fibrotic changes due to sarcoid. Most of the fibrosis can be seen to radiate from the hila to the lung periphery along the bronchovascular bundles.

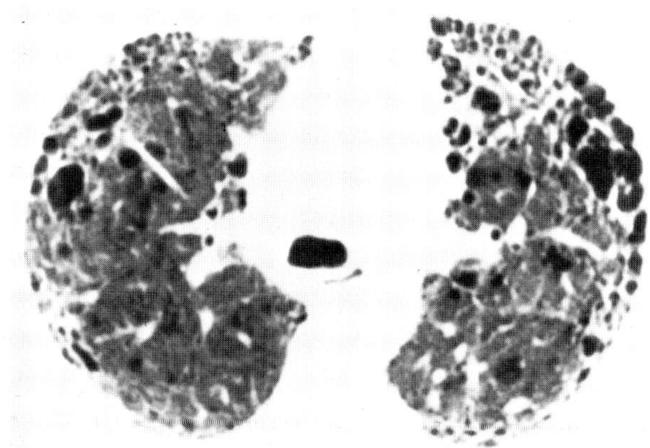

Figure 2–8 CT scan at the level of the tracheal carina in a patient with severe UIP. Extensive honeycomb cyst formation involves predominantly the subpleural lung regions.

diagnosis without requiring open lung biopsy. In others, we use CT to determine whether transbronchial or open lung biopsy is required and to guide the surgeon to the optimal site for biopsy. Traditionally, the lingula and right middle lobe have been considered to be poor sites for open lung biopsy because of the presence of nonspecific fibrosis. However, in a review of the results of open lung biopsy in 73 patients, we found that these sites were as likely to be representative as any other lung region in both immunocompromised and nonimmunocompromised patients (Miller et al, 1987). CT gives an accurate assessment of disease distribution and thus allows selection of areas most likely to be diagnostic and representative.

REFERENCES

Adamson IYR, Bowden DH. The pathogenesis of bleomycin-induced pulmonary fibrosis in mice. Am J Pathol 1974; 77:185–197.

Anderson WR, Engel RR. Cardiopulmonary sequelae of reparative stages of bronchopulmonary dysplasia. Arch Pathol Lab Med 1983; 107:603–608.

Banks DE, Salvaggio JE, Goetzl EJ. Eosinophilic syndromes and eosinophilic granuloma. In: Murray JF, Nadel JA, eds. Textbook of respiratory medicine. Philadelphia: WB Saunders, 1988:1515–1534.

Basset F, Ferrans V, Soler P, et al. Intraluminal fibrosis in interstitial lung disease. Am J Pathol 1986; 122:443–461.

Bergin, CJ, Müller NL, Vedal S, Chan-Yeung M. CT in silicosis: correlation with plain films and pulmonary function tests. AJR 1986;146:477–483.

Bergin CJ, Müller NL. CT of interstitial lung disease: a diagnostic approach. AJR 1987; 148:8–15.

Bertrand J-M, Riley SP, Popkin K, Coates AL. The long-term pulmonary sequelae of prematurity: the role of familial airway hyperreactivity and the respiratory distress syndrome. N Engl J Med 1985; 312:742–745.

Bitterman BP, Rennard SI, Keogh BA, et al. Familial idiopathic pulmonary fibrosis: evidence of lung inflammation in unaffected family members. N Engl J Med 1986; 314:1343–1347.

Carrington CB, Gaensler EA. Clinical-pathologic approach to diffuse infiltrative lung disease. In Thurlbeck WM, Abell MR, eds. The lung: structure, function and disease. Baltimore: Williams & Wilkins, 1978:58.

Churg AC, Golden J, Fligiel S, Hogg JC. Bronchopulmonary dysplasia in the adult. Am Rev Respir Dis 1983; 127:117–120.

Colby TV, Lombard C. Histiocytosis X in the lung. Hum Pathol 1983; 14:847–856.

Cooper JAD Jr, White DA, Matthay RA. Drug-induced pulmonary disease, part 1: cytotoxic drugs. Am Rev Respir Dis 1986a; 133:321–340.

Cooper JAD Jr, White DA, Matthay RA. Drug-induced pulmonary disease, part 2: noncytotoxic drugs. Am Rev Respir Dis 1986b; 133:488–505.

CPC 21-1986: Pulmonary veno-occlusive disease. N Engl J Med 1986; 314:1435–1445.

CPC 24-1988: Lymphangioleiomyomatosis. N Engl J Med 1988; 318:1601–1610.

CPC 30-1988: Idiopathic pulmonary hemosiderosis. N Engl J Med 1988; 319:227–237.

Crystal RG, Bitterman PB, Rennard SI, et al. Interstitial lung diseases of unknown cause: disorders characterized by chronic inflammation of the lower respiratory tract (second of two parts). N Engl J Med 1984; 310:235–244.

Crystal RG, Gadek JE, Ferrans VJ, et al. Interstitial lung disease: current concepts of pathogenesis, staging, and therapy. Am J Med 1981; 70:542–568.

Davis PB, di Sant'Agnese PA. Diagnosis and treatment of cystic fibrosis: an update. Chest 1984; 85:802–809.

DeRemee RA. Diffuse interstitial pulmonary disease from the perspective of the clinician. Chest 1987; 92:1068–1073.

Dickey BF, Myers AR. Pulmonary Manifestations of collagen-vascular diseases. In Fishman AP, ed. Pulmonary diseases and disorders. 2nd ed. Vol. 1. New York: McGraw-Hill, 1988:645–666.

Epler GR, Colby TV, McLoud TC, et al. Bronchiolitis obliterans organizing pneumonia. N Engl J Med 1985; 312:152–158.

Epler GR, McLoud TC, Gaensler EA, et al. Normal chest roentgenograms in chronic diffuse infiltrative lung disease. N Engl J Med 1978; 298:934–939.

Fanburg BL, Pitt EA. Sarcoidosis. In: Murray JF, Nadel JA, eds. Textbook of respiratory medicine. Philadelphia: WB Saunders, 1988:1486–1500.

Felson B. Chest roentgenology. Philadelphia: WB Saunders, 1973:314–349.

Felson B. A new look at pattern recognition of diffuse pulmonary disease. AJR 1979; 133:183–189.

Fraser RG, Paré JAP. Diagnosis of diseases of the chest. Philadelphia: WB Saunders, 1977.

Fulmer JD, Crystal RG. Interstitial lung disease. In Simmons DH, ed. Current pulmonology. Chicago: Year Book, 1979:1–65.

Genereux GP. The end-stage lung: pathogenesis, pathology, and radiology. Radiology 1975; 116:279–289.

Grammar LC, Patterson R. Occupational immunologic lung disease. Ann Allergy 1987; 58:151–160.

Hay JG, Turner-Warwick M. Interstitial pulmonary fibrosis. In Murray JF, Nadel JA, eds. Textbook of respiratory medicine. Philadelphia: WB Saunders, 1988:1445–1461.

Jederlinic PJ, Sicilian L, Gaensler EA. Chronic eosinophilic pneumonia: a report of 19 cases and a review of the literature. Medicine 1988; 67:154–162.

Johns CJ. Sarcoidosis. In Fishman AP, ed. Pulmonary diseases and disorders. 2nd ed. Vol. 1. New York: McGraw-Hill, 1988:619–644.

Kapanci Y, Weibel ER, Kaplan HP, et al. Pathogenesis and reversibility of the pulmonary lesions of oxygen toxicity in monkeys. II: ultrastructural and morphometric studies. Lab Invest 1969; 20:101–118.

Katzenstein AL, Bloor CM, Liebow AA. Diffuse alveolar damage: the role of oxygen, shock and related factors. Am J Pathol 1976; 85:210-224.

Lacronique J, Roth C, Battesti J-P, et al. Chest radiologic features of pulmonary histiocytosis X: a report based on 50 adult cases. Thorax 1982; 37:104-109.

Lakshminarayan S, Stanford RE, Petty TL. Prognosis after recovery from adult respiratory distress syndrome. Am Rev Respir Dis 1976; 113:7-16.

Lopez M, Salvaggio JE. Hypersensitivity pneumonitis. In Murray JF, Nadel JA, eds. Textbook of respiratory medicine. Philadelphia: WB Saunders, 1988:1606-1616.

Mathieson JR, Mayo JR, Stapler CA, Müller NL. Chronic diffuse infiltrative lung disease: diagnostic accuracy of computed tomography versus chest radiography. Radiology 1989; 171:111-116.

McLoud TC, Carrington CB, Gaensler EA. Diffuse infiltrative lung disease: a new scheme for description. Radiology 1983; 149:353-363.

Miller RR, Nelems B, Müller NL, et al. Lingular and right middle lobe biopsy in the assessment of diffuse lung disease. Ann Thorac Surg 1987; 44:269-273.

Müller NL, Miller RR, Webb WR, et al. Fibrosing alveolitis: CT-pathologic correlation. Radiology 1986; 160:585-588.

Müller NL, Staples CA, Miller RR, et al. Disease activity in idiopathic pulmonary fibrosis: computed tomographic-pathologic correlation. Radiology 1987; 165:731-734.

Müller NL, Kullnig P, Miller RR. The CT findings of pulmonary sarcoidosis: Analysis of 25 patients. AJR 1989; 152:1179-1182.

Munk PL, Müller NL, Miller RR, Ostrow DN. Pulmonary lymphangitic carcinomatosis: CT and pathologic findings. Radiology 1988; 166:705-709.

Naidich DP, Zerhouni EA, Hutchins GB, et al. Computed tomography of the pulmonary parenchyma. Part 1: distal airspace disease. J Thorac Imag 1985; 1:39-53.

Patterson R, Greenberger PA, Radin RC, Roberts M. Allergic bronchopulmonary aspergillosis: staging as an aid to management. Ann Intern Med 1982; 96:286-291.

Pimentel JC. Tridimensional photographic reconstruction in a study of the pathogenesis of honeycomb lung. Thorax 1967; 22:444-452.

Prakash UBS, Barham SS, Carpenter HA, et al. Pulmonary alveolar phospholipoproteinosis: experience with 34 cases and a review. Mayo Clin Proc 1987; 62:499-518.

Prakash UBS, Barham SS, Rosenow EC III, et al. Pulmonary alveolar microlithiasis: a review including ultrastructural and pulmonary function studies. Mayo Clin Proc 1983; 58:290-300.

Prophet D. Primary pulmonary histiocytosis-X. Clin Chest Med 1982; 3:643-653.

Rosenow EC III. Drug-induced pulmonary disease. In Murray JF, Nadel JA, eds. Textbook of respiratory medicine. Philadelphia: WB Saunders, 1988a:1681-1702.

Rosenow EC III. Primary pulmonary histiocytosis X. In Fishman AP, ed. Pulmonary diseases and disorders. 2nd ed. Vol. 1. New York: McGraw-Hill, 1988b: 813-818.

Ryan SF, Bell ALL Jr, Barrett CR Jr. Experimental acute alveolar injury in the dog: morphologic-mechanical correlations. Am J Pathol 1976; 82:353-372.

Salvaggio JE. Hypersensitivity pneumonitis. J Allergy Clin Immunol 1987; 79:558-571.

Schraufnagel DE, Claypool WC, Fahey PJ, et al. Interstitial pulmonary fibrosis. Am Rev Respir Dis 1987; 136: 1281-1284.

Schwarz MI, King TE Jr., eds. Interstitial lung disease. Toronto: BC Decker, 1988.

Smith P, Heath D. The ultrastructure and sequence of the early stages of paraquat lung in rats. J Pathol 1974; 114:177-184.

Staples CA, Müller NL, Vedal S, et al. Usual interstitial pneumonia: correlation of CT with clinical, functional, and radiologic findings. Radiology 1987; 162: 377-381.

Stein MG, Mayo J, Müller NL, et al. Pulmonary lymphangitic spread of carcinoma: appearance on CT scans. Radiology 1987; 162:371-375.

Stokes LT, Turner-Warwick M. Lungs and Connective Tissue Disorders. In Murray JF, Nadel JA, eds. Textbook of respiratory medicine. Philadelphia: WB Saunders, 1988:1462-1485.

Thomas PD, Hunninghake GW. Current concepts of the pathogenesis of sarcoidosis. Am Rev Respir Dis 1987; 135:747-760.

Turner-Warwick M. General principles and diagnostic approach. In Murray JF, Nadel JA, eds. Textbook of respiratory medicine. Philadelphia: WB Saunders, 1988a:1435-1444.

Turner-Warwick M. Widespread pulmonary fibrosis. In Fishman AP, ed. Pulmonary diseases and disorders. 2nd ed. Vol. 1. New York: McGraw-Hill, 1988b: 755-772.

Wasserman K, Mason GR. Pulmonary alveolar proteinosis. In Murray JF, Nadel JA, eds. Textbook of respiratory medicine. Philadelphia: WB Saunders, 1988: 1535-1547.

Weill H, Jones RN. Occupational pulmonary diseases. In Fishman AP, ed. Pulmonary diseases and disorders. 2nd ed. Vol. 1. New York: McGraw-Hill, 1988:819-860.

Wilson CB. Immunologic diseases of the lung and kidney (Goodpasture's syndrome). In Fishman AP, ed. Pulmonary diseases and disorders. 2nd ed. Vol. 1. New York: McGraw-Hill, 1988:675-682.

Zerhouni EA, Naidich DP, Stitik FP, et al. Computed tomography of the pulmonary parenchyma. Part 2: interstitial disease. J Thorac Imag 1985; 1:54-64.

CHAPTER 3

PRACTICAL CONSIDERATIONS OF LUNG BIOPSY

All too often the surgeon, chest physician, radiologist, pathologist, and microbiologist use their knowledge and skills independently of each other. Infiltrative lung disease is a relatively uncommon problem and, other than in large centers, only a few open lung biopsies are performed per year. Thus diagnostic experience may be limited, particularly in the hands of general surgical pathologists, general radiologists, general internists, and nonthoracic surgeons. It, therefore, behooves all interested parties to be fully aware of all the features of a given case. Transbronchial biopsies may be misleading in many types of chronic infiltrative lung disease (Wall et al, 1981). Lesions are often not uniformly distributed through the lung, and the input of the radiologist may be critical in the choice of technique and site to be biopsied. The physician in charge of the case should consult fully with colleagues and should be aware of the limitations and the diagnostic potential of various radiologic examinations and of biopsy.

The chest radiograph is usually the first and foremost investigation performed on patients with diffuse lung disease. It is the cornerstone in the assessment of both acute and chronic conditions.

A number of imaging techniques may be used to complement the chest radiograph. The main ones to consider are computed tomography (CT), magnetic resonance imaging (MRI), radionuclide scanning, and pulmonary angiography. Investigations that may be performed under radiologic guidance include fine needle aspiration biopsy and fiberoptic bronchoscopy.

CHEST RADIOGRAPH

The optimal chest radiograph is performed in the radiology department with the patient standing. Both posteroanterior (PA) and lateral projections are required in the assessment of diffuse lung disease. The radiograph should be obtained at total lung capacity with the X-ray beam properly centered, and using an adequate exposure. These parameters can easily be checked by noting that the dome of the right hemidiaphragm lies between the anterior fifth and sixth ribs, that the medial ends of the clavicles lie equidistant to the spinous processes of the fourth dorsal vertebra, and that the thoracic spine and intervertebral disks are faintly visible behind the heart shadow. Failure of the radiograph to fulfill any of these criteria will make interpretation more difficult and often unreliable. The majority of institutions use high kilovoltage technique (120 to 150 kVp) because this allows better assessment of the mediastinum, retrocardiac structures, and pulmonary vascularity than do lower kilovoltage techniques. A grid is used to decrease scatter radiation (noise).

In the seriously ill patient, the standard radiograph must often be substituted by the anteroposterior (AP) portable chest radiograph. This is obtained at bedside using portable radiographic equipment. The quality of the portable radiograph is always inferior to the standard one because it is usually performed at low kilovoltage, without a grid, and in a poorly cooperative patient. Low kilovoltage (80 to 90 kVp) results in poor visualization of mediastinal and retrocardiac structures and difficulty in differentiating normal parenchyma from mild reticular or nodular infiltrates. Technical considerations preclude the use of a grid in most portable radiographs. They therefore have more scatter and thus a much lower signal-to-noise ratio than do standard radiographs. The sick patient is often unable to make an adequate inspiratory effort. This results in crowding of the bronchovascular markings and artifactual appearance of cardiac enlargement and reticulonodular changes. The portable radiograph is therefore easily, and often, overcalled. It is of limited value in the initial assessment of diffuse lung disease but is helpful in determining the position of various tubes, the presence of complications such as pneumomediastinum and pneumothorax, and the assessment of serial changes in the pattern and extent of disease.

COMPUTED TOMOGRAPHY

Recently, several reports have demonstrated the usefulness of CT in the diagnosis and management of patients with acute and chronic diffuse lung disease (Bergin and Müller, 1987; Miller et al, 1987). CT provides a two-dimensional representation of a section whose thickness is 1 cm or less. It may be seen as a series of contiguous radiographs, each obtained in the transverse plane along the long axis of the body. As a conventional radiograph, the image is based on the quantity of X-ray photons absorbed by the different tissues in the body. By measuring the amount of radiation absorbed around a section of body, the computer can calculate the attenuation within each area and thus produce a cross-sectional image. Because a narrow beam is used, the image is almost free of scatter radiation (noise). The decreased superimposition of parenchymal structures on CT allows a better estimation of the type, distribution, and severity of parenchymal changes than is possible on the chest radiograph.

The main advantages of CT over the radiograph are a much higher signal-to-noise ratio, superior contrast resolution, and the lack of superimposition of parenchymal structures. The disadvantages include lower spatial resolution, high cost, and radiation exposure. We therefore limit its use to the initial assessment of patients with diffuse lung disease and whenever open lung biopsy is being considered. Adequate assessment of lung parenchyma requires high spatial resolution, and this is obtained only with state-of-the-art CT scanners. Assessment of diffuse lung disease requires that besides the use of routine 1-cm-thick CT slices, additional 1.5-mm-thick slices also be obtained. In these patients, we routinely perform CT scans without intravenous contrast material, using 1-cm collimation scans and additional 1.5-mm scans at three levels: aortic arch, tracheal carina, and 1 cm above the right hemidiaphragm. The additional cost is small and the increase in information great.

MAGNETIC RESONANCE IMAGING

MRI is based on the property of certain atomic nuclei, when placed in a magnetic field and stimulated by radiowaves of a particular frequency, to re-emit some of the absorbed energy in the form of radio signals. The magnetic resonance images depict the location and behavior of nuclei emitting these radio signals. Unlike chest radiographs or CT scans, which essentially measure a single parameter (i.e., X-ray beam attenuation), the MR scan may provide different kinds of information, depending on the technique used. It has several advantages over CT, including the ability to produce images in the sagittal and coronal planes and the lack of ionizing radiation. It has been shown to be equal or superior to CT in the assessment of the central nervous system, mediastinum, and heart. However, MRI has several major limitations in the assessment of bronchopulmonary disease. These include a low spatial resolution, long scanning time and thus the presence of motion artifacts, as well as a very poor signal-to-noise ratio. These limitations are slowly being overcome but, as yet, MRI plays no role in the assessment of diffuse lung disease.

RADIONUCLIDE SCANNING

The two main techniques to consider in the assessment of diffuse lung disease are ventilation-perfusion scans and gallium scanning. Ventilation-perfusion radionuclide scanning is used mainly in the diagnosis of pulmonary embolism. The perfusion scan is performed using an intravenous injection of radioisotope-labeled albumin. Areas of decreased or absent perfusion are detected as defects in perfusion. These are seen not only in pulmonary embo-

lism but also in other conditions leading to focal areas of hypoperfusion such as vasculitis, chronic obstructive airway disease, and pneumonia. The specificity of the test is improved by complementing it with a ventilation scan. The ventilation scan is performed by inhaling a radioisotope-labeled gas, usually xenon. Pulmonary embolism characteristically leads to defects in the perfusion scan but a normal ventilation scan, i.e., ventilation-perfusion mismatch. The presence of multiple segmental areas of ventilation-perfusion mismatch is virtually pathognomonic of pulmonary embolism.

Radioactive gallium scanning (^{67}Ga) has been used in the diagnosis and follow-up of patients with certain inflammatory or neoplastic diseases. It localizes in the lung in a variety of diffuse diseases including sarcoidosis, fibrosing alveolitis, pneumonia, tuberculosis, and drug toxicity. The degree of gallium uptake has been said to correlate with the severity of disease activity in fibrosing alveolitis and sarcoidosis. However, there is much controversy over its usefulness in these conditions.

Gallium-67 scintigraphy has been most useful in the detection of *Pneumocystis carinii* pneumonia, particularly in patients with AIDS. In these patients *Pneumocystis carinii* pneumonia is often associated with more subtle symptoms than in other immunocompromised patients (Kovacs et al, 1984), and 10 to 24 percent of patients may have normal chest radiographs and abnormal gallium scans (Murray et al, 1984; Woolfenden et al, 1987). Diffusely increased lung uptake in patients with AIDS is seen most commonly with *Pneumocystis carinii* pneumonia but also with other inflammatory conditions such as cytomegalovirus and cryptococcal pneumonia. Focal uptake corresponding to hilar lymph nodes is seen most commonly with *Mycobacterium avium intracellulare* but also may be seen with lymphoma (Kramer et al, 1987). Localized intrapulmonary uptake in patients with AIDS may be seen in bacterial pneumonias. Although gallium-67 scans are sensitive in detecting pneumocystis pneumonia and other pulmonary infections in patients with AIDS, they are not useful for localizing Kaposi's sarcoma (Woolfenden et al, 1987).

Gallium-67 scanning is not only useful in the early diagnosis of pneumocystis pneumonia but may also be used for monitoring treatment. Patients with pneumocystis pneumonia should be continued on treatment as long as the follow-up gallium scan is positive (Bekerman and Hoffer, 1987).

Besides the use in the assessment of pulmonary infection, gallium-67 scintigraphy has also been recommended for the early detection of interstitial pneumonitis associated with bleomycin (Richman et al, 1975), amiodarone pneumonitis (van Rooij et al,

1984), and nitrofurantoin-induced pulmonary reaction (Crook et al, 1982).

PULMONARY ANGIOGRAPHY

The technique is simple: A catheter is passed through a vein, usually the femoral, and advanced into the pulmonary artery, and contrast material is injected. Usually, the right and left arteries are injected separately. This allows visualization of the pulmonary arterial tree in exquisite detail. It is an invasive technique, but the rate of complication is small. Although it is often performed in critically ill patients, the mortality is less than 0.5 percent.

The main indication is in the assessment of pulmonary embolism, where angiography remains the gold standard in the diagnosis. It should be performed within 48 hours of the onset of the clinical episode; otherwise, extensive thrombolysis may have occurred, resulting in a false-negative result. Less common indications include the assessment of various congenital and acquired pulmonary vascular diseases, particularly arteriovenous malformations. At one time, angiography was used in the preoperative evaluation of bullous lung disease. In this setting, it has been largely replaced by the CT scanner.

PERCUTANEOUS NEEDLE BIOPSY OF THE LUNG

Needle biopsy is performed by passing a fine (20- or 22-gauge) needle into the lung under fluoroscopic or CT guidance. A small sample is aspirated by attaching a syringe and applying suction. It is a simple technique to obtain diagnostic cytologic material. The main indication is in the assessment of lung nodules, where accuracy rates of 90 to 95 percent have been reported. It can be performed safely in most patients, the main complication being pneumothorax. In a review of 422 patients, Westcott observed pneumothorax in 21 percent, 13 percent of whom required treatment (Westcott, 1981). Although it has been reported to have a high yield in the diagnosis of such diverse conditions as pneumocystis infection and lymphangitic carcinomatosis (Weisbrod et al, 1985), we do not use it in the assessment of diffuse lung disease at the Vancouver General Hospital.

PRACTICAL ASPECTS OF LUNG BIOPSY

Basic Patient Considerations

Many patients with diffuse lung disease will ultimately require tissue diagnosis. A major responsibility of the clinicians to the patient is to establish a diagnosis in a noninvasive manner (see Chapter 2). Once this has failed and it is evident that obtaining tissue is necessary, the type of biopsy, site of biopsy, and laboratory procedures all depend on a few basic clinical and radiologic questions:

1. Is the patient immunocompromised or non-immunocompromised? If immunocompromised, are there disorders of clotting?
2. Is the process acute or chronic?
3. Is the process central or peripheral?
4. Is the process localized or diffuse?
5. How critically ill is the patient, and how quickly is a laboratory diagnosis required?
6. Has the cost-to-benefit ratio been taken into account and explained to the patient and family?

Acute Infiltrative Lung Disease

Immunocompromised Patient

Because of the frequent use of immunosuppressive agents in the treatment of malignancy, autoimmune diseases, and transplant recipients, as well as the epidemic proportions of the acquired immunodeficiency syndrome (AIDS), lung disease in the immunocompromised host has become common. These patients ordinarily present acutely, and the important differential diagnoses are infection, drug reaction, recurrent malignancy, and pulmonary hemorrhage. Approximately 15 to 20 percent of patients will develop two or three of these. The cited yield of different diagnostic techniques is variable. Induced sputum and bronchoalveolar lavage (BAL) are highly sensitive in detecting *Pneumocystis carinii* pneumonia in patients with AIDS (Ognibene et al, 1984); the use of monoclonal antibodies in BAL fluid is also effective in the diagnosis of cytomegalovirus (CMV) infection and herpes infection in patients with AIDS (Clark and Crawford, 1987). Transbronchial lung biopsy is said to be even more sensitive than BAL (Mones et al, 1986) in the diagnosis of *Pneumocystis carinii* in patients with AIDS. Thus, open biopsy is seldom indicated in this particular population (Stulbarg, 1987). In immunocompromised patients with pneumocystis pneumonia who do not also have AIDS, BAL and transbronchial biopsy are not so sensitive. Milburn et al (1987) reported a yield of 80 percent for BAL in the diagnosis of infection in marrow transplant patients. Cordonnier et al (1986) were slightly less successful, with a diagnostic yield of 66 percent. However, marrow transplant patients suffer from a variety of noninfectious pulmonary infiltrates also, and open lung biopsy is required for diagnosis in a greater proportion of patients (Clark and Crawford, 1987). Transbronchial lung biopsy, usually in conjunction with BAL and brushing, is a reasonably sensitive method of diagnosing infection in non-AIDS, non–bone marrow transplant immunocompromised hosts (Canham et al, 1983). However, open lung biopsy is still the major means of diagnosing noninfectious infiltrates in the immunocompromised host (Wetstein, 1986). If an open lung biopsy is required, the biopsy site in these patients should ordinarily be from the area of worst involvement, as this increases the probability of finding diagnostic abnormalities (Miller et al, 1987). Preliminary bacteriologic results, fluorescence studies for viral antigens, and histologic examination for pattern of reaction, viral inclusions, and fungal or *Pneumocystis carinii* organisms should be available within 24 hours.

There is incontrovertible evidence (Robin and Burke, 1986; Warner et al, 1988) that the precise diagnostic information afforded by open lung biopsy does not statistically translate into improved patient survival, because of the limitations of treatment options. Nevertheless, every patient should be considered individually with all the risk factors and beneficial effects of this invasive procedure taken into account. Many clinicians elect to treat patients with empirical use of antibiotics and proceed to biopsy only if this fails.

Nonimmunocompromised Patient

Occasionally, an apparently nonimmunocompromised patient will present with acute infiltrative lung disease, the etiology of which eludes less invasive diagnostic techniques than open biopsy. Considerations of site of biopsy and laboratory procedure, in general, are similar to those pertaining to the immunocompromised host. One is likely to find nonspecific diffuse alveolar damage, presumably due to viral infection in many instances, but one may be surprised on occasion to find lymphangitic carcinoma, or *Legionella* pneumonia, or an unusual infection in an unsuspected patient with AIDS.

Chronic Infiltrative Lung Disease

In a nonimmunocompromised patient with chronic infiltrative lung disease, the principles of type and site of biopsy and laboratory procedure are different. Transbronchial lung biopsy (TBB) is likely to be fruitful only in patients with sarcoidosis and lymphangitic carcinoma, and most such patients are so diagnosed (Wall et al, 1981). It should be noted, however, that in this study, seven of 20 patients found to have sarcoidosis had normal or nonspecific findings on TBB and the diagnosis was only made on open lung biopsy. In most other causes of chronic

---

TABLE 3–1

COMPARISON OF TRANSBRONCHIAL AND OPEN BIOPSY ON THE SAME PATIENT*

TRANSBRONCHIAL BIOPSY	OPEN LUNG BIOPSY
Normal (10 patients)	Chronic interstitial pneumonia (4) Sarcoid (4) Eosinophilic granuloma (1) Fibrosis of uncertain significance (1)
Nonspecific inflammation (11)	Chronic interstitial pneumonia (5) Eosinophilic granuloma (2) Sarcoid (1) Lymphoma (1) Nondiagnostic (2)
Chronic interstitial pneumonia (9)	Chronic interstitial pneumonia (2) Eosinophilic granuloma (2) Bronchiolitis (1) Sarcoid (1) Honeycomb lung (1) Pulmonary hypertension (1) Nondiagnostic (1)
Inadequate biopsy (3)	Chronic interstitial pneumonia (2) Sarcoid (1)
Specific diagnosis (20)(37.7%)	Not done

*Modified with permission from Wall CP, Gaensler EA, Carrington CB, Hayes JA. Comparison of transbronchial and open biopsies in chronic infiltrative lung diseases. Am Rev Respir Dis 1981; 123: 280–285.

infiltrative lung disease, TBBs are normal or nonspecific. Further, it should be recognized that TBB may be misleading in chronic infiltrative lung disease (Table 3–1), and the diagnosis of interstitial fibrosis (usual interstitial pneumonia) or desquamative interstitial pneumonia should ordinarily not be made (Wall et al, 1981). This widely quoted paper referred to early experience with TBB when the size and number of pieces of tissue were small. It also does not include examples of alveolar proteinosis, bronchiolar-alveolar carcinoma, eosinophilic pneumonia, or bronchiolitis obliterans–organizing pneumonia (cryptogenic organizing pneumonia), in which conditions we have confidently and correctly made these diagnoses. TBB may be more sensitive and specific with current biopsy techniques in patients with a wide range of causes of chronic infiltrative lung diseases.

Should open lung biopsy be required, the objective, contrary to the acute situation, is to sample areas of "average" involvement rather than areas of worst involvement because of the likelihood of obtaining end-stage lung in the latter sites (Miller et al, 1987). Recent advances in CT of the lungs play a major role in the preoperative evaluation of these patients. It can be useful in distinguishing sarcoidosis and lymphangitic carcinoma (Munk et al, 1988) from other types of chronic infiltrative lung disease, thus assisting in the decision of whether or not to attempt a TBB (Mathieson et al, 1989). CT is also useful in assessing the distribution of disease, thus directing the surgeon to the area of accessible "average" involvement (Miller et al, 1987). While routine avoidance of the lingula and right middle lobe was once the recommended policy, this no longer seems to be necessary, especially in view of the additional information provided by CT (Miller et al, 1987). Frozen section is rarely indicated in chronic infiltrative lung disease, microbiologic studies may be done on a routine rather than "stat" basis, and special stains for organisms may also be performed routinely on paraffin sections. In the largest reported series of open lung biopsies in chronic infiltrative lung disease (Carrington and Gaensler, 1978), no diagnosis was made in five of 490 patients (1 percent) and 40 (8.2 percent) had nonspecific diagnoses.

TECHNICAL CONSIDERATIONS

Bronchoalveolar Lavage

The actual technique of performing BAL has been extensively reviewed in several series (Crystal et al, 1986; Reynolds, 1987; Daniele et al, 1985). The procedure can be done in almost any cooperative patient and is performed through the fiberbronchoscope after the usual application of topical anesthesia. This has not been found to affect the results. A seal is obtained by gently wedging the tip of the adult-sized bronchoscope into either the right middle lobe or the lingular orifice. The upper lobes are almost never used unless it is for a very specific process, and the lower lobes are rarely used. Sterile saline (0.9 percent) solution is the fluid used for lavage, either at room temperature or warmed to 37°C. Usually the segment is infused with five to seven 20-ml aliquots or two to three 50-ml aliquots for a total of 100 to 150 ml; rarely is more than 300 ml used. Following the slow (5 ml per second) instillation of each aliquot, gentle suction is applied. Because of sampling errors, most investigators pool two or three separate sites.

Bronchoalveolar lavage is a safe procedure as long as the investigator follows reasonable guidelines. The most common complication is fever, occurring in 10 to 15 percent of the patients. This increases with the use of total lavage volume greater than 250 to 300 ml per segment lavaged. Approximately 10 to 15 percent of patients develop minor reductions in the vital capacity following the procedure.

The number and type of cells is determined using a hemacytometer or centrifuge preparation stained with either Wright-Giesma or "Diff-Quick." This method, though, may produce an artifact with an underestimate of the actual number of lymphocytes recovered. Use of a Millipore filter appears to overcome this artifact (Crystal et al, 1986). In addition to assessing the number and type of cells recovered, a multitude of other substances such as interleukin-1, various proteases, proteins, chemotactic factors, and the use of monoclonal antibodies to assess other types of cells and even viruses can be used.

The total number of cells averages 15×10^6, with the differential showing 85 to 90 percent macrophages, 7 to 12 percent lymphocytes, and 1 to 2 percent polymorphonuclear leukocytes (PMNs). Lymphocyte subsets disclosed that 70 percent of the lymphocytes are T cells, with a T_H/T_S ratio of 1.5 to 1.8. In smokers the number of PMNs increases up to 10 percent.

Transbronchial Biopsy

Transbronchoscopic lung biopsy is an attempt to obtain a small piece of representative lung tissue through the bronchoscope at minimal risk to the patient as well as low morbidity. Most procedures are done under topical anesthesia using 4 percent lidocaine. Preparations include administration of meperidine (50 mg intramuscularly) and glycopyrrolate (0.3 to 0.4 mg intramuscularly). During the procedure, midazolam (1 to 3 mg in titrated doses intravenously) is often used to obtain maximal relaxation as well as amnesia for the procedure. Most patients undergoing transbronchoscopic lung biopsy will have a soft latex orotracheal tube placed in the trachea, using a flexible bronchoscope as a guide. Or, the bronchoscope is passed through the nose and supplemental oxygen is delivered throughout the procedure via a side-port.

Before the procedure is started, the patient is instructed to point with his or her fingers to the area in the chest at the time of the transbronchoscopic lung biopsy if there is pain. If the patient indicates pain, a biopsy is not attempted. If diagnostic BAL is also requested, this is accomplished before proceeding with transbronchoscopic lung biopsy. Ideally, the use of biplane fluoroscopy is desirable to obtain optimal biopsies. The tip of the bronchoscope is introduced as far as possible into the bronchus leading to the pulmonary infiltrates. Many bronchoscopists wedge the bronchoscope into the bronchus in an effort to tamponade the bronchus, should there be serious hemorrhage following the biopsy.

Either a cup forceps or an alligator forceps is advanced beyond the tip of the bronchoscope and into the area from which biopsies are to be taken. The forceps is opened and the instrument advanced until resistance is met. At this point the biopsy forceps is closed, and if the patient does not complain of pain, the forceps is withdrawn, leaving the bronchoscope wedged in the bronchus. Studies have shown that it does not make any difference whether the biopsies are obtained during end-inspiration or end-expiration. It is also true that there is not much difference in the size of the biopsy sample or the complications whether a cup forceps or an alligator forceps is used.

After several biopsies are taken and hemostasis is assured, the bronchoscope is gently withdrawn. Usually the endoscopist examines the apices in the periphery of the lung with fluoroscopy during end-expiration to make sure there is no evidence of pneumothorax. Routine chest radiographs are not obtained after transbronchoscopic lung biopsy, unless the procedure was complicated, the patient was uncooperative, or the patient complained of chest pain during the procedure. In the absence of severe bleeding and pneumothorax, most patients are sent home the same day.

To avoid the crush artifact, it is important not to squeeze the biopsy specimens with pickup forceps or other means. In most diffuse lung diseases, four to six biopsy specimens are obtained. Biopsies from different lobes and segments of the same side can be done, but bilateral transbronchoscopic lung biopsy is not advisable. The major complication of transbronchoscopic lung biopsy is pneumothorax, seen in 1 to 3 percent of patients undergoing the procedure. Significant hemorrhage is unusual unless the biopsies were done in the face of thrombocytopenia or renal failure.

Open Lung Biopsy

The side and site of biopsy depend on the particular features of the case. However, an anterior subpectoral incision with access through the fourth interspace allows sampling of the lingula/right middle lobe and lower lobe, and is our preferred procedure provided that these sites are appropriately involved radiologically (Miller et al, 1987). If excess pleural fluid is present, a sample is collected for laboratory studies. The lung is gently palpated for nodules or areas of particular induration. The tissue to be biopsied is brought up toward the wound using atraumatic grasping forceps (Fig. 3-1). The base of

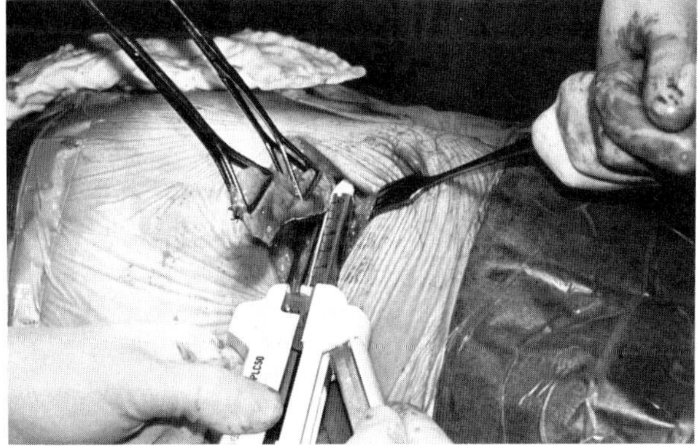

Figure 3-1 A forceps brings the lung wedge toward the thoracotomy site.

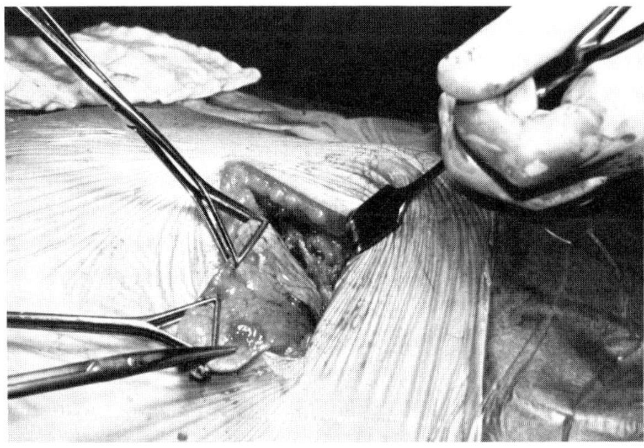

Figure 3-2 A stapling device transects the lung at the base of the biopsy sample.

the wedge is transected with a surgical stapling device (Fig. 3–2), which seals the parent lung and leaves a staple line at the base of the wedge. We believe that this procedure with subsequent inflation of the biopsy by the pathologist is superior to the method suggested by Carrington and Gaensler (1978) as described below. It is certainly simpler and easier on the patient.

Handling of Biopsied Tissue

Transbronchial Biopsy

All of the tissue is embedded in paraffin or plastic. Routine blind sampling for electron microscopy is not particularly useful. Serial sections should be obtained for hematoxylin and eosin (H&E) staining as indicated; and unstained slides should also be prepared in order to have additional use of the limited amount of tissue at a later time if necessary.

Open Lung Biopsy

It is of the utmost importance that open lung biopsies be fixed in the inflated state for adequate interpretation. There are two methods of doing this.

Carrington and Gaensler (1978) described the technique of taking a biopsy of the lung while it is inflated with air by the anesthetist, maintaining closure of the cut surface by clamps, and then immersing the clamped sample into fixative, relying on transpleural diffusion for adequate fixation. This technique necessitates additional sampling for cultures, electron microscopy, mineral analysis, and snap freezing. We use the alternative approach as described above whereby the lung sample is wedged out in the partially inflated state using a stapler. The staple line of the specimen is excised and used for microbiologic examination. The remainder of the wedge can be sampled as desired for frozen section, electron microscopy, etc. Inflation of the remaining lung sample is then achieved by gentle infusion of fixative into the cut surface via a small-bore syringe (Fig. 3–3). Fixation in inflation should be allowed for at least 2 to 3 hours before sectioning into blocks, and all of the tissue should be processed. Uninflated lung may render diagnosis difficult or even impossible since the general architecture of the lung will be obscured (Fig. 3–4).

Patterns of Lung Reaction

As will be apparent from the following sections in this book, different diseases give rise to different architectural patterns. Usually these are easily recognized using a scanning objective, and all available

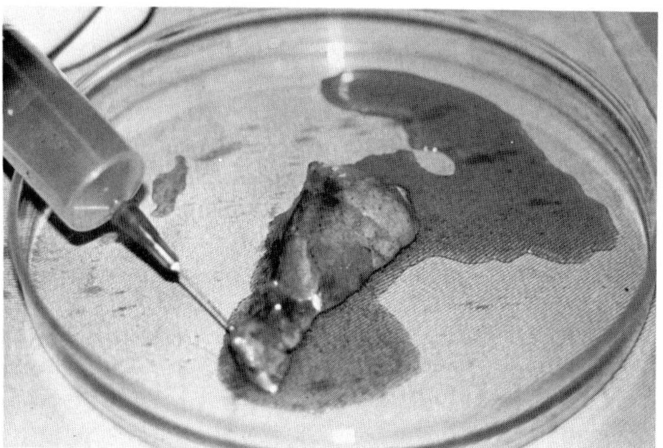

Figure 3–3   Syringe inflation of open lung biopsy sample.

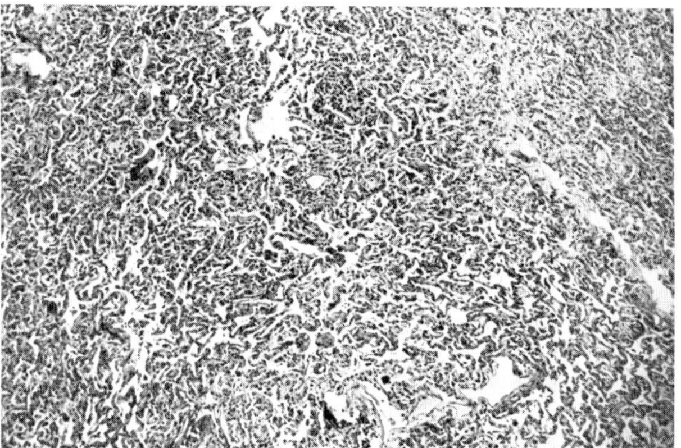

A

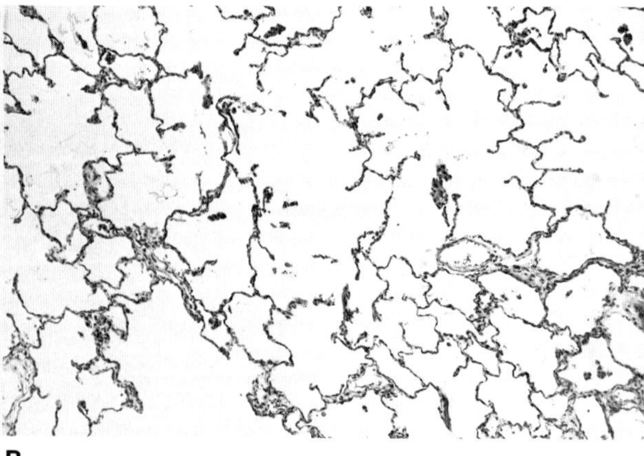

B

Figure 3–4   A, Uninflated lung biopsy, normal area (H&E, × 100). B, Inflated lung biopsy, normal area (H&E, × 100).

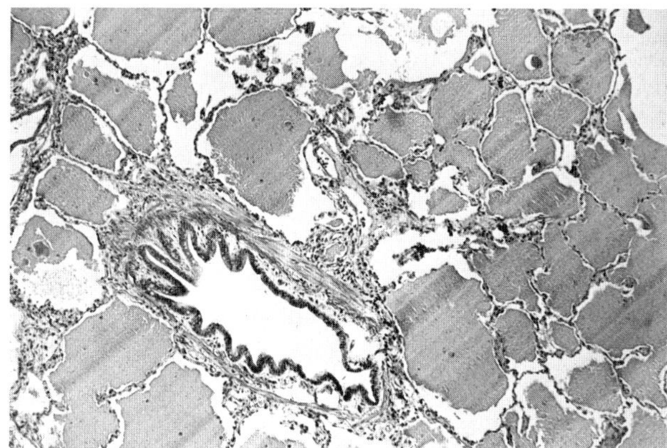

Figure 3–5 Pulmonary alveolar proteinosis: intra-alveolar process (H&E, × 100).

sections should be systematically scanned. This survey is essential to determine the general architectural pattern, and a formal analysis should be given to the components of the lung: alveoli, airways, arteries, veins, lymphatics, lobular septa, and pleura.

The most important questions are as follows:

1. Is the process primarily intra-alveolar or interstitial (Figs. 3–5 and 3–6)?
2. Is there preferential involvement of the lymphatic tissue of the lobular septa and bronchovascular bundle (Figs. 3–7 and 3–8)?
3. Are nodules randomly distributed through the lobule? What is the shape of the nodules (Figs. 3–9 and 3–10)?

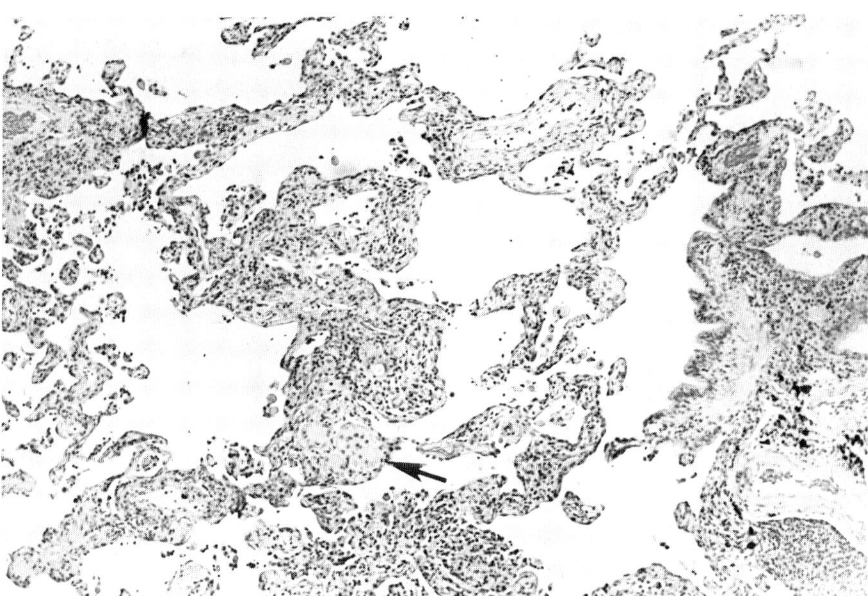

Figure 3–6 Extrinsic allergic alveolitis: interstitial process with granuloma (*arrow*) (H&E, × 100).

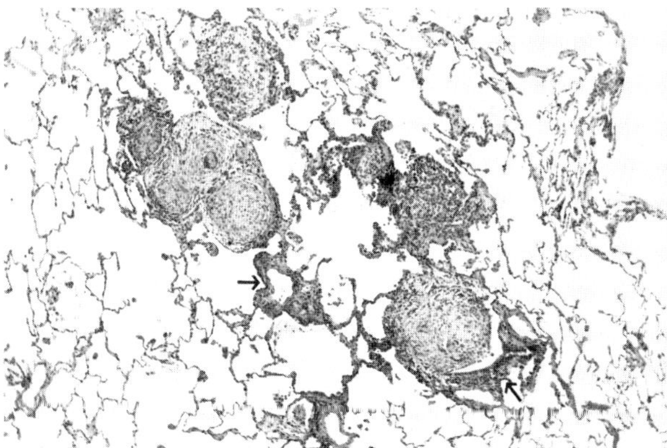

Figure 3–7 Sarcoidosis: granulomas along respiratory bronchioles (*arrows*) without alveolitis (H&E, × 63).

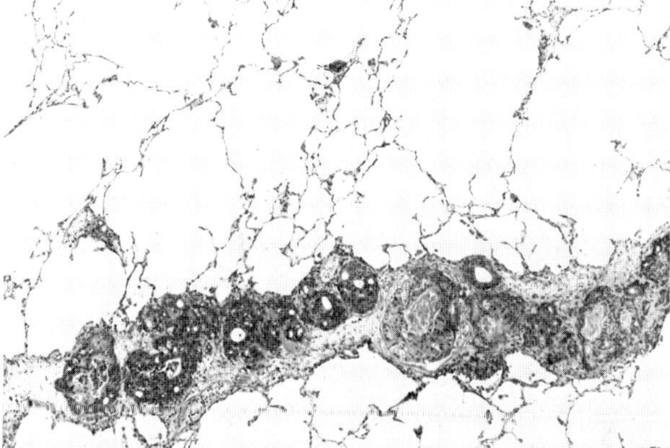

Figure 3–8 Lymphangitic carcinoma: expansion of septal lymphatics by malignant cells (H&E, × 63).

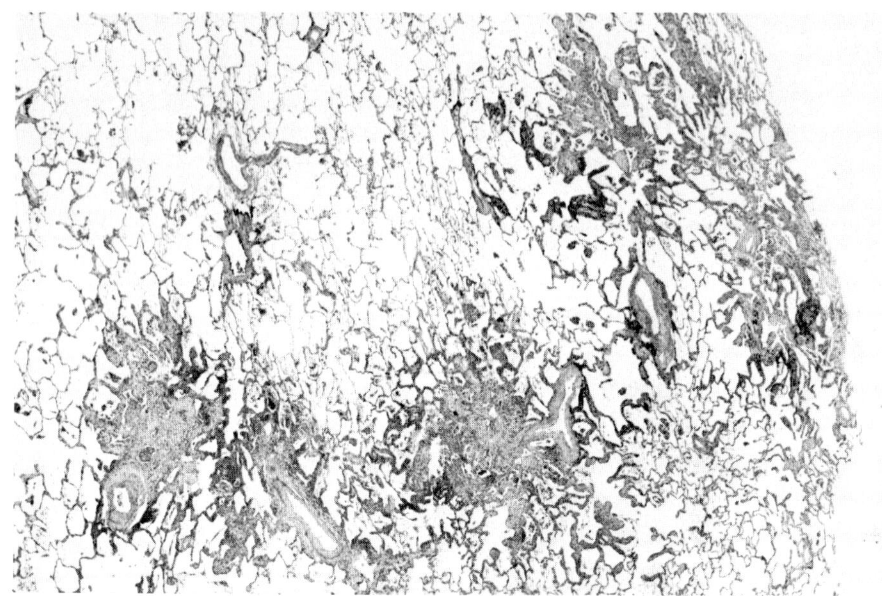

Figure 3–9 Eosinophilic granuloma: randomly distributed stellate nodules (H&E, × 25).

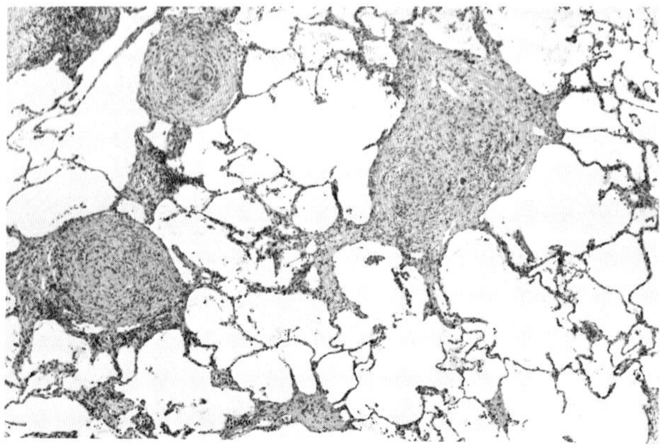

Figure 3–10 Coccidioidomycosis: randomly distributed round granulomas (H&E, × 63).

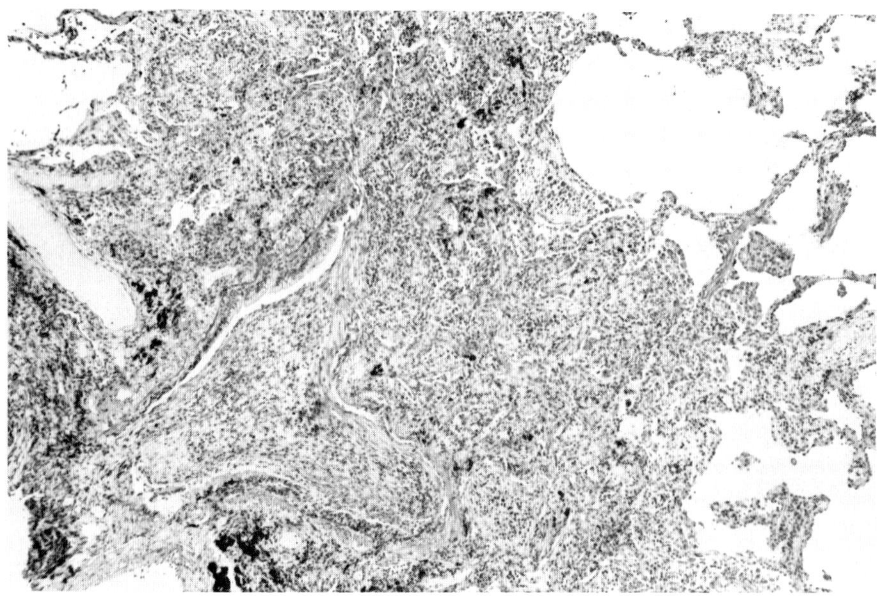

Figure 3–11 Bronchiolitis obliterans: disease centered on proximal respiratory bronchiole (H&E, × 63).

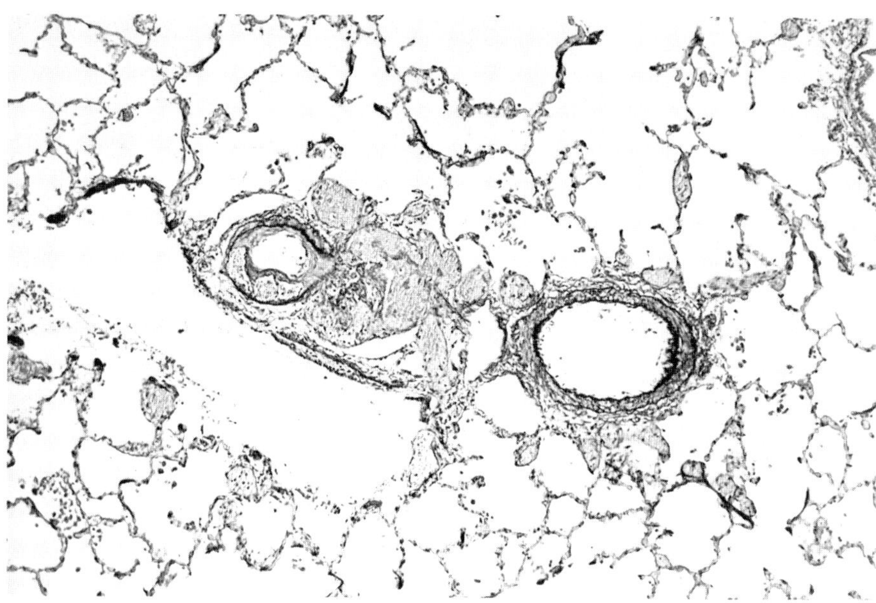

Figure 3–12   Primary pulmonary hypertension: plexiform lesion (VVG, × 100).

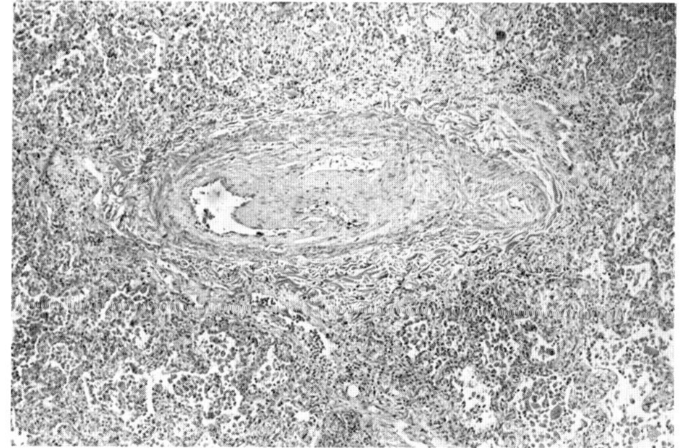

Figure 3–13   Veno-occlusive disease: thrombosis and recanalization of venous lumen (H&E, × 100).

4. Is there particular involvement of the bronchioles (Fig. 3–11)?
5. What is the status of the pulmonary arteries and veins (Figs. 3–12 and 3–13)?
6. What is the nature of the cellular infiltrate? Is it inflammatory or neoplastic?

Polarized light microscopy should always be performed, and various special stains for organisms, elastin, fibrous tissue, etc. should be applied as indicated. Some observers believe that an iron stain should be routinely used, as this facilitates recognition of asbestos bodies.

REFERENCES

Bekerman C, Hoffer PB. The role of gallium-67–citrate imaging in the clinical evaluation of pulmonary disorders. In Loken MK, ed. Pulmonary nuclear medicine. Norwalk CT: Appleton & Lange, 1987:257–289.

Bergin CJ, Müller NL. CT of interstitial lung disease: a diagnostic approach. AJR 1987; 148:8–15.

Canham EM, Kennedy TC, Merrick TA. Unexplained pulmonary infiltrates in the compromised patient. Cancer 1983; 52:325–329.

Carrington CB, Gaensler EA. Clinical-pathologic approach to diffuse infiltrative lung disease. In Thurlbeck WM, Abell MR, eds. The lung: structure, function and disease. Baltimore: Williams & Wilkins, 1978:58.

Clark JG, Crawford SW. Diagnostic approaches to pulmonary complications of marrow transplantation. Chest 1987; 91:477–479.

Cordonnier C, Bernaudin J-F, Brerling P, et al. Pulmonary complications occurring after allogeneic bone marrow transplantation: a study of 130 consecutive transplanted patients. Cancer 1986; 58:1047–1054.

Crook, MJ, Kaplan, PD, Adatepe MH. Gallium-67 scanning in nitrofurantoin-induced pulmonary reaction. J Nucl Med 1982; 23:690–692.

Crystal RG, Reynolds HY, Kalica AR. Bronchoalveolar lavage: the report of an international conference. Chest 1986; 90:122–131.

Daniele RP, Elias JA, Epstein PE, Rossman MD. Bronchoalveolar lavage: the pathogenesis, diagnosis, and management of interstitial lung disease. Ann Intern Med 1985; 102:93–108.

Epler GR, McLoud TCC, Gaensler EA, et al. Normal chest roentgenograms in chronic diffuse infiltrative lung disease. N Engl J Med 1978; 298:934–939.

Kovacs JA, Hiemenz JW, Macher AM, et al. *Pneumocystis*

carinii pneumonia: a comparison between patients with the acquired immunodeficiency syndrome and patients with other immunodeficiencies. Ann Intern Med 1984; 100:663–671.

Kramer EL, Sanger JJ, Garay SM, et al. Gallium-67 scans of the chest in patients with acquired immunodeficiency syndrome. J Nucl Med 1987; 28:1107–1114.

Mathieson JR, Mayo JR, Staples CA, Müller NL. Chronic diffuse infiltrative lung disease: diagnostic accuracy of computed tomography versus chest radiography. Radiology 1989; in press.

McLoud TC, Carrington CB, Gaensler EA. Diffuse infiltrative lung disease: a new scheme for description. Radiology 1983; 149:353–363.

Milburn HJ, Prentice HG, du Bois RM. Role of bronchoalveolar lavage in the evaluation of interstitial pneumonitis in recipients of bone marrow transplants. Thorax 1987; 42:766–772.

Miller RR, Nelems B, Müller NL, et al. Lingular and right middle lobe biopsy in the assessment of diffuse lung disease. Ann Thorac Surg 1987; 44:269–273.

Mones JM, Saldana MJ, Oldham SA. Diagnosis of *Pneumocystis carinii* pneumonia. Chest 1986; 89:522–526.

Müller NL, Miller RR, Webb WR, et al. Fibrosing alveolitis: CT-pathologic correlation. Radiology 1986; 160:585–588.

Munk PL, Müller NL, Miller RR, Ostrow DN. Pulmonary lymphatic spread of tumor: CT and pathologic findings. Radiology 1988; 166:705–709.

Murray JF, Felton CP, Garay SM, et al. Pulmonary complications of the acquired immunodeficiency syndrome: report of a National Heart, Lung and Blood Institute Workshop. N Engl J Med 1984; 310:1682–1688.

Ognibene FP, Shelhamer J, Gill V, et al. The diagnosis of *Pneumocystis carinii* pneumonia in patients with the acquired immunodeficiency syndrome using subsegmental bronchoalveolar lavage. Am Rev Respir Dis 1984; 129:929–932.

Reynolds HY. Bronchoalveolar lavage. Am Rev Respir Dis 1987; 135:251–261.

Richman SD, Levenson SM, Bunn PA, et al. Gallium-67 accumulation in pulmonary lesions associated with bleomycin toxicity. Cancer 1975; 36:1966–1972.

Robin ED, Burke CM. Lung biopsy in immunosuppressed patients. Chest 1986; 89:276–277.

Stulbarg MS, Golden JA. Open lung biopsy in the acquired immunodeficiency syndrome (AIDS). Chest 1987; 91:639–640.

van Rooij WJ, van der Meer SC, van Royen EA, et al. Pulmonary gallium-67 uptake in amiodarone pneumonitis. J Nucl Med 1984; 25:211–213.

Wall CP, Gaensler EA, Carrington CB, Hayes JA. Comparison of transbronchial and open biopsies in chronic infiltrative lung diseases. Am Rev Respir Dis 1981; 123:280–285.

Warner DO, Warner MA, Divertie MB. Open lung biopsy in patients with diffuse pulmonary infiltrates and acute respiratory failure. Am Rev Respir Dis 1988; 137:90–94.

Weisbrod GL, Stoneman HR, Tao LC. Diagnostic of diffuse malignant infiltration of lung (lymphangitic carcinomatosis) by percutaneous fine-needle aspiration biopsy. J Can Assoc Radiol 1985; 36:238–243.

Westcott JL. Percutaneous needle biopsy of hilar and mediastinal masses. Radiology 1981; 141:323–328.

Wetstein L. Sensitivity and specificity of lingular segmental biopsies of the lung. Chest 1986; 90:383–386.

Woolfenden JM, Carrasquillo JA, Larson SM, et al. Acquired immunodeficiency syndrome: Ga-67 citrate imaging. Radiology 1987; 162:383–387.

CHAPTER 4

ACUTE INFILTRATIVE LUNG DISEASE IN THE NONIMMUNOCOMPROMISED HOST

This chapter and the following three have divided the topic of infiltrative lung disease into somewhat arbitrary categories. This chapter will deal with acute infiltrative lung disease in the normal host and will be followed in order by disease in the immunocompromised host, then diffuse alveolar hemorrhage, and finally chronic infiltrative lung disease. The great majority of lung biopsies are done for these conditions. Diffuse pulmonary hemorrhage is generally acute but may be chronic, as in idiopathic pulmonary hemosiderosis. Also, diffuse alveolar hemorrhage is primarily an alveolar filling disease, but it may enter into the differential diagnosis of acute infiltrative lung disease. The definition of acute is not clear, but the course of most of the diseases is usually measured in days or weeks, whereas the chronic infiltrative lung diseases have a course over months or years. Acute idiopathic interstitial pneumonia (Katzenstein et al, 1986) is an obvious problem. All the patients in that study developed respiratory failure that required mechanical ventilation within 1 to 2 weeks of onset, and the course of the disease was short, generally being fatal within a few months. However, this topic is discussed in relation to the chronic interstitial pneumonias, and as described there it may be an example of accelerated usual interstitial pneumonia.

Another problem is that infections that present acutely in the normal host can and do occur in the immunocompromised host. It is also true that it may not be clear whether a patient is immunologically competent or not. The subdivision into the four chapters is done primarily on clinical grounds since each of them represents, in general, a distinct clinical presentation.

THE ADULT RESPIRATORY DISTRESS SYNDROME OR SEVERE ACUTE PARENCHYMAL LUNG INJURY

First described by Ashbaugh et al in 1967, the concept of the adult respiratory distress syndrome (ARDS) has been controversial and the need for the term was questioned (Murray 1975). A case has been made for ARDS representing oxygen toxicity (Pratt, 1974, 1978). The point was well made by Murray that ARDS was multifactorial and that it was important to consider the various causes separately, since management and outcome might be different depending on the cause.

No agreed definition for ARDS exists, but the simplest one is the rapid development of respiratory failure in a patient who previously had apparently normal lungs. Murray et al (1988) have expanded this definition and used the term "acute parenchymal

lung injury." They point out that the degree of lung injury and its outcome can be quite variable. In some, the injury and its complications may resolve quickly if the patient survives the initial day or two following it. Typical causes associated with a usually benign course include pulmonary edema due to heroin overdose, neurogenic causes, high altitude, near-drowning, fat embolism, pulmonary contusion, acute nitrofurantoin toxicity, leukoagglutinin transfusion reactions, some infectious pneumonias, and air embolism. All of these are diagnosed by virtue of their occurrence in the proper clinical setting; thus there should be no need for a biopsy. In other patients, the disease is progressive and runs a subacute course, with development of parenchymal injury, multisystem organ failure, and death usually within 5 to 7 days. The common associations are sepsis, nonthoracic trauma with shock, and multiple transfusions. Murray et al therefore advocate a scoring system for lung injury and confine the term "ARDS" to severe lung injury (Table 4–1). They also suggest that acute parenchymal lung injury be defined by three parts (Table 4–2), according to the time course of the injury, its severity, and cause.

An all-encompassing definition of ARDS obscures analysis of outcome and treatment. For example, corticosteroids may be beneficial in lung injury due to fat embolism (Flick and Murray, 1984), ineffective in ARDS associated with the sepsis syndrome (fever and hypotension), and worsen the severity of lung injury and increase the incidence of infectious complications in surgical patients with acute lung injury (Weigelt et al, 1985). Further, the expanded definition emphasizes that diffuse lung injury *due to* various causes may be clinically different from that *associated with* various conditions. Those due to the causes listed in Table 4–2 mainly have injury localized to the lung, whereas lung injury associated with the listed conditions often have multiorgan failure involving kidneys, liver, and central nervous system.

In the usual case, a previously well person, or one with apparently normal lungs, suffers a sudden insult such as nonthoracic trauma, generally with shock and multiple blood transfusions. After an apparently stable period, dyspnea occurs and the chest radiograph becomes abnormal. Respiratory failure ensues, requiring ventilatory assistance and varying concentrations of inspired oxygen. The syndrome has been described in patients who have not had high levels of inspired oxygen (Bachofen and Weibel, 1977). About half of the patients recover from this episode with gradual radiologic clearing; the remainder experience a falling arterial oxygen tension (PaO_2), requiring progressively more aggressive ventilation, with higher ventilator end expiratory pressures, and higher concentrations of oxygen.

The lung becomes progressively stiffer, chest infiltrates progress, ventilation is more difficult, and the patient dies. It is a common condition: Although precise figures are not available, it has been estimated that there are 150,000 cases per year in the United States.

ARDS may be divided into four phases: preclinical, exudative, proliferative, and healing. The preclinical phase of ARDS is the stage in which the patient has suffered one of the causes of ARDS (see Table 4-2), but respiratory symptoms and evidence of respiratory failure have not appeared. Attempts have been made to predict those who will develop ARDS and those that will not, but no clear cut predictors have yet emerged. Factor VIII–related antigen may be predictive in the sepsis syndrome but not in other situations (Murray et al, 1988). Most of the data about this stage are derived from experimental animals, but a remarkable study in human trauma (Joachim et al, 1978) has shown that lung weight and hemoglobin content doubles in the lung in patients who die up to 1 hour after trauma, compared with those who die immediately. Experimental studies have shown that the initial phase is subtle endothelial and alveolar epithelial damage associated with capillary leak. The damage is probably due to aggregation of polymorphonuclear leukocytes (PMNs) after activation of the complement cascade. The PMNs produce damage to the endothelium by release of their lysosomal enzymes or generation of free radicals. Another remarkable study has shown aggregations of PMNs in capillaries in lung biopsies performed in humans in the acute phase (Schlag et al, 1980). More florid edema now occurs, and survival after 1 hour is accompanied by a further increase in lung weight.

TABLE 4–1

LUNG INJURY SCORE*

COMPONENT		VALUE
Chest roentgenogram score		
No alveolar consolidation		0
Alveolar consolidation confined to 1 quadrant		1
Alveolar consolidation confined to 2 quadrants		2
Alveolar consolidation confined to 3 quadrants		3
Alveolar consolidation in all 4 quadrants		4
Hypoxemia score		
PaO_2/FiO_2[†]	$\geq$300	0
PaO_2/FiO_2	225–299	1
PaO_2/FiO_2	175–224	2
PaO_2/FiO_2	100–174	3
PaO_2/FiO_2	<100	4
PEEP[‡] score (when ventilated)		
PEEP	$\leq$5 cm H_2O	0
PEEP	6–8 cm H_2O	1
PEEP	9–11 cm H_2O	2
PEEP	12–14 cm H_2O	3
PEEP	$\geq$15 cm H_2O	4
Respiratory system compliance score (when available)		
Compliance	$\geq$80 ml/cm H_2O	0
Compliance	60–79 ml/cm H_2O	1
Compliance	40–59 ml/cm H_2O	2
Compliance	20–39 ml/cm H_2O	3
Compliance	$\leq$19 ml/cm H_2O	4

The final value is obtained by dividing the sum of the scores by the number of components that were used:

	SCORE
No lung injury	0
Mild-to-moderate lung injury	0.1–2.5
Severe lung injury (ARDS)	>2.5

---

*Reprinted with permission from Murray JF, Matthay MA, Luce JM, Flick MR. Pulmonary perspectives: an expanded definition of the adult respiratory distress syndrome. Am Rev Respir Dis 1988; 138:720–723.

[†]PaO_2/FiO_2: Ratio of arterial oxygen tension to inspired oxygen fraction

[‡]PEEP: Positive end-expiratory pressure

TABLE 4–2

THREE-PART DEFINITION OF PARENCHYMAL LUNG INJURY*

Part 1   Acute or subacute, depending on course
Part 2   Mild to moderate lung injury (ARDS), depending on lung injury score
Part 3   *Caused by*
    Aspiration pneumonitis
    Fat embolism
    Drug (e.g., heroin, paraquat) ingestion
    Toxic gases (e.g., phosgene, smoke) inhalation
    Infectious agents (e.g., influenza A, *Pneumocystis carinii*)
    Near-drowning
  or associated with
    Sepsis
    Trauma usually with multiple blood transfusions
    Acute pancreatitis
    Disseminated intravascular coagulation

---

*Modified from Murray JF, Matthay MA, Luce JM, Flick MR: Pulmonary perspectives: an expanded definition of the adult respiratory distress syndrome. Am Rev Respir Dis 1988; 138:720–723.

The next phase is the *exudative phase* and is characterized morphologically by acute diffuse alveolar damage, with less obvious edema, epithelial necrosis, and hyaline membrane formation (Fig. 4–1). Clinically, respiratory failure occurs. This phase merges into the next one, the *proliferative phase*, in which alveolar injury is more prominent and cellular reaction becomes apparent, with type-II cell metaplasia of the airspaces and fibroblastic proliferation and fibrosis (Fig. 4–2). Functionally, the lungs become stiff. The process is apparently reversible for some period and leads to the final phase, the *healing phase*, which has not been observed in any detail morphologically. Patients who recover generally have normal pulmonary function (Petty, 1988) and presumably relatively normal lung structure. Alternatively, at some stage fibrosis becomes progressive and leads to a condition similar to bronchopulmonary dysplasia of neonates (Churg et al, 1983) (Fig. 4–3).

During the latent period the chest radiograph is usually normal unless ARDS is caused by a pulmonary process such as aspiration or infection. Airspace consolidation, the radiologic hallmark of ARDS, usually appears 12 to 24 hours after onset of the clinical

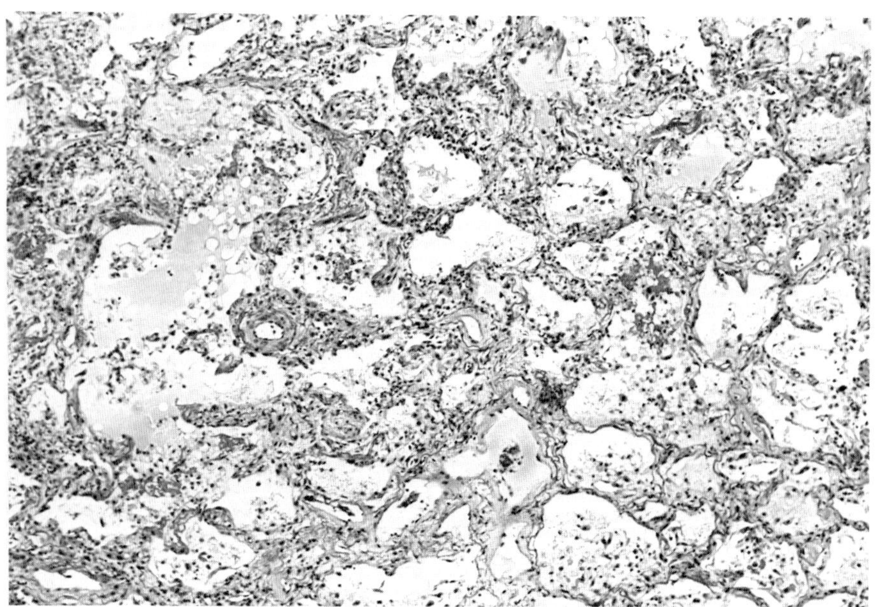

Figure 4–1 Diffuse alveolar damage, largely exudative phase, with edema and fibrinocellular debris in alveolar spaces. The patient was a 78-year-old immunologically intact female with influenza (H&E, × 96).

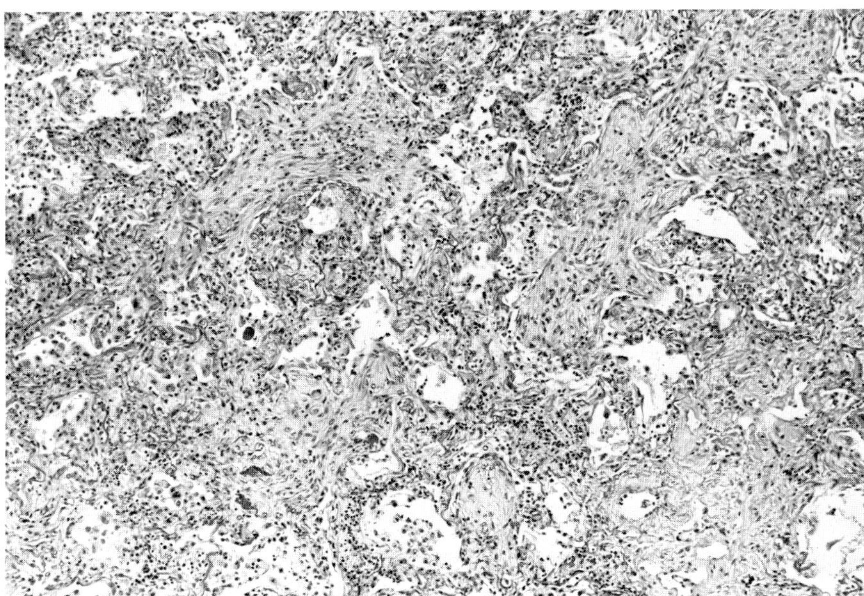

Figure 4–2 Diffuse alveolar damage, proliferative phase, with type-II cell enlargement and obvious intra-alveolar fibrosis. This is the same patient as in Figure 4–1, but a different site of biopsy. (H&E, × 96).

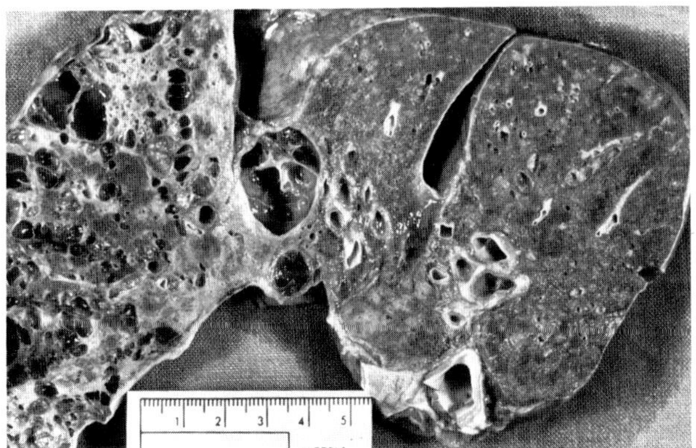

Figure 4–3 Bronchopulmonary dysplasia in a 22-year-old previously healthy man with ARDS due to influenza B. The patient had required mechanical ventilation for 26 days prior to death.

symptoms (Joffe, 1974). The consolidation is initially patchy and indistinct, becoming confluent over the following 1 to 5 days. The consolidation may involve the entire lung parenchyma ("white-out") but tends to be more marked peripherally (Milne, 1986); it is characteristically associated with air bronchograms. On computed tomography (CT), the consolidation is often patchy and predominantly in the dependent lung regions, even if it appears uniform on the radiograph (Greene, 1987). The extent of the radiographic abnormalities correlates with the amount of extra-vascular lung water and, thus, with the severity of pulmonary permeability edema (Sibbald et al, 1983).

As indicated below, ARDS may complicate infections in the immunocompromised host and most lung biopsies in ARDS are performed under these circumstances. Biopsy may be performed in nonimmunocompromised patients to exclude other conditions or to establish the presence of infection, which may complicate and aggravate ARDS.

INFECTIONS OF THE LUNG

In the immunocompromised host, opportunistic infection is a major differential diagnostic consideration of pulmonary infiltrates (see Chapter 5). Viral, bacterial, fungal, protozoal, or mixed organisms may also be responsible for acute lung disease in the nonimmunocompromised host. The morphologic reactions often differ between the two groups since the immunocompromised host may be unable to mount an appropriate inflammatory response.

Bacterial Infections

The usual bacterial pathogens are the single most important cause of acute infiltrative lung disease. They rarely present as a diagnostic problem in the nonimmunocompromised hosts. Pneumococcal lobar pneumonia is one such example. *Mycobacterial infections*, either typical or atypical (Kaplan et al, 1974; Wolinsky, 1979; CPC 23-1989), are an occasional surprise in the nonimmunocompromised patient (Fig. 4-4).

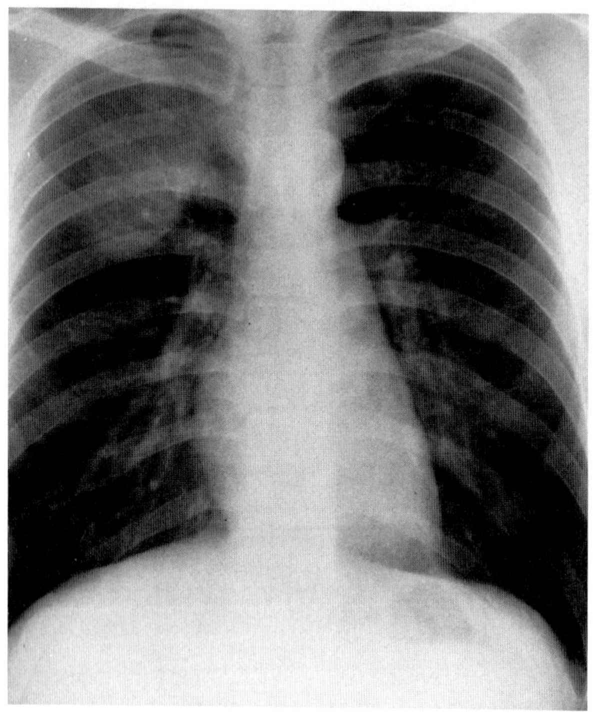

A

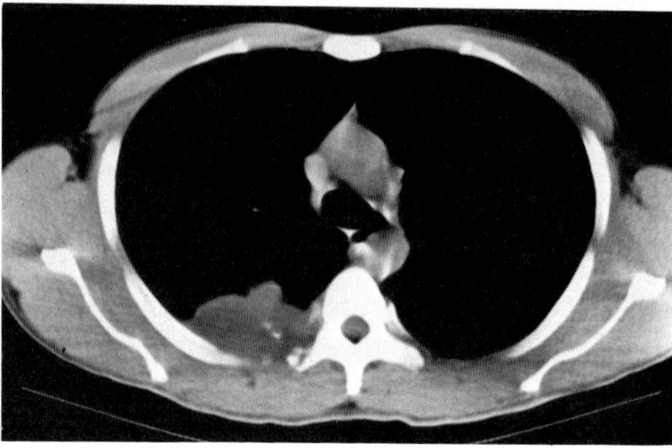

B

Figure 4–4   The patient was a 32-year-old man with a 2-month history of dry cough, right chest pain, and 7-pound weight loss. *A*, Chest radiograph shows pleural-based mass in the right upper chest associated with localized destruction of the inferior margin of the posterior fifth rib. *B*, CT scan better delineates the localized rib destruction. Preoperative fine-needle aspiration biopsy and intraoperative large-gauge-needle biopsies showed only necrosis. Chest wall resection and wedge resection of the involved area of the right upper lobe were performed. Pathologically the mass had caseating necrosis, and cultures grew *Mycobacterium tuberculosis hominis*.

Miliary Tuberculosis

Miliary tuberculosis may be a manifestation of primary or reactivation tuberculosis. Diffuse hematogenous dissemination of mycobacteria is common in primary tuberculosis, but miliary disease is rare. In less than 2 percent of patients with active disease, a large number of bacilli overwhelm the host defense mechanisms, resulting in miliary disease. Although in prior decades miliary disease was most commonly seen in children, in North America it is now more common in the elderly population (Munt, 1971; Gelb et al, 1973; Geppert and Leff, 1979).

The radiographic hallmark of miliary tuberculosis is the presence of nodules of 1 to 3 mm in diameter throughout the lung parenchyma. It is important to note that patients may initially present with a normal chest radiograph or with a pattern indistinguishable from that of acute interstitial pneumonia (Berger and Samortin, 1970; Geppert and Leff, 1979) (Fig. 4–5).

Legionnaires' Disease

Legionnaires' disease is an acute respiratory infection caused by *Legionella pneumophila*, so named because it was found to be responsible for the 1976 epidemic with numerous fatalities at an American Legion convention in Philadelphia. In retrospect, the same organism was found to have caused earlier outbreaks of respiratory disease in Pontiac, Michigan, Washington, D.C., and Philadelphia (Winn and Myerowitz, 1981). The organism needs complex media for growth, stains best in tissue with the Diderle stain, and has at least six antigenically different serogroups that can be differentiated by direct fluorescence. Serotype I is the most common. This organism is notable for being a pathogen in community-acquired pneumonia, nosocomial pneumonia, and pneumonia in the immunocompromised host.

The radiographic findings in *Legionella pneumophila* pneumonia include segmental or lobar consolidation, diffuse patchy consolidation, or poorly marginated, rounded consolidation that rarely cavitates (Lake et al, 1979; Fairbank et al, 1982) (Fig. 4–6). Pleural effusion occurs in one third of patients.

A related organism, *Legionella micdadei* occurs apparently exclusively in the immunocompromised host (Winn and Myerowitz, 1981). On gross examination, the lungs have lobular or confluent lobular consolidation, with abscesses in about 25 percent of cases. Lobar pneumonia is less frequently seen. *Legionella micdadei* may cause nodular, segmental, or bilateral infiltrates. Lobar pneumonia is a less

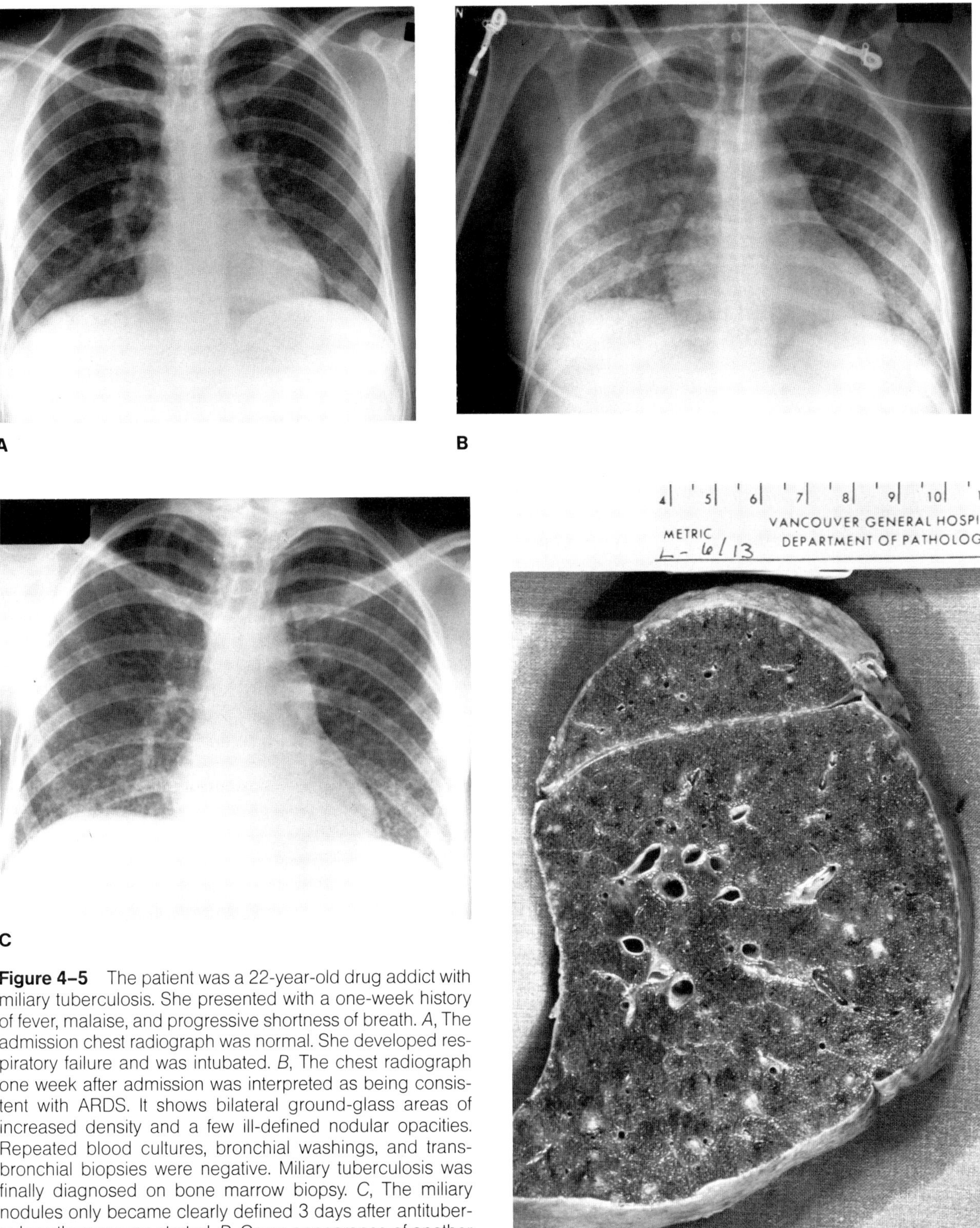

Figure 4–5 The patient was a 22-year-old drug addict with miliary tuberculosis. She presented with a one-week history of fever, malaise, and progressive shortness of breath. *A*, The admission chest radiograph was normal. She developed respiratory failure and was intubated. *B*, The chest radiograph one week after admission was interpreted as being consistent with ARDS. It shows bilateral ground-glass areas of increased density and a few ill-defined nodular opacities. Repeated blood cultures, bronchial washings, and transbronchial biopsies were negative. Miliary tuberculosis was finally diagnosed on bone marrow biopsy. *C*, The miliary nodules only became clearly defined 3 days after antituberculous therapy was started. *D*, Gross appearance of another case of miliary tuberculosis at autopsy. The patient had been on an alcoholic binge since his wife's death several weeks earlier.

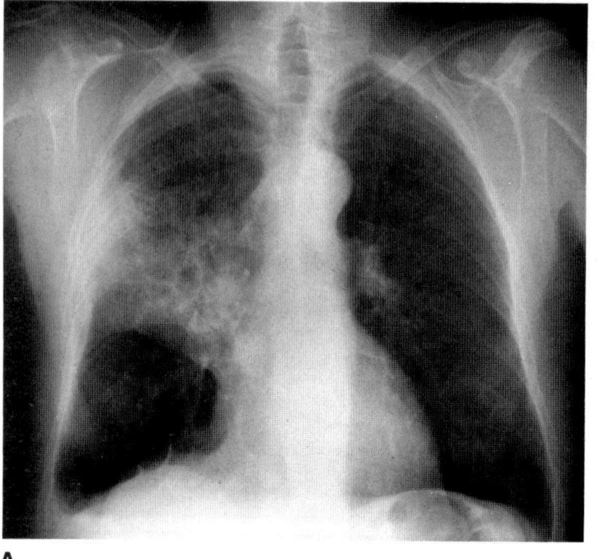

A

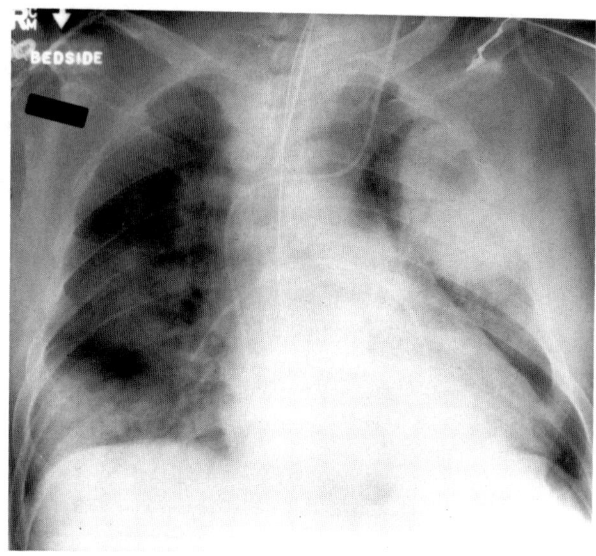

B

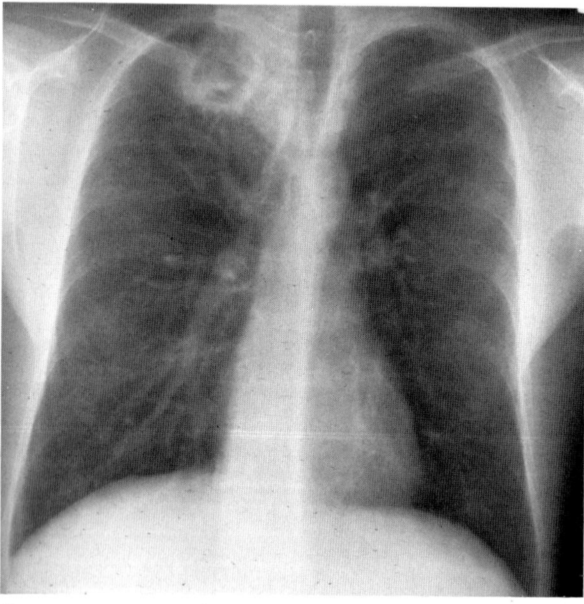

C

Figure 4–6 *A*, A 77-year-old man with right upper lobe pneumonia and a small pleural effusion due to *Legionella pneumophila*. *B*, A 45-year-old man with extensive bilateral *Legionella* pneumonia. Note the dense consolidation in the left upper lobe. The diagnosis was proved by percutaneous fine-needle aspiration biopsy of the left upper lobe. *C*, A 25-year-old man, after renal transplantation, with cavitating *Legionella* pneumonia in the apex of the right upper lobe. Cavitation of *Legionella* pneumonia has been described only in immunocompromised patients.

frequent manifestation. Not only is the radiologic pattern nonspecific, but the radiographic severity does not correlate with the severity of underlying disease, immune status, or outcome (Muder et al, 1984).

Microscopically, alveolar filling by an exudate of fibrin is seen with PMNs and macrophages. Leukocytoclasis with resultant nuclear dust is thought to be characteristic. Bronchitis and bronchiolitis are common (Hernandez et al, 1980), but there is some evi-dence that the changes begin in the distal acinus and involve larger airways secondarily (Hicklin et al, 1980). The appearance is nonspecific and the diagnosis *must* be confirmed by a Diderle stain, direct fluorescence, culture, or serology. Diffuse alveolar damage has been described in a few cases, but this reaction pattern may be related to oxygen therapy rather than to the primary infection (Hernandez et al, 1980). It is in the setting of diffuse alveolar damage that a biopsy is most likely to be performed.

Other Bacterial Pathogens

A variety of other organisms may cause acute infiltrative lung disease, particularly as seen on the chest radiograph. They rarely require lung biopsy. *Chlamydia psittaci* causes "ornithosis" as a result of inhalation of excreta from birds (usually pets), and often parrots (in which case it is called "psittacosis"). *Coxiella burnetii* causes Q fever; its hosts are farm animals and thus the human disease occurs in farm workers and meat packers. *Mycoplasma pneumoniae* causes primary atypical pneumonia characterized by an insidious onset, relatively slight respiratory symptoms, and severe systemic symptoms (Mansel et al, 1989). *Mycoplasma pneumoniae* infection is typically a disease of otherwise healthy adolescents and young adults and is a common pathogen in this population (Clyde, 1983). The radiographic findings in *M. pneumoniae* pneumonia are variable. The most common abnormality is lower lobar, segmental consolidation that may be unilateral or bilateral (Dean, 1981; Linz et al, 1984; MacFarlane et al, 1984). Upper lobe infiltrates are seen in approximately 20 percent of cases (Dean, 1981; Linz et al, 1984); diffuse reticular interstitial infiltrates are seen in 10 to 20 percent of cases (Dean, 1981; Izumikawa and Hara, 1983; Linz et al, 1984). Pleural effusions, usually small, and hilar adenopathy are seen in approximately 20 percent of cases (MacFarlane et al, 1984). Cases examined at autopsy have shown primarily bronchiolitis with microatelectasis, and interstitial and patchy alveolar pneumonia.

Viral Infections

The viruses that may cause lower respiratory tract infection and that may be seen in lung biopsy material are summarized in Table 4–3 (Miller, 1988). They are seen in nonimmunocompromised hosts, but are more common as a diagnostic problem in immunocompromised hosts. In the nonimmunocompromised hosts they come as a surprise, usually in patients with ARDS.

Influenza

Influenza is the most common cause of viral pneumonia in the nonimmunocompromised adult. Various patterns of reaction may be seen: viral pneumonia followed by bacterial superinfection; influenza and bacterial pneumonia occurring together; and "pure" influenza pneumonia. The latter is characterized by a combination of diffuse alveolar damage and necrotizing bronchitis/bronchiolitis (Fig. 4–7). Concurrent and subsequent bacterial infection show intra-alveolar PMNs with or without visible bacteria by Gram's stain. There are no specific influenza virus inclusions. The radiologic findings are nonspecific and variable, depending on the severity of the pneumonia and the presence of superinfection. Influenza most often presents with small areas of consolidation that rapidly become confluent (Galloway and Miller, 1959). It may be unilateral or bilateral, and in more severe cases it may lead to diffuse bilateral airspace consolidation with air bronchograms (Noble et al, 1973). Unilateral pleural effusions are seen in approximately 10 percent of patients (Galloway and Miller, 1959).

Measles

Radiologic infiltrates and pneumonia are common in nonimmunocompromised patients with measles (rubeola) infection (Gremillion and Crawford,

---

TABLE 4–3

VIRAL PNEUMONIAS

VIRUS	USUAL PATIENT
RNA	
Influenza	NIH,[*] adult
Measles	ICH[†]
Respiratory syncytial virus	NIH, infant
DNA	
Adenovirus	NIH, children, recruits, institutions
	ICH
Herpes simplex	ICH
Herpes varicella-zoster	NIH, adult
	ICH
Cytomegalovirus	ICH

[*]NIH, Nonimmunocompromised host
[†]ICH, Immunocompromised host

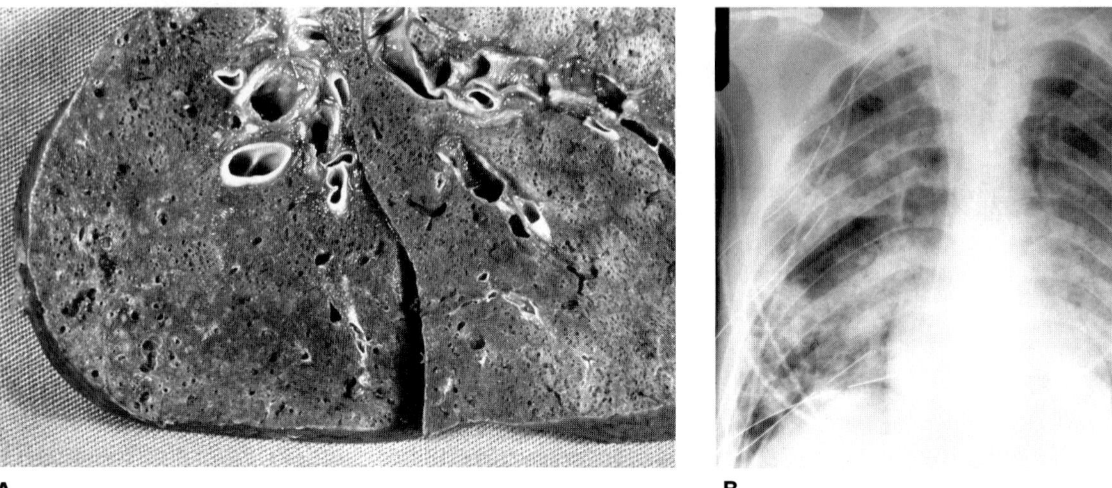

A   **B**

Figure 4–7   *A*, Gross appearance of influenza pneumonia with superinfection in the form of bronchiolar-based abscesses. This is the same patient as in Figures 4–1 and 4–2; death occurred 2 weeks following biopsy. *B*, This previously healthy 25-year-old man developed fatal influenza virus pneumonia. Chest radiograph shows extensive bilateral airspace consolidation.

1981). Life-threatening measles pneumonia is rare in nonimmunocompromised patients but is well recognized in immunocompromised children (Haram and Jacobsen, 1973). An absent rash, persistence of culturable virus, and a poor antibody response suggest an immunocompromised host and indicate a poor prognosis. The morphologic patterns of reaction include bronchitis, bronchiolitis, and diffuse alveolar damage. In contrast to influenza, inclusions are found easily in submucosal glands and alveolar epithelium. The cells are characteristically multinucleated (Hecht's giant cell pneumonia) (Fig. 4–8).

Intranuclear and intracytoplasmic inclusions occur and are usually easy to recognize.

Respiratory Syncytial Virus

Respiratory syncytial virus (RSV) is a very common cause of lower respiratory tract infection in children under one year of age. Rarely, RSV may cause life-threatening pneumonia in immunologically intact adults. The typical histologic appearance is that of obvious bronchiolitis with epithelial necrosis, acute inflammatory debris in bronchiolar lumina, and a mono-

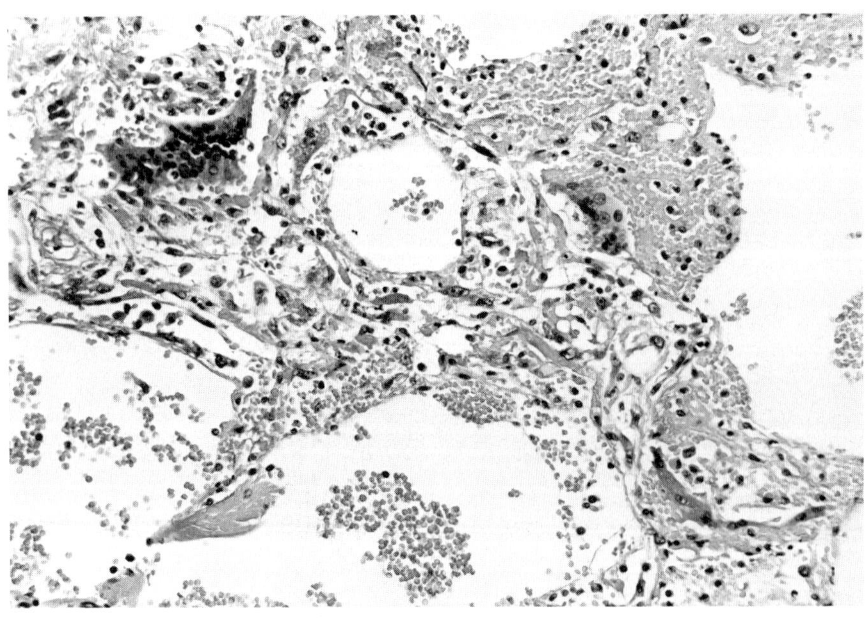

Figure 4–8   Diffuse alveolar damage due to measles virus, with inclusion-bearing multinucleated giant cells (H&E, × 265).

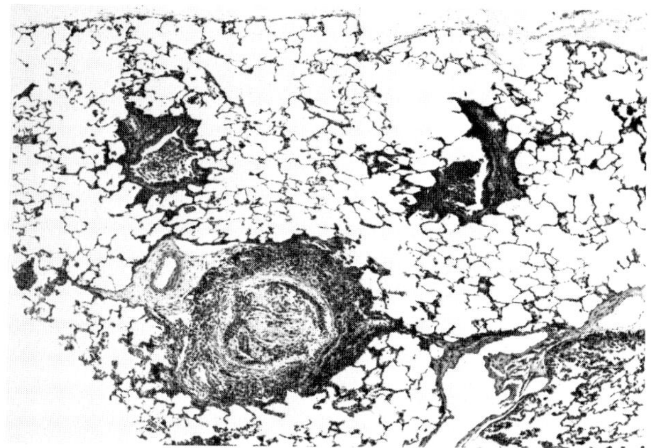

Figure 4–9 Respiratory syncytial virus bronchiolitis in an infant with prominent bronchiolar inflammation and little alveolitis (H&E, × 63). (Courtesy of Dr. Richard Sobonya.)

nuclear cell peribronchiolitis. The epithelial organization appears disturbed. There is little alveolitis so that the bronchiolar lesions are particularly prominent (Fig. 4–9). Inclusions can be seen in the bronchiolar epithelium early in the course of the disease. These are small intracytoplasmic eosinophilic structures that are difficult to find but may be made more obvious by Giemsa stain or specific fluorescence.

Adenovirus

Adenovirus is an important cause of lower respiratory tract infection in children, as it carries a high risk of long-term sequelae such as bronchiecta-

sis. Most adult cases occur in the immunocompromised host or, surprisingly, in closed populations such as military recruits. The lesions of adenoviral pneumonia include necrotizing bronchitis, necrotizing bronchiolitis, and diffuse alveolar damage. Two types of inclusions are found. The smaller, less numerous, and earlier-formed inclusion is an intranuclear, irregular, granular inclusion surrounded by a halo. This inclusion by itself can be mistaken for a herpes simplex virus inclusion, but it is accompanied by larger, basophilic, and more numerous "smudge" cells (Fig. 4–10), in which the nuclear membrane is disrupted and the entire nucleoplasm and cytoplasm are packed with virus particles. Electron microscopy is helpful, since the virions form a characteristic crystalline array.

Fungal Infections

Fungal infections give rise to granulomatous pulmonary inflammation with variable degrees of caseous necrosis, acute inflammation, fibrosis, and lymph node involvement. They all may cause significant disease in nonimmunocompromised patients, but lesions are usually localized, are not acute, and come to biopsy more often as an undiagnosed coin lesion than as diffuse infiltrative lung disease. More serious disease and, more commonly, diffuse lung disease occur in immunocompromised hosts (see Chapter 5). The exact diagnosis depends on morphology and culture of the offending organism, and the differential diagnostic considerations include *Histoplasma capsulatum* (Goodwin and Des Prez, 1978; Wheat et al, 1981; Sathapatayavonga et al, 1983), *Cryptococcus*

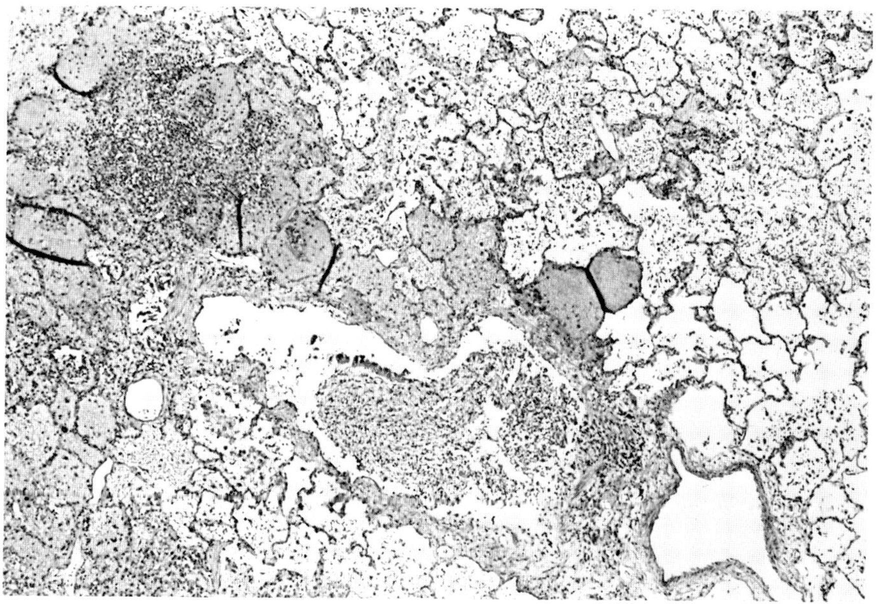

Figure 4–10 *A*, Adenovirus bronchiolitis with neutrophil response (H&E, × 63).

Continued **A**

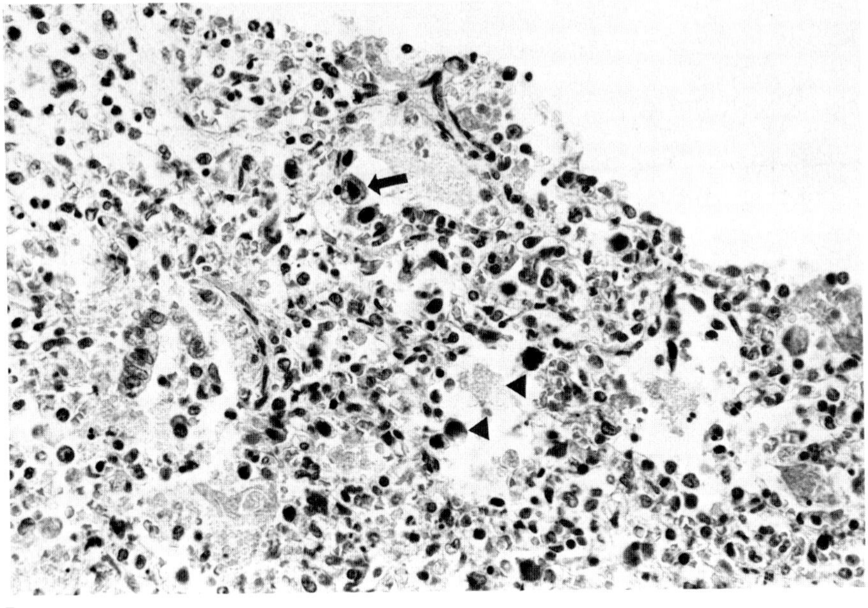

B

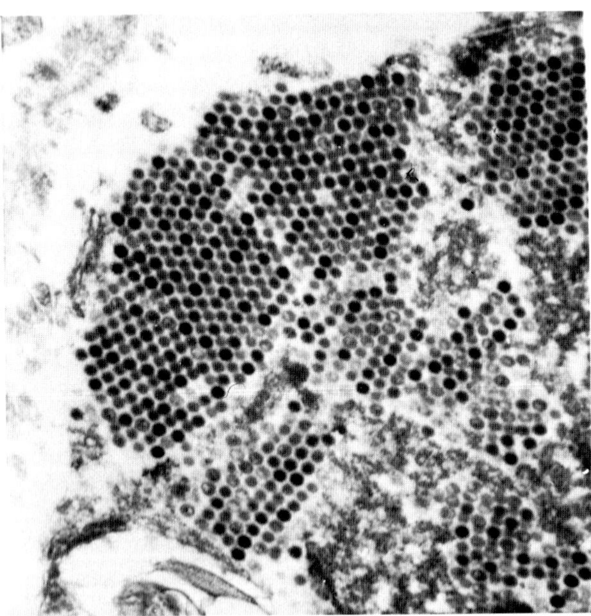

C

Figure 4–10 cont'd   *B*, Intranuclear (*arrow*) and smudge (*arrowhead*) inclusions (H&E, × 63). *C*, Electron micrograph of crystalline array of adenovirus (× 42,000).

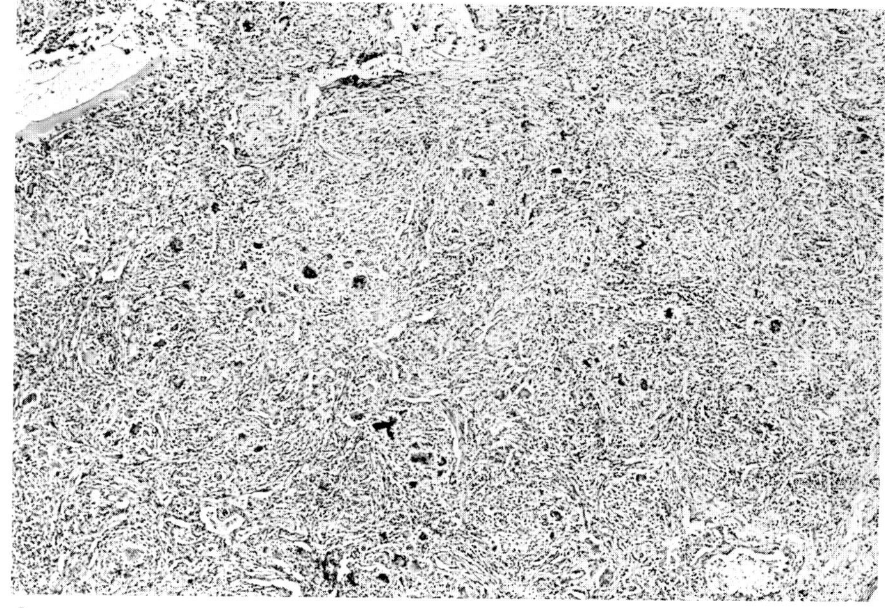

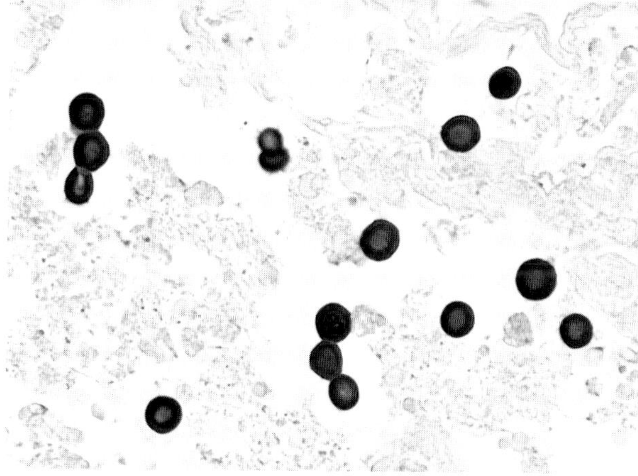

Figure 4–11   *A*, Granulomatous inflammation with minimal necrosis in an immunologically intact patient with cryptococcosis (H&E, × 63). *B*, Mucin stain demonstrates organism with mucinous capsule (Mucicarmine, × 265).

neoformans (Fig. 4-11) (CPC 37-1978), coccidioidomycosis (Beller et al, 1979; (CPC 3-1980), *Blastomyces dermatitidis* (Sarosi and Davies, 1979; Atkinson and McCurley, 1983), and *Sporothrix schenckii* (England and Hochholzer, 1985).

Aspergillus

Aspergillus infection may occur as allergic bronchopulmonary aspergillosis (ABPA) (Greenberger and Patterson, 1987; Boskin et al, 1988). The diagnostic criteria for ABPA include asthma, radiologic pulmonary infiltrates, peripheral blood eosinophilia, elevated serum IgE, and hypersensitivity to *Aspergillus*. Cases with straightforward clinical and laboratory findings of ABPA do not undergo biopsy. Bronchial biopsy in patients with an acute exacerbation of ABPA shows eosinophilic infiltration of the bronchial wall and "allergic mucin," composed of laminated mucin and eosinophil debris. *Aspergillus* hyphal segments may be identified in the mucin by appropriate silver stains. Resected specimens of ABPA show a combination of mucoid impaction of bronchi and bronchocentric granulomatosis of bronchi and bronchioles (Fig. 4-12). Intraluminal noninvasive hyphae and varying degrees of tissue eosinophils are the rule. *Aspergillus* may also cause fungus balls ("aspergillomas") in the nonimmunocompromised host, in which fungi colonize pre-existent pulmonary cavities (Fig. 4-13). Invasive pulmonary aspergillosis occurs almost exclusively in the immunocompromised host.

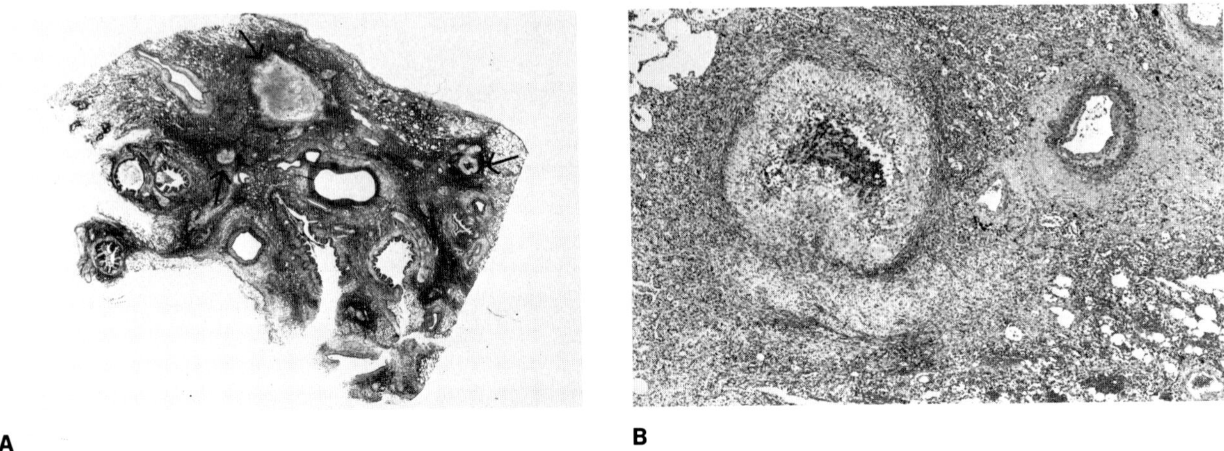

Figure 4–12   Bronchocentric granulomatosis in a patient with allergic bronchopulmonary aspergillosis. *A*, Several bronchi occluded by granulomatous inflammation (*arrows*). *B*, Bronchial wall and lumen replaced by granuloma.

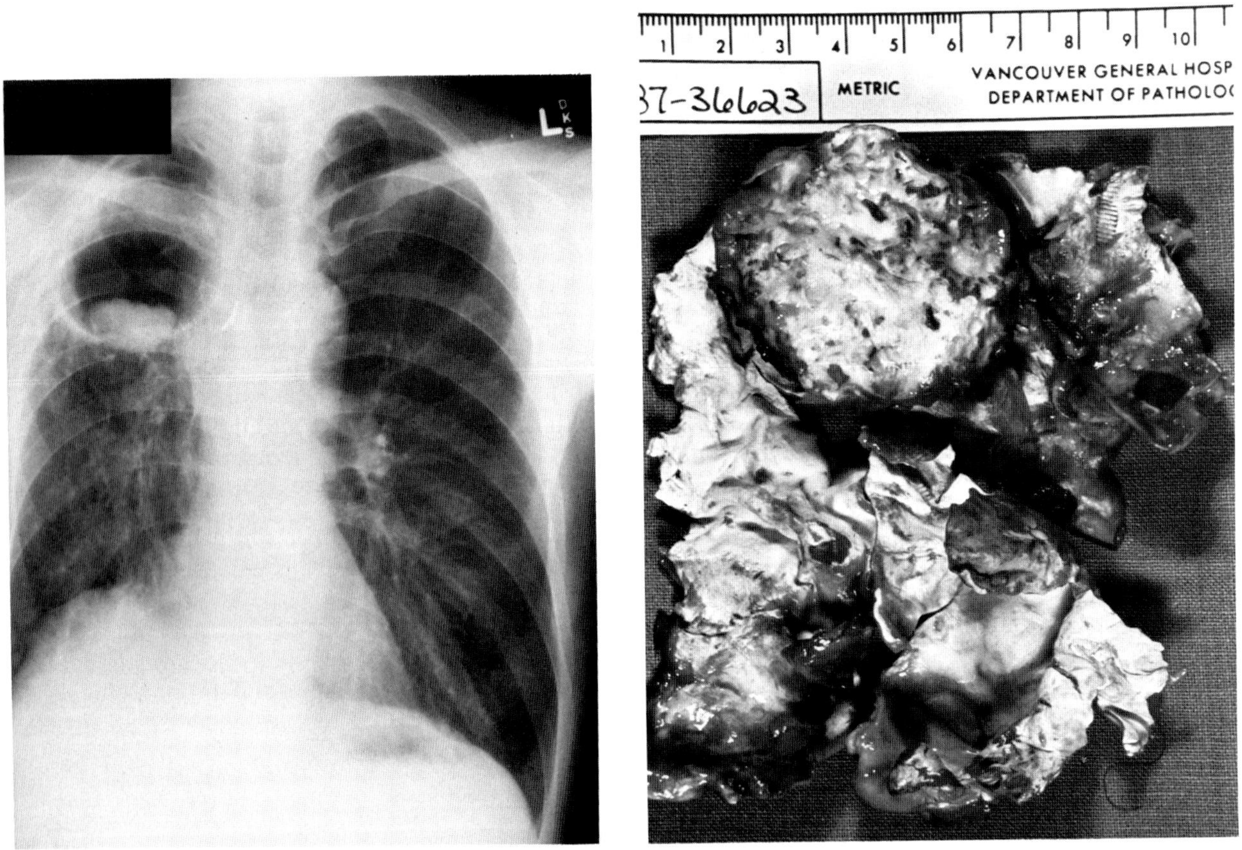

Figure 4–13   *A*, Chest radiograph of a 45-year-old man with apical fungus ball developing in an area of postradiation bronchiectasis. *B*, The fungus ball itself consists entirely of organisms without tissue invasion or incorporation. The surface is covered with white mold.

IATROGENIC AND NON-ANTINEOPLASTIC DRUGS

Toxic Agents

Oxygen Poisoning

Lung toxicity to increased oxygen levels has been known for many years in animals, and physiologic effects on lung function have been documented in healthy volunteers for some years. That lesions follow prolonged inhalation of high levels of oxygen is not disputed, and they are well documented in retrospective autopsy studies (Nash et al, 1967; Pratt, 1974; Hogg and Katzenstein, 1988). However, prospective studies have suggested that normal lungs are relatively resistant to oxygen and that damaged lungs are particularly susceptible (Jackson, 1985; Hogg and Katzenstein, 1988).

Experimental studies have shown that alveolar endothelial cells are first affected by oxygen poisoning. Experimentally, and in human cases, the fibrosis is often exquisitely interstitial with relative preservation of alveolar architecture so that the fibrotic phase may contrast with the lesions of paraquat poisoning and of ARDS in some instances. An interesting lesion has been ascribed to oxygen poisoning (Pratt, 1978): fibroblastic proliferation within alveolar ducts and sacs with relative preservation of alveolar wall architecture. It differs from the lesions of paraquat toxicity in that there are often central spaces within the fibrous tissue, sometimes filled with blood, and structures are seen that superficially resemble blood vessels (Fig. 4–14). Another difference is that in oxygen toxicity there is not the complete continuity between alveolar wall and exudate that is seen in paraquat poisoning, and there is irregularity of the alveolar wall-exudate contact.

Paraquat (1,1'-dimethyl-4,4'-dipyridylium dichloride)

Paraquat is an herbicide that releases hydrogen peroxide and the free radical superoxide during its cyclic oxidation and reduction. In plants it is thought to act on chloroplasts, and in animals by damage to cell membranes. Paraquat in high concentrations is very irritating, and the initial lesion in humans may be an ulcerative oropharyngitis. Transient renal and hepatic dysfunction follow in the next few days, and the patient appears to be recovering when, 5 to 7 days after ingestion, respiratory distress and a radiologic pattern of patchy pulmonary edema develops. Evidence of lung restriction and diminished diffusing capacity may precede the pulmonary symptoms. The delayed effect on the lung is thought to be due to the fact that the concentration of paraquat is high in the lungs for several days, whereas in other organs there is a rapid fall 24 to 36 hours after ingestion (Rose et al, 1976). Once pulmonary symptoms appear, the course is usually rapidly progressive. Lung involvement was considered to be always fatal, but cases have now been reported in which clinical recovery has occurred, and a case has also been described in which a patient was found to have pulmonary fibrosis radiologically after having had a previously

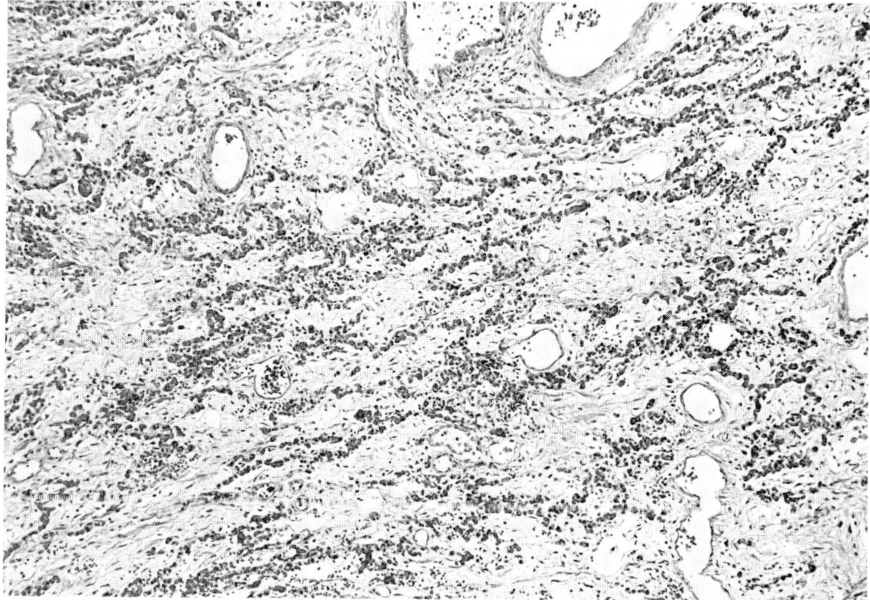

Figure 4–14   Fibroblastic proliferation in alveolar ducts and alveoli ducts due to oxygen toxicity. This patient had been mechanically ventilated with high oxygen concentrations for nearly 4 weeks.

normal chest film. He was found to have ingested paraquat in the intervening period (Anderson, 1970). Paraquat lung lesions probably do not occur in sprayers of paraquat (Fairshter, 1978). The issue of lesions in smokers of marijuana that had been sprayed with paraquat has been raised, since inhaled paraquat in rabbits produces lung disease (Zavala and Rhodes, 1978). There is no convincing evidence that lung disease due to paraquat occurs in marijuana smokers.

Experimentally the first pulmonary lesions appear in the type-I cells of the alveolar epithelium (Dearden et al, 1978). Degenerative changes occur within 12 to 18 hours, and necrosis by 24 hours. Alveolar edema and congestion are seen. Type-II cell and endothelial damage then occur, and the appearance is of acute diffuse alveolar damage. Fibroblastic proliferation and fibrosis follow. In a patient who dies, or on whom a biopsy is performed 1 week to 10 days after ingestion, a striking pattern is seen (Rebello and Mason, 1978). There is distortion of the lung architecture, dilation of bronchioles and alveolar ducts, and alveolar collapse and fibrosis. Quite large cysts may form, which may be lined by alveolar walls (Rebello and Mason, 1978). A distinctive form of fibrosis has been described that may be characteristic of paraquat (Copland et al, 1974; Thurlbeck and Thurlbeck, 1976). The lung structure remains intact, but the distal airspaces are filled with loose fibrous tissue (Fig. 4–15). The skeletons of alveolar walls remain and are emphasized by the congested alveolar capillaries. This may represent organization of fibrin-rich "reticulated" edema fluid (Rebello and Mason, 1978). Both the acute and the subacute phases may be irregularly distributed through the lung.

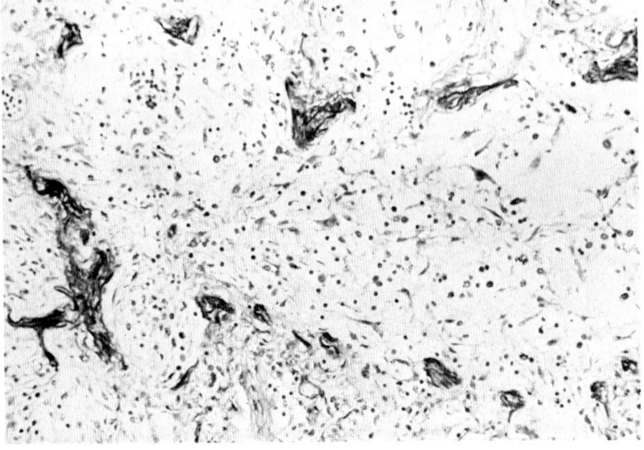

Figure 4–15 Paraquat poisoning, resulting in obliteration of the distal airway lumina by loose fibrous tissue.

Drug Reactions

Parenterally or orally introduced substances may produce a variety of lesions within the lung (Gillett and Ford, 1978; Cooper, 1986a, 1986b; Rosenow and Martin 1988). These include diffuse alveolar damage, pulmonary edema, asthma, eosinophilic pneumonia, and usual interstitial pneumonia.

Many drugs have been associated with pulmonary lesions. Because there is a general lack of distinctive clinical or pathologic features, the best method of diagnosing drug-induced lesions is the combination of a high index of suspicion with a good clinical history. Drug-related injury can be approached as a classification of the drugs involved (Rosenow, 1972; Cooper et al, 1986a, 1986b), a classification of reaction involved such as allergic, idiosyncratic or overdosage, or a classification of target-organ effects (Cole, 1977).

Nitrofurantoin

Nitrofurantoin is a bacteriostatic agent used mainly to treat urinary tract infection. Acute or chronic reactions can occur (Sovijarv et al, 1977; Holmberg et al, 1980; Holmberg and Boman, 1981; Cooper, 1986b); there is no overlap. Acute reactions appear within one hour to 2 weeks after administration, and there is usually fever, dyspnea, bilateral infiltrates on the chest radiograph, and often peripheral eosinophilia. Wheezing occurs in one third of patients. Approximately 20 percent of the patients also have gastrointestinal symptoms, headaches, or muscle pain. Histologically, mild interstitial inflammation and vasculitis are present; occasionally, granulomas can be identified. Intra-alveolar eosinophils and macrophages are seen, and an appearance closely resembling desquamative interstitial pneumonia may occur (Bone et al, 1976). The chronic reactions appear after months to years of treatment (Robinson, 1983). Dyspnea is quite variable in severity; systemic reactions are rare. Autoantibodies are occasionally present (Lundgren et al, 1975). There may be fibrosis and vascular sclerosis.

Amphophilic Drugs

This category includes amiodarone as well as the antihistamine chlorcyclizine; haloperidol; chloroquine; the anorectic substances chlorphentermine, cloforex, and fenfluramine; and tricyclic antidepressants prindole, amitriptyline hydrochloride, imipramine, and clomipramine (Kruban, 1976; Martin and Rosenow, 1988a, 1988b). The underlying abnormality is the deposition of phospholipid in many cells, especially alveolar macrophages and type-2 pneumocytes. Interstitial edema occurs, and interstitial macrophages become prominent. Type-II pneumonocytes become hyperplastic and have large secretory vacuoles. Foam cells and amorphous material are present in alveoli, and this appearance closely resembles alveolar proteinosis (p. 128). In addition, numerous lamellar inclusions are identified ultrastructurally, both free and within macrophages. The drugs may impair metabolism in phagosomes by forming complexes with phospholipids.

Analgesics and Opiates

A common, serious drug reaction is produced by heroin overdosage (Siegel, 1972). Methadone and propoxyphene produce similar lesions (Rosenow, 1977; Glassroth et al, 1987), as does aspirin (Davis and Burch, 1974; Heffner and Sahn, 1981; Thisted et al, 1987; McGuigan, 1987), but probably by a different mechanism. Pulmonary edema results and may be complicated by aspiration. Granulomas containing birefringent material may be found in the interstitium in patients who inject mixtures of drugs with a talc filler (Fig. 4–16) (Crouch and Churg, 1983; Radow et al, 1983).

Miscellaneous

Patients receiving crysotherapy (gold treatment) for rheumatoid arthritis may develop diffuse, pulmonary lesions. There is interstitial pneumonitis, with an infiltrate of lymphocytes and plasma cells accompanied by interstitial fibrosis (Winterbauer et al, 1976; Cooper et al, 1986b; Evans et al, 1987). Granulomas or vasculitis are not seen. There may be blood eosinophilia with elevated IgE levels, suggesting hypersensitivity (Geddes and Brostoff, 1976). We

have seen a case of pulmonary interstitial eosinophilia due to crysotherapy. Since a wide spectrum of pulmonary complications of rheumatoid arthritis is recognized (see Chapter 9), the distinction between rheumatoid lung disease and crysotherapy-related lung disease can be difficult. Rheumatoid pneumonitis tends to be irreversible, whereas gold pneumonitis is reversible with discontinuation of the drug and, if necessary, adding corticosteroids. This, plus the finding of lymphocytes in bronchoalveolar lavage fluid, discriminate between the two entities.

Cytotoxic Drugs and Radiation Pneumonitis

These are discussed in the following chapter since they are part of the differential diagnosis of pulmonary infiltrates in the immunocompromised host.

REFERENCES

Anderson CG. Paraquat and the lung. Aust Radiol 1970; 14:409–411.

Ashbaugh DG, Bigelow DB, Petty TL, et al. Acute respiratory distress in adults. Lancet 1967; 2:319–323.

Atkinson JB, McCurley TL. Pulmonary blastomycosis: filamentous forms in an immunocompromised patient with fulminating respiratory failure. Hum Pathol 1983; 14:186–188.

Bachofen A, Weibel ER: Alterations of the gas-exchange apparatus in adult respiratory insufficiency associated with septicemia. Am Rev Respir Dis 1977; 116:589–615.

Beller TA, Mitchell DM, Sobonya RE, Barbe RA. Large airway obstruction secondary to endobronchial coccidiomycosis. Am Rev Respir Dis 1979; 120:939–942.

Berger HW, Samortin TG. Miliary tuberculosis: diagnostic methods with emphasis on the chest roentgenogram. Chest 1970; 58:586–589.

Bone RC, Fisher CJ, Clemmer TP, Slutman GJ, Metz CA. Methylprednisolone Severe Sepsis Group: early methylprednisolone treatment for the septic shock syndrome and the adult respiratory distress syndrome. Am J Med 1976; 60:697–701.

Bone RC, Wolfe J, Sobonya RE, et al. Desquamative interstitial pneumonia following chronic nitrofurantoin therapy. Chest 1976; 69 | suppl 2 |:296–298.

Boskin CH, Myers JL, Greenberger PA, Katzenstein ALA. Pathologic features of allergic bronchopulmonary aspergillosis. Am J Surg Pathol 1988; 12:216–222.

Churg A, Golden J, Fliegel S, Hogg JC. Bronchopulmonary dysplasia in the adult. Am Rev Respir Dis 1983; 127:117–120.

Clyde WA Jr. *Mycoplasma pneumoniae* respiratory disease symposium: summation and significance. Yale J Biol Med 1983; 56:523–527.

Cole P. Drug-induced lung disease. Drugs 1977; 13:422–444.

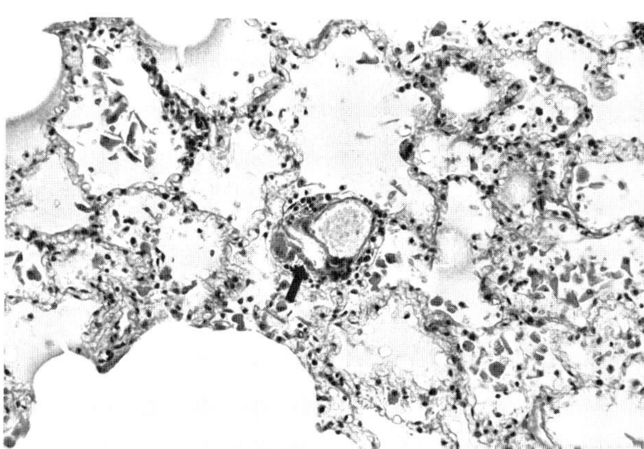

Figure 4–16 Pulmonary edema and interstitial foreign body reaction (*arrow*) in a drug addict who died of overdose.

Cooper JAD Jr, White DA, Matthay RA. Drug-induced pulmonary disease, part I: cytotoxic drugs. Am Rev Respir Dis 1986a; 133:321-340.

Cooper JAD Jr, White DA, Matthay RA. Drug-induced pulmonary disease, part II: non-cytotoxic drugs. Am Rev Respir Dis 1986b; 133:488-505.

Copland GM, Kolin A, Schulman HS. Fatal pulmonary intra-alveolar fibrosis after paraquat ingestion. N Engl J Med 1974; 291:290-292.

CPC 37-1978. N Engl J Med 1978; 299:644-650.

CPC 3-1980. N Engl J Med 1980; 302:218-223.

CPC 23-1989. N Engl J Med 1989; 320:1540-1549.

Crouch E, Churg A. Progressive massive fibrosis of the lung secondary to intravenous injection of talc: a pathologic and mineralogic analysis. Am J Clin Pathol 1983; 80:520-526.

Davis PR, Burch RE. Pulmonary edema and salicylate intoxication. Ann Intern Med 1974; 80:553-554.

Dean NL. Mycoplasma pneumonias in the community hospital: the "unusual" manifestations become common. Clin Chest Med 1981; 2:121-131.

Dearden LC, Fairshter RD, McRae DM, et al. Pulmonary ultrastructure of the late aspects of human paraquat poisoning. Am J Pathol 1978; 93:667-680.

England DM, Hochholzer L. Primary pulmonary sporotrichosis. Am J Surg Pathol 1985; 9:193-204.

Evans RB, Ettensohn DB, Fawaz-Estrup F, et al. Gold lung: recent developments in pathogenesis, diagnosis and therapy. Semin Arthritis Rheum 1987; 16:196-205.

Fairbank JT, Mamoiurian AC, Dietrich PA, Girod JC. The chest radiograph in legionnaires' disease: further observations. Radiology 1982; 147:33-34.

Fairshter RD. Paraquat poisoning: an update. West J Med 1978; 128:56-58.

Flick MR, Murray JF. High dose corticosteroid therapy in the adult respiratory distress syndrome. JAMA 1984; 251:1054-1056.

Galloway RW, Miller RS. Lung changes in recent influenza epidemic. Br J Radiol 1959; 32:28-31.

Geddes P, Brostoff J. Letter to editor. N Engl J Med 1976; 295:506-507.

Gelb AF, Leffler C, Brewin A, et al. Miliary tuberculosis. Am Rev Respir Dis 1973; 108:1327-1333.

Geppert EF, Leff A. The pathogenesis of pulmonary and miliary tuberculosis. Arch Intern Med 1979; 139:1381-1383.

Gillett DG, Ford GT. Drug-induced lung disease. In Thurlbeck WM, Abell MR, eds. The lung: structure, function and disease. Baltimore: Williams & Wilkins, 1978:21-42.

Glassroth J, Adams GD, Schnoll S. The impact of substance abuse on the respiratory system. Chest 1987; 91:596-602.

Goodwin RA, Des Prez RM: State of the art: histoplasmosis. Am Rev Respir Dis 1978; 117:929-956.

Greenberger PA, Patterson R. Allergic bronchopulmonary aspergillosis. Chest 1987; 91:165S-171S.

Greene R. Adult respiratory distress syndrome: acute alveolar damage. Radiology 1987; 163:57-66.

Gremillion DH, Crawford GE. Measles pneumonia in young adults. Am J Med 1981; 71:539-542.

Haram K, Jacobsen K. Measles and its relationship to giant cell pneumonia (Hecht pneumonia). Acta Pathol Microbiol Scand [A] 1973; 81:761-769.

Heffner JE, Sahn SA. Salicylate-induced pulmonary edema: clinical features and prognosis. Ann Intern Med 1981; 95:405-409.

Hernandez FJ, Kirby BD, Stanley TM, Edelstein PH. Legionnaires' disease: postmortem pathologic findings of 20 cases. Am J Clin Pathol 1980; 73:488-495.

Hicklin MD, Thomason BM, Chandler FW, Blackman JA. Pathogenesis of acute legionnaires' disease pneumonia: immunofluorescent microscopic study. Am J Clin Pathol 1980; 73:480-487.

Hogg JC, Katzenstein A-LA. Pulmonary edema and diffuse alveolar injury. In Thurlbeck WM ed. Pathology of the lung. New York: Thieme, 1988:263-282.

Holmberg I, Boman G. Pulmonary reactions to nitrofurantoin: 447 cases reported to the Swedish Adverse Drug Reaction Committee 1966-1976. Eur J Respir Dis 1981; 62:180-189.

Holmberg I, Boman G, Bottiger IE, et al. Adverse reactions to nitrofurantoin: analysis of 921 reports. Am J Med 1980; 69:733-738.

Izumikawa K, Hara K. Clinical features of mycoplasmal pneumonia in adults. Yale J Biol Med 1983; 56:505-510.

Jackson RM. Pulmonary oxygen toxicity. Chest 1985; 88:900-905.

Joachim H, Riede UN, Mittenmeyer CH. The weight as a diagnostic criterion (distinction of normal lungs from shock lungs by histologic, morphometric and biochemical investigations). Pathol Res Pract 1978; 162:24-40.

Joffe N. The adult respiratory distress syndrome. Am J Roentgenol Radium Therapy Nucl Med 1974; 122:719-732.

Kaplan MH, Armstrong D, Rosen P. Turberculosis complicating neoplastic disease: a review of 201 cases. Cancer 1974; 33:850-858.

Katzenstein A-LA, Myers JL, Mazur MT. Acute interstitial pneumonia: a clinicopathologic, ultrastructural and cell kinetic study. Am J Surg Pathol 1986; 10:256-267.

Kruban Z. Pulmonary changes induced by amphophilic drugs. Environ Health Perspect 1976; 16:111-126.

Lake KB, Van Dyke JJ, Gerberg E, Browne PM. Legionnaires' disease and pulmonary cavitation. Arch Intern Med 1979; 139:485-486.

Linz DH, Tolle SW, Elliot DL. *Mycoplasma pneumoniae* pneumonia: experience at a referral center. West J Med 1984; 140:895-900.

Lundgren R, Back O, Wiman LG. Pulmonary lesions and autoimmune reactions after long-term nitrofurantoin treatment. Scan J Respir Dis 1975; 56:208-216.

MacFarlane JT, Miller AC, Roderick-Smith WH, et al. Comparative radiographic features of community-acquired legionnaires' disease, pneumococcal pneumonia, mycoplasma pneumonia, and psittacosis. Thorax 1984; 39:28-33.

Mansel JK, Rosenow EC III, Smith TF, Martin JW. Today's practice of cardiopulmonary medicine: *Mycoplasma pneumoniae* pneumonia. Chest 1989; 95:639–646.

Martin WJ, Rosenow EC III. Amiodarone pulmonary toxicity: recognition and pathogenesis (part 1). Chest 1988a; 93:1067–1075.

Martin WJ, Rosenow EC III. Amiodarone pulmonary toxicity: recognition and pathogenesis (part 2). Chest 1988b; 93:1242–1248.

McGuigan MA. A two-year review of salicylate deaths in Ontario. Arch Intern Med 1987; 147:510–512.

Miller RR. Viral infections of the respiratory tract. In Thurlbeck WM, ed. Pathology of the lung. New York: Thieme, 1988:147–179.

Milne ENC. A physiological approach to reading critical care unit films. J Thorac Imag 1986; 1:60-90.

Muder RR, Reddy SC, Yu VL, Kroboth FJ. Pneumonia caused by Pittsburgh pneumonia agent: radiologic manifestations. Radiology 1984; 150:633-637.

Munt PW. Miliary tuberculosis in the chemotherapy era: with a clinical review in 69 American males. Medicine 1971; 51:139–155.

Murray JF. The adult respiratory distress syndrome (may it rest in peace). Am Rev Respir Dis 1975; 111:716–718.

Murray JF, Matthay MA, Luce JM, Flick MR. Pulmonary perspectives: an expanded definition of the adult respiratory distress syndrome. Am Rev Respir Dis 1988; 138:720-723.

Nash G, Blennerhassett JB, Pontoppidan H. Pulmonary lesions associated with oxygen therapy and artificial ventilation. N Engl J Med 1967; 276:368–374.

Noble RL, Lillington GA, Kempson RL. Fatal diffuse influenzal pneumonia: premortem diagnosis by lung biopsy. Chest 1973; 63:644–647.

Petty TL. ARDS: refinement of concepts and redefinition. Am Rev Respir Dis 1988; 138:724.

Petty TL, Ashbaugh DG. The adult respiratory distress syndrome: clinical features, factors influencing prognosis and principles of management. Chest 1971; 60:233–239.

Pratt PC. Pathology of pulmonary oxygen toxicity. Am Rev Respir Dis 1974; 110:51–57.

Pratt PC: Pathology of adult respiratory distress syndrome. In Thurlbeck WM, Abell MR, eds. The lung, structure, function and disease. Baltimore: Williams & Wilkins, 1978:43–57.

Radow SK, Nachamkin I, Morrow G, et al. Foreign body granulomatosis: clinical and immunologic findings. Am Rev Respir Dis 1983; 127:575–580.

Rebello G, Mason JK. Pulmonary histological appearances in fatal paraquat poisoning. Histopathology 1978; 2:53–66.

Robinson BWS. Nitrofurantoin-induced interstitial pulmonary fibrosis. Med J Aust 1983; 1:72–76.

Rose MS, Lock A, Smith LL, et al. Paraquat accumulation: tissue and species specificity. Biochem Pharmacol 1976; 25:419–423.

Rosenow EC III, Martin WJ II. Drug-induced interstitial lung disease. In Schwarz MI, King TE Jr, eds. Interstitial lung disease. Toronto: BC Decker, 1988:123–137.

Rosenow EC III. The spectrum of drug-induced pulmonary disease. Ann Intern Med 1972; 77:977–991.

Rosenow EC. Drug-induced pulmonary disease. Clin Notes Respir Dis 1977; 16:3–11.

Sarosi GA, Davies SF. Blastomycosis. Am Rev Respir Dis 1979; 120:911–938.

Sathapatayovonga B, Batteiger BE, Wheat J, et al. Clinical and laboratory features of disseminated histoplasmosis during two large urban outbreaks. Medicine 1983; 62: 263–270.

Schlag G, Voight WH, Redl H, Glatzel A. Vergleichende Morphologie des posttraumatischen Lungenversagens. Anaesth Intensivther Notfallmed 1980; 15:315–389.

Sibbald WJ, Warshawski FJ, Short AK, et al. Clinical studies of measuring extravascular lung water by the thermal dye technique in critically ill patients. Chest 1983; 83:725–731.

Siegel H. Human pulmonary pathology associated with narcotic and other addictive drugs. Hum Pathol 1972; 3:55–66.

Sovijarvi A, Lemola M, Stenius B, Idanpaan-Heikkila J. Nitrofurantoin-induced acute, subacute and chronic pulmonary reactions. Scand J Respir Dis 1977; 58: 41–50.

Thisted B, Krantz T, Strom J, Sorensen MB. Acute salicylate self-poisoning in 177 consecutive patients treated in ICU. Acta Anaesthesiol Scand 1987; 31:312–316.

Thurlbeck WM, Thurlbeck SM. Pulmonary effects of paraquat poisoning. Chest 1976; 69[suppl 2]:276–280.

Weigelt JA, Norcross JF, Borman KR, Snyder WH. Early steroid therapy for respiratory failure. Arch Surg 1985; 120:536–540.

Wheat LJ, Slama TG, Eitzen HE, et al. A large urban outbreak of histoplasmosis: clinical features Ann Intern Med 1981; 94:331–337.

Winn WC Jr, Myerowitz RL. The pathology of the Legionella pneumonias: a review of 74 cases and the literature. Hum Pathol 1981; 12:401–422.

Winterbauer RH, Wilske KR, Wheelis RF. Diffuse pulmonary injury associated with gold treatment. N Engl J Med 1976; 294:919–921.

Wolinsky E. State of the art: nontuberculous mycobacteria and associated diseases. Am Rev Respir Dis 1979; 119:107–159.

Zavala DC, Rhodes ML. An effect of paraquat on the lungs of rabbits: its implication in smoking contaminated marihuana. Chest 1978; 74:418–420.

CHAPTER 5

ACUTE INFILTRATIVE LUNG DISEASE IN THE IMMUNOCOMPROMISED HOST

As indicated in the previous chapter, acute diffuse lung disease may occur in the nonimmunocompromised host. The same agents, as well as others, may also involve the immunocompromised host (Nash, 1982). Some organisms are almost never opportunistic: *Actinomyces*, most RNA viruses, anaerobes, spirochetes, *Mycoplasma*, and *Chlamydia*. This chapter emphasizes those conditions that most commonly only involve the immunocompromised host, or involve the immunocompromised host in unusual ways.

ROLE OF BIOPSY IN THE IMMUNOCOMPROMISED HOST

Table 5-1 outlines the differential diagnosis of pulmonary disease in immunocompromised patients.

TABLE 5-1

DIFFERENTIAL DIAGNOSIS OF PULMONARY DISEASE IN THE IMMUNOCOMPROMISED HOST

---

1. Opportunistic Infection
2. Recurrence of underlying disease
     Lymphoma, leukemia
     Connective tissue disease (e.g., systemic lupus erythematosus)
     Neoplasm
3. Transplant: rejection, fibrosis, graft-vs-host disease, bronchiolitis obliterans, edema
4. Drug effect

CYTOTOXIC	NONCYTOTOXIC
Bleomycin	Methotrexate
Cyclophosphamide	Ara-C (cytosine arabinoside)
Mitomycin-C	Procarbazine
Busulfan	Bleomycin
Chlorambucil	
Melphalan	
Nitrosoureas	
Azathioprine	
Vinblastine	
Etoposide (VP-16)	

5. Opportunistic neoplasm (Kaposi's sarcoma in AIDS, lymphoma, connective tissue tumors)
6. Nonspecific diffuse alveolar damage and fibrosis (?drug and/or radiation)
7. "Unrelated"
     Congestive heart failure
     Pulmonary emboli
     Adult respiratory distress syndrome
     Oxygen toxicity
     Community-acquired pneumonia
8. Unusual complications
     Pulmonary veno-occlusive disease
     Alveolar proteinosis
     Sarcoid-like reaction
     Diffuse pulmonary hemorrhage (penicillamine)
9. 2 or more of the above

It is worth referring to a table such as this when approaching an immunocompromised host with a pulmonary lesion, because obtaining a number of different facts can quickly narrow the differential diagnosis. Infection accounts for 75 percent of the conditions affecting the lung in the immunocompromised host, but this means that 25 percent of instances are noninfectious. It is also important to keep in mind that even at autopsy a definitive diagnosis cannot be made in 15 percent of the cases, with the final diagnosis being "fibrosis" (Wilson et al, 1985; Singer et al, 1979; Rosenow, 1985, 1989). In this setting, the fibrosis may well be a valid final diagnosis if it is related to an adverse drug or radiation effect.

Infections are the primary concern and must be aggressively sought because many are treatable, especially in the earlier stages if the host has reasonable defense mechanisms. Usually, but not always, the diagnosis can be established without resorting to invasive procedures, such as transbronchial lung biopsy and open lung biopsy.

Recurrence of underlying disease is a significant problem in the patient with hematologic malignancies, especially lymphoma. A rule of thumb is that a patient with lymphoma and a new pulmonary infiltrate has a 50 percent chance that the infiltrate is due to lymphoma (Greenman et al, 1975). This can be a problem, since establishing a diagnosis of lymphoma involving the lung can be very difficult short of performing an open lung biopsy.

Connective tissue diseases rarely recur acutely and seldom mimic infection or acute or subacute drug reaction, but systemic lupus erythematosus occasionally can and must also be considered, especially when such a patient is responding poorly to immunosuppressive therapy.

In patients with AIDS, infection accounts for most pulmonary lesions, but Kaposi's sarcoma occurs in enough of these patients to warrant its consideration if positive diagnosis of the usual opportunistic organisms is not obtained (Ognibene and Shelhamer, 1988; Hanson et al, 1987; Meduri et al, 1986). Kaposi's sarcoma also is very difficult to diagnose without an open lung biopsy.

Patients with solid neoplasms often are immunocompromised as a result of immunosuppressive chemotherapeutic agents or radiation. When a carcinoma or sarcoma involves the lungs, it is usually insidious, not often associated with fever, and usually, but not always, has a characteristic reticulonodular (lymphangitic) or "cannonball" appearance.

The transplant patient may have a whole spectrum of disorders that are not found in the other entities mentioned here, namely rejection, increased incidence of fibrosis (especially in the bone marrow transplant patient), complications of graft-versus-host disease (GVHD) in the bone marrow transplant patient (Krowka et al, 1985; Weiner et al, 1986), and bronchiolitis obliterans in the heart-lung transplant patients (Glenville et al, 1987). Pulmonary edema is not uncommon in the first month following renal and bone marrow transplantation (Dickout et al, 1987) and can mimic almost any other disorder including infection because of the occasional association with fever. It is a challenge at times to avoid doing an open lung biopsy for this.

Drug reactions account for 15 to 20 percent of diffuse pulmonary disease in some series and is difficult to diagnose with bronchoalveolar lavage, transbronchoscopic lung biopsy, or other means (Cooper and Matthay, 1987; Rosenow, 1989). It is a condition of exclusion and, for the diagnosis to be made, the patient needs to be on or have recently been on a drug that is known to be toxic to the lung (see Table 5-1), to have typical cytopathologic histology, and to have other disorders excluded. Certain drugs such as Ara-C produce an unusual reaction that results in acute noncardiac pulmonary edema that is fatal in nearly half the patients and almost impossible to diagnose without an open lung biopsy (Jehn et al, 1988). Mitomycin-C, when given in conjunction with 5-fluorouracil and/or a leukocyte transfusion, can produce a hemolytic uremia syndrome with noncardiac pulmonary edema due to thrombi obstructing the vessels (Verweij et al, 1987). Usually there is systemic presentation with neurologic sequelae, but an open lung biopsy may be required.

Secondary or "opportunistic" neoplasms are a significant problem in the chronically immunosuppressed host (Tucker et al, 1988). These include non-Hodgkin's lymphoma, sarcomas, and lung cancers, all of which may be difficult to diagnose without thoracotomy.

A category of "unrelated" must also always be considered because many of these patients are prone to additional disease processes. For example, elderly patients with "silent" coronary artery disease and congestive failure may develop signs and symptoms mimicking diffuse lung disease of many varieties. Immunocompromised patients are also subject to pulmonary emboli, the adult respiratory distress syndrome (ARDS), oxygen toxicity, community-acquired pneumonias, and aspiration.

Some unusual complications can occur as a consequence of therapy for many of these disorders. These include pulmonary veno-occlusive disease, alveolar proteinosis, "sarcoidosis," and Goodpasture's syndrome secondary to penicillamine. Pulmonary veno-occlusive disease is usually associated with bleomycin, mitomycin, or the nitrosoureas, and cannot be diagnosed without an open lung biopsy (Lombard et al, 1987). Alveolar proteinosis can be

diagnosed from bronchoalveolar lavage if the diagnostic PAS-positive intra-alveolar material is recovered (Bedrossian et al, 1980). "Sarcoidosis" has been diagnosed in a number of patients on chemotherapy, but this almost certainly represents drug-induced granulomas. Methotrexate, mineral oil, nitrofurantoin, and a few other drugs can incite granulomatous reaction. There are at least a dozen cases of well-documented penicillamine-induced Goodpasture's syndrome (Devogelaer et al, 1987).

Finally, in 10 to 20 percent of immunocompromised hosts, there is the possibility that two or more of the above entities may occur together. One should not be satisfied with a single diagnosis without thinking of the possibility that two or more other conditions may be present.

The approach to the immunocompromised host must be thorough. The clinician must do a complete review of systems and physical examination in the hopes of finding a clue. A minimally invasive biopsy with culture from a skin lesion, lymph node, enlarged liver, or other source may reflect the pulmonary process. Funduscopic examination can be helpful in determining the presence of cytomegaloviral infection, disseminated histoplasmosis or toxoplasmosis, or *Candida* infection. The finding of characteristic changes in the fundus does not necessarily reflect the nature of the lung lesion, but it may. Gram's stains of sputum are probably more important than cultures, but both should be done in every patient and repeatedly so. Blood cultures must always be done, as well as urine cultures and cultures of lesions. If all of these are negative, it is unlikely that serologic tests will be rewarding but they should be considered. Seroconversion in *Legionella* infection usually does not occur soon enough to be of value in establishing an immediate diagnosis, nor do other serologic studies, with the exception of perhaps cytomegalovirus.

There are a number of variables that must be considered in deciding which, if any, diagnostic and therapeutic options should be pursued. For example, what is the stage of the underlying disease? Is the patient in remission with a good outlook or in his or her third relapse with no further chance of receiving an appropriate chemotherapeutic agent or radiation? What is the status of the transplanted organ? Is it being rejected with little hope of retransplantation? Has the patient been given an empiric trial of antibiotics? If so, this will influence the yield of cultures obtained in any invasive procedure, including bronchoalveolar lavage. Are there other organ system failures such as renal failure, cardiac failure, or bone marrow suppression from drugs? Even with an exact diagnosis, will it alter therapy (25 to 60 percent of the time) or outcome (5 to 20 percent)? What is the biologic age of the patient? What is the rate of progression of the disease? Is there time to wait for the initial cultures? Finally, what are the wishes of the patient and family? One would obviously be more aggressive in a 20-year-old with Hodgkin's disease in remission on treatment than an 80-year-old with a hematologic malignancy who is hypoxic, on corticosteroids, is neutropenic and septic, and has an elevated serum creatinine level. It is between these two extreme examples that the clinician will be called upon to make most of his or her decisions.

At this point the clinician may either proceed with bronchoscopy—including bronchial brushings, bronchoalveolar lavage (BAL), and transbronchoscopic lung biopsy—or go directly to an open lung biopsy. Most clinicians would choose the least invasive procedure, and bronchoscopy is almost noninvasive if transbronchoscopic lung biopsy is not done. Thus it is "easy" to proceed right to fiberbronchoscopy, BAL, and brushing of a diffuse pulmonary process in the immunocompromised host. Table 5–2 lists a review of the literature of bronchoalveolar lavage in the immunocompromised host with

the reported yields. The results are quite variable, and most clinicians should be very uncomfortable with sensitivity and specificity of anything less than 80 to 85 percent. The clinician and pathologist must also ask themselves, "Do the data from bronchoscopy and bronchoalveolar lavage fit the clinical pattern?"; if they do not, an open lung biopsy must be considered.

The complications of bronchoscopy and BAL are minimal. Transient fever and/or pulmonary infiltrate in the region of lavage occur in 15 to 30 percent of the patients and have no long-term sequelae. Transbronchoscopic lung biopsy may increase the diagnostic information, but in the immunocompromised host with clotting disorders, bleeding can be fatal, as can a tension pneumothorax. Thus there are fewer and fewer reports of transbronchoscopic lung biopsy being added to, or included in, the procedure of bronchoscopy.

Table 5–3 is a compilation of these various series of the anticipated yield of BAL in the non-AIDS patient, including "more than 80 percent sensitive and specific"; to "borderline," which includes 55 to

TABLE 5–2

RESULTS OF BRONCHOALVEOLAR LAVAGE

REFERENCE		FINDINGS	PERCENT
Crawford		Cytomegalovirus	96%
Ann Intern Med 1988; 108:180			
Schulman			63%
Chest 1988; 93:960			
Stover			
Ann Intern Med 1984; 101:1			66%
Malignancy	45%		
Drug	40%		
Hemorrhage	78%		
Nonbacterial infection	82%		
Young		General*	
J Clin Pathol 1984; 37:390		Cytology	70%
		with Microbiol	93%
deBlic		General*	60%
Thorax 1987; 42:759		Children	
Saito		Leukemia	17%
Chest 1988; 94:745			
Levy		Malignancy	100%
Chest 1988; 94:1028			
Xaubet		General*	49%
Chest 1989; 95:130		TPC†	69%
Cordonnier		Bone marrow transplants	50%
Am Rev Respir Dis 1985; 132:1118			
Cancer 1986; 58:1047			
Several series		Pneumocystis pneumonia in AIDS	95%
Several series		Non-AIDS	66%
		Pneumocystis pneumonia	55–70%

*General: wide spectrum of immunocompromised hosts
†TPC: Telescoped plug-catheter

TABLE 5–3

BRONCHOALVEOLAR LAVAGE IN NON-AIDS PATIENTS

\>80% SENSITIVE AND SPECIFIC
    Bacteria
        Usual gram-positive or gram negative
        Legionella
        Mycobacteria
    Parasites
        Toxoplasmosis
        Strongyloides
    Viruses
        Cytomegalovirus
        Herpes

BORDERLINE (55–80% SENSITIVE AND SPECIFIC)
    Nocardia
    Pneumocystis
    Aspergillus/Mucor
    Candida
    Cryptococcus
    Neoplasm
    (Yields further reduced if already on antibiotics)

DOUBTFUL (<55% SENSITIVE AND SPECIFIC)
    Drugs and treatment, especially cytosine arabinoside
    Mitomycin (hemolytic uremic syndrome)
    Oxygen
    Blood (leukoagglutinin reaction)
    Hemorrhage
    Nonspecific diffuse alveolar damage and fibrosis (15% at autopsy; bone marrow transplant; drug?)
    Radiation
    Edema (renal transplant; rejection; congestive heart failure; other)
    Patients with:
        Lyphoma
        Leukemia
            Leukemic infiltrate
            Leukemic cell lysis pneumonopathy
            Hyperleukocytic phenomenon
    Graft-vs-host disease
    Opportunistic neoplasm
    Pulmonary emboli
    Adult respiratory distress syndrome
    Connective tissue diseases, especially systemic lupus erythematosus
    Rare complications
        Pulmonary veno-occlusive disease
        Alveolar proteinosis
        Diffuse pulmonary hemorrhage
        "Sarcoidosis"
        Fat emboli
    Second or third process

80 percent sensitivity; and finally "least sensitive and specific," which would be less than 55 percent sensitivity and specificity.

Open lung biopsy is the best way of making a definitive diagnosis when everything else has failed. It should be recognized, however, that open lung biopsy (or even autopsy) does not invariably provide a diagnosis more specific than fibrosis or diffuse alveolar damage. In many instances this is probably a drug or radiation effect without the typical cytotoxic changes seen.

One of us reviewed all of the series of open lung biopsies in the immunocompromised host, which total 30 separate reports since 1976 including four abstracts (Rosenow, unpublished data). This includes approximately 1,000 patients, but a few of these series include nonimmunocompromised patients. A specific diagnosis was made in about 80 percent of the patients (range, 55 to 90 percent), which is consistent with the final diagnosis at autopsy as mentioned above. The established diagnosis from open lung biopsy altered treatment in approximately 45 percent of the patients (range, 25 to 60 percent), although in many of these the "treatment alteration" was merely discontinuation of medications when certain entities were ruled out. From about five of these series the reviewer could establish a percentage in which the authors thought the results of the open lung biopsy altered the outcome, and this ranged from 5 to 50 percent, with an average estimate of about 20 percent. Thus in only a small percentage of the patients does open lung biopsy affect the outcome in a beneficial way. This partly reflects the fact that our ability to diagnose exceeds our ability to treat at this time.

Interestingly, of these nearly 1,000 patients in which an open lung biopsy was performed, the reviewer could find mention of only five deaths immediately or within 24 hours of the procedure. This is less morbidity than has been reported with transbronchoscopic lung biopsy. Theoretically, the surgical procedure must accelerate respiratory failure and the need of intubation in many of these

patients, thereby possibly accelerating their demise. Nevertheless, it is a surprisingly "safe" procedure considering that many, if not most, of these patients are extremely ill and are poor risks for general anesthesia.

It is important to stress that there must be a single individual or a single team responsible for the patient's care, including writing all the orders. The surgeon must not be bridled with taking over the management of the patient during the usual postoperative period that occurs in the immunocompromised host setting. The surgeon's only responsibility is the care of the patient during the surgical procedure and immediately after, and he or she should not be responsible for handling of the tissue obtained at the time of the procedure. There should be a protocol within every institution that deals with the handling of tissue from the immunocompromised host. Table 5–4 outlines the procedure of handling of tissue obtained at the time of open lung biopsy specimen at the Mayo Clinic. The microbiologist and pathologist must be made aware ahead of time that this tissue is coming and have a plan for calling the primary service (and *only* the primary service) with these results as soon as they become available. The primary service should relay the working diagnosis

---

TABLE 5–4

HANDLING OF OPEN LUNG BIOPSY SPECIMEN

CLINICAL MICROBIOLOGY			SURGICAL PATHOLOGY	
Stain*		Cultures (days)	Fixed	Frozen
Gram	General	1–10	Hematoxylin and eosin (H&E)	Tumor, drug Hemorrhage
	Strongyloides (not cultured)		Gram	Edema Nonspecific pneumonitis
KOH/calcofluor	Fungi	3–40	Methenamine silver	
Methenamine silver	*Pneumocystis* (not cultured)	–	Methenamine silver	
Auramine-rhodamine	Mycobacteria	7–40	Auramine-rhodamine	
Modified Kinyoun	*Nocardia*	5–7	Modified Kinyoun	
Fluorescent antibodies	*Legionella*	4–7	Fluorescent antibodies	
Monoclonal antibody to	Cytomegalovirus	1–14	H&E (inclusions) FA[†],ISH[‡]	
viruses (<16 hrs)		3–14	H&E (inclusions)	
Touch prep	*Chlamydia*	2–3	Fluorescent antibodies	
Wright-Giemsa	Toxoplasmosis	–	Giemsa	

*Stains are completed in 10 to 60 minutes
[†]FA: fluorescent antibodies
[‡]ISH: in-situ hybridization

to the pathologist and microbiologist, as this will help them make some of their interpretations.

It is very important to re-emphasize that the clinician must approach every one of these patients individually and take into account the risks and benefits of all the procedures, including the use of empiric antibiotics in their care. The patient cannot simply be entered into an algorithm and decisions made from that without taking into account all of the variables that have been discussed up to this point.

VIRAL INFECTIONS

Measles

In the pediatric age group, most cases of life-threatening measles pneumonia occur in the immunocompromised host with depressed cellular immunity (Becroft and Osborne, 1980). The occurrence of fatal measles pneumonia in adults is virtually always found in a setting of immunodeficiency (Sobonya et al, 1978), although the nature of the immune abnormality may be a poorly characterized overlap of humoral and cellular dysfunction. The pathologic findings of fatal measles pneumonia are similar in the immunocompromised host and the nonimmunocompromised host, specifically bronchitis, bronchiolitis and alveolitis with inclusion-bearing multinucleated epithelial giant cells (see Fig. 4-8). Giant cells are generally more numerous in the more severely immunocompromised patients.

Herpes Simplex Virus

Herpes simplex virus (HSV) pneumonia is usually seen in immunocompromised hosts. Two patterns of reaction are seen. HSV tracheobronchitis begins as an ulcerative lesion in the upper airways and extends distally to reach the bronchioles and parenchyma. This pattern of reaction is seen in a wide variety of seriously ill patients, notably in patients with burns (Nash, 1972) and ARDS (Tuxen et al, 1982). The other type of HSV infection occurs specifically in immunosuppressed patients and consists of hemorrhagic, variably inflamed, miliary nodules (Fig. 5-1). It is often found with multisystem herpetic infection and is thought to represent disseminated viremic seeding. Clinically the diagnosis may be suspected if the patient has associated facial, oral, or esophageal lesions (Williams et al, 1976b). The radiographic findings are nonspecific and consist of interstitial infiltrates or a bronchopneumonia (Williams et al, 1976b; Douglas et al, 1969). The hemorrhagic nodules observed pathologically are usually difficult to identify on the chest radiograph.

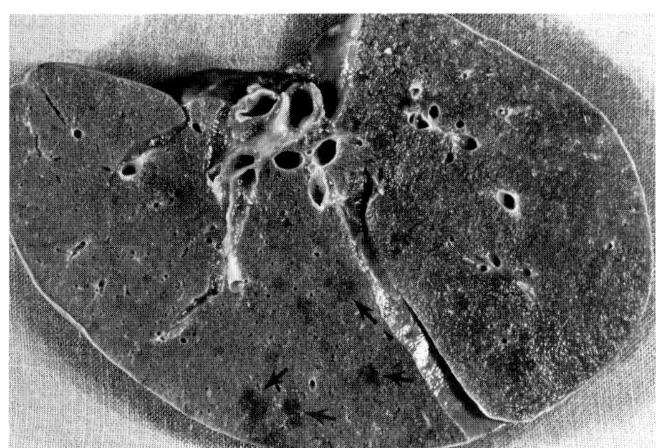

Figure 5-1 Hemorrhagic nodules in patient with herpes simplex viremia.

However, on CT the hemorrhagic nodules are seen as 2- to 10-mm-diameter, poorly marginated, nodular densities (Fig. 5-2). Confluence of the nodules and airspace consolidation often progress rapidly. The presence of nodules on CT in an immunocompromised patient is most characteristic of herpes simplex and cytomegalovirus pneumonia. Both herpetic ulcers and hemorrhagic nodules contain the characteristic nuclear herpetic inclusions. Enlargement and a basophilic, diffuse ground-glass appearance of the nucleus is first seen. The intranuclear material coalesces into a eosinophilic inclusion surrounded by a halo. Multinucleated inclusion cells are seldom seen in histologic sections but may appear in cytologic specimens (Vernon, 1982). The inclusions may be difficult to identify with certainty, and either immunoperoxidase stains or electron microscopy may be useful in verifying the diagnosis (Fig. 5-3).

Herpes Varicella-Zoster

Varicella infection (chickenpox) usually occurs in childhood; in immunocompetent subjects, serious pulmonary complications are unusual. Primary varicella infection in adults is associated with radiologic evidence of pneumonia in about 15 percent of cases (Triebwasser et al, 1967). Herpes varicella-zoster (HVZ) pneumonia is seen particularly in cancer patients who are on chemotherapy at the time of exposure to the virus (Miliauskas and Webber, 1984). The radiologic findings include peribronchovascular consolidation, miliary nodules, or diffuse acinar densities (Greene, 1980). Acinar densities—which are rosette-like, and are 5- to 10-mm-diameter nodular densities with ill-defined margins—are the most characteristic finding in HVZ pneumonia. A presumptive diagnosis can be made when acinar

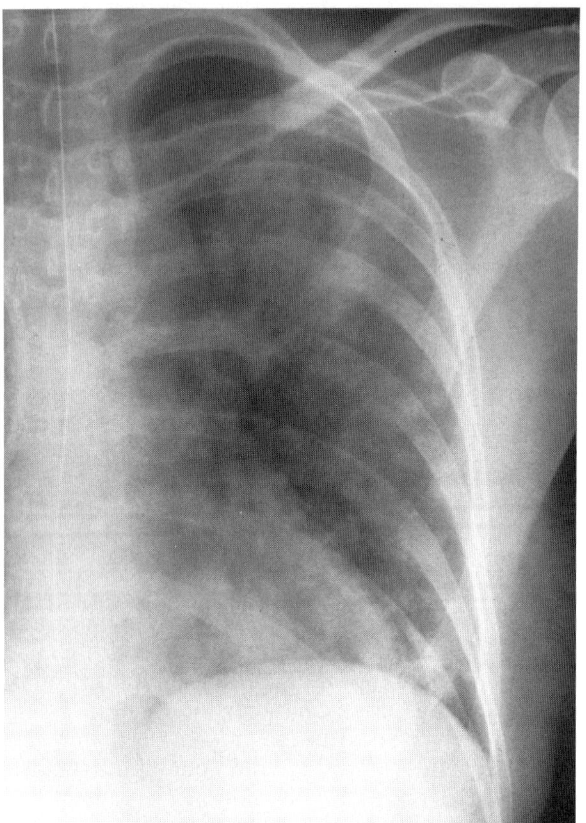

A

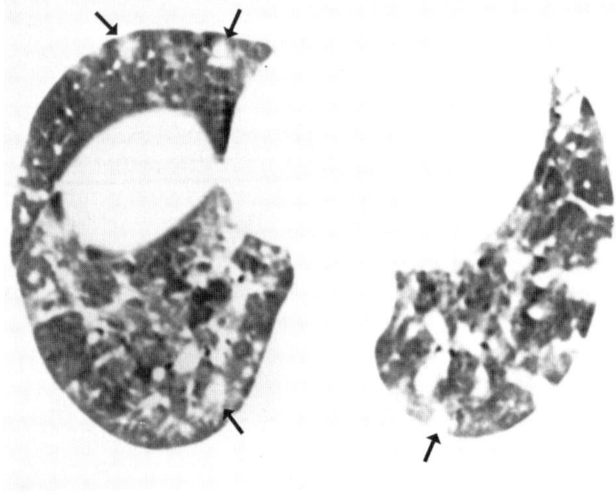

B

Figure 5–2   The patient is a 41-year-old woman with herpes simplex pneumonia. *A*, Magnified view of the left lung shows patchy areas of airspace consolidation and a few ill-defined nodular densities. *B*, 1.5-mm collimation CT scan through the lower lung zones better delineates the nodular densities (*arrows*). Pathologically these correspond to hemorrhagic nodules with or without surrounding edema. Patchy areas of ground-glass density are also present, which may represent hemorrhage or edema.

densities are present in a patient with a coexistent skin rash. Reactivation of varicella infection occurs as zoster, which is a very painful cutaneous vesicular rash, distributed along dermatomes. In immunologically intact patients, primary varicella and zoster seldom cause life-threatening respiratory illness. In immunocompromised patients, both types of infections may cause pneumonia, which is morphologically similar to the hemorrhagic nodules described above for HSV. Ulcers of the conducting airways are much less common in HVZ than in HSV infection.

Cytomegalovirus

Cytomegalovirus (CMV) pneumonia is seen almost exclusively in immunocompromised patients. Patients with renal transplants or bone marrow transplants are particularly prone to this illness; it is catastrophic in bone marrow transplants and has a mortality of over 80 percent. Radiologically, CMV may produce interstitial infiltrates or airspace consolidation, which is usually extensive and bilateral but which may also be lobar in distribution (Abdallah et al, 1976; Schulman, 1987). A characteristic radiologic pattern of CMV pneumonia is the rapid progression of radiographic findings from a predominantly "interstitial" to an airspace pattern (Fig. 5–4). The characteristic hemorrhagic nodules pathologically are difficult to appreciate on the radiograph but can be seen on computed tomography (CT) (Fig. 5–5). The pattern of reaction in CMV pneumonia may be hemorrhagic nodules similar to those of HSV and HVZ pneumonia; more often CMV presents as an interstitial pneumonia. The hemorrhagic nodules are accompanied by diffuse alveolar damage to a variable degree (Fig. 5–6). Usually there is no involvement of bronchi and bronchioles. CMV infection is often accompanied by *Pneumocystis carinii* pneumonia, and the interstitial pneumonia may be a response to *Pneumocystis*. Whenever characteristic CMV inclusions are seen, careful search for *Pneumocystis* organisms should be made. CMV inclusions are usually easily recognized by dramatic nuclear and cytoplasmic cellular enlargement, hence the virus' name.

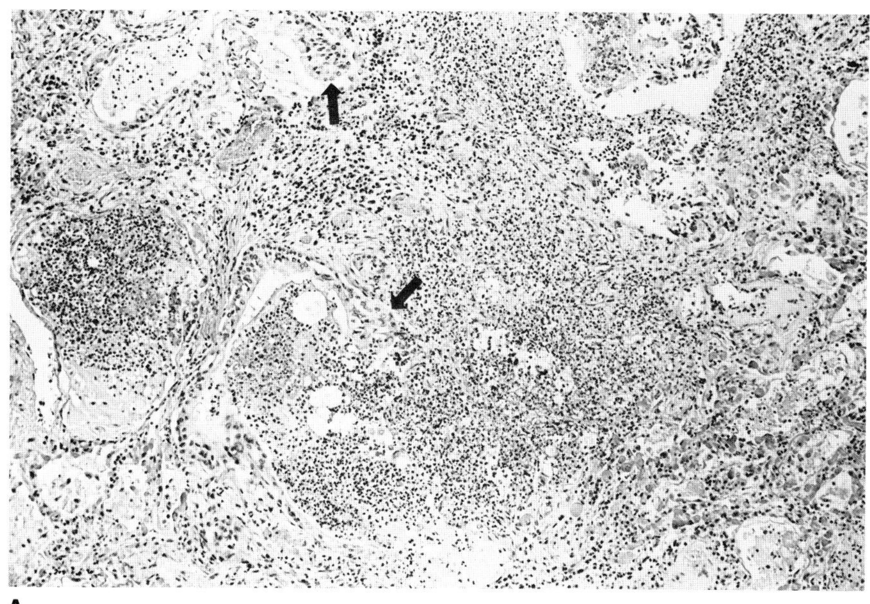

A

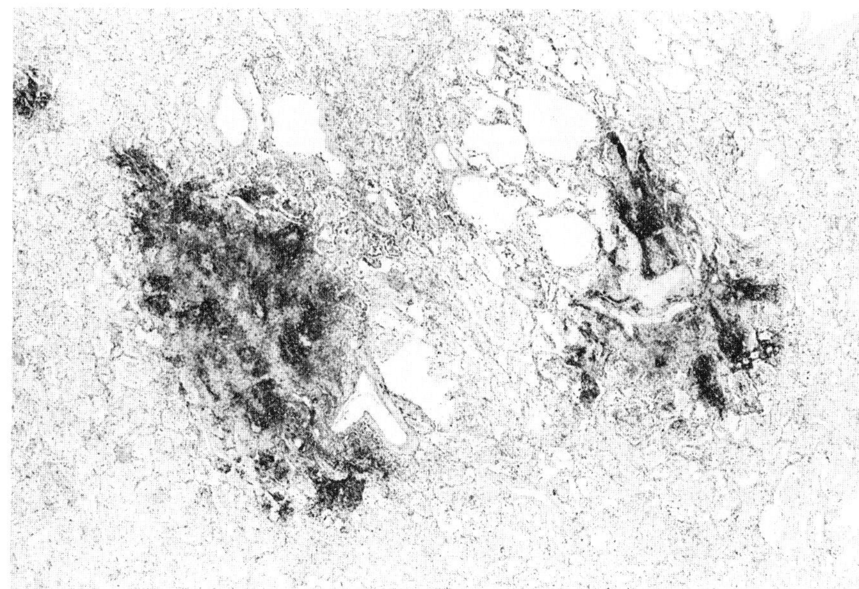

B

Figure 5–3 Mechanically ventilated patient with herpetic bronchitis and bronchiolitis. *A*, Purulent bronchiolitis with epithelium (*arrows*) suggestive of herpetic inclusions. *B*, Immunoperoxidase reaction showing strong positivity in the involved bronchioles.

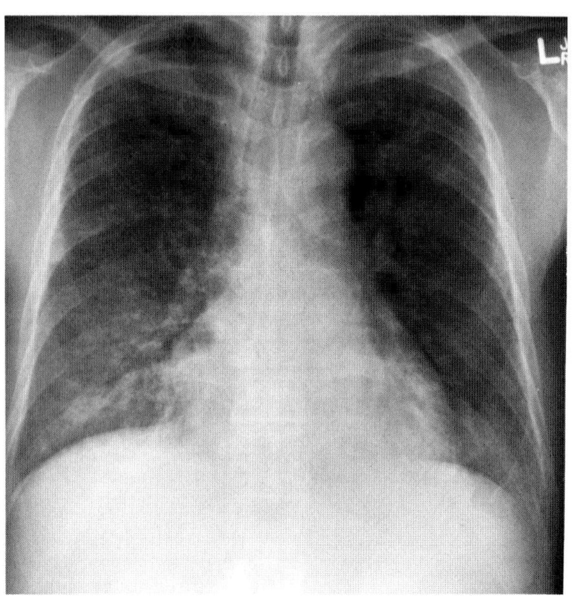

A

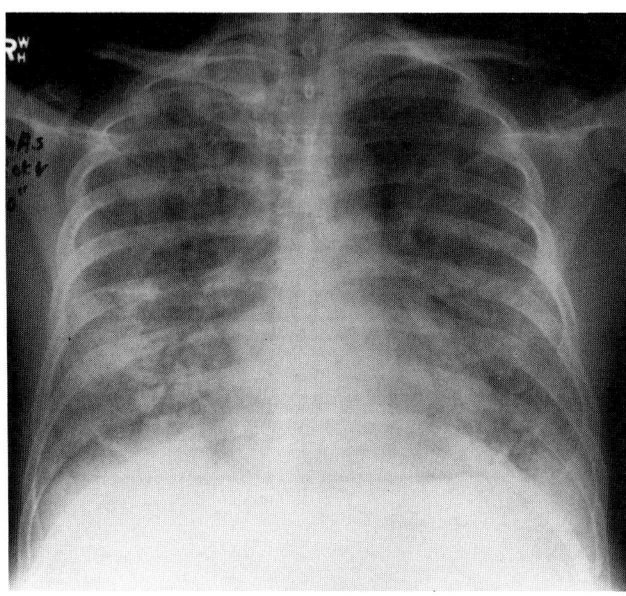

B

Figure 5–4 The patient is a 53-year-old man with cytomegalovirus pneumonia. *A,* Chest radiograph shows irregular linear opacities and ill-defined areas of ground-glass density, particularly in the lower lung zones. *B,* Within one week the findings progressed to extensive bilateral airspace consolidation.

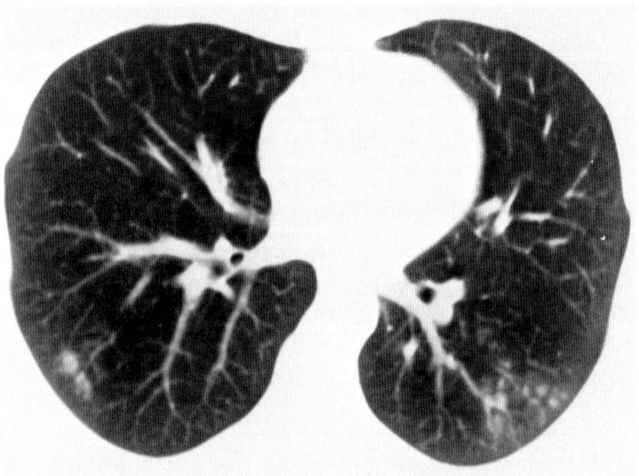

Figure 5–5 CT scan at the level of the inferior pulmonary veins in a patient with CMV pneumonia shows small nodular densities. These presumably represent hemorrhagic nodules.

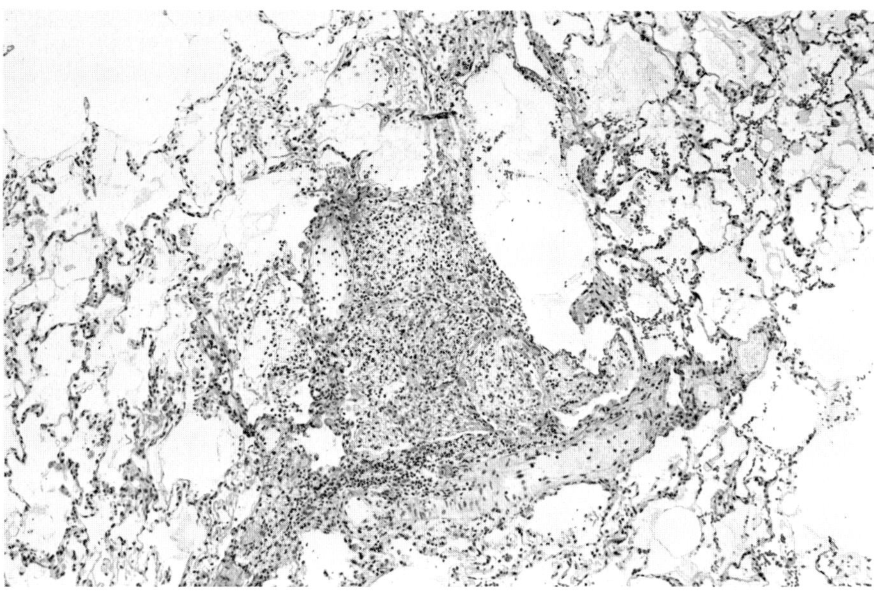

Figure 5–6 Hemorrhagic, acutely inflamed nodule due to hematogenous CMV. Surrounding lung shows early diffuse alveolar damage with edema and fibrinous exudate.

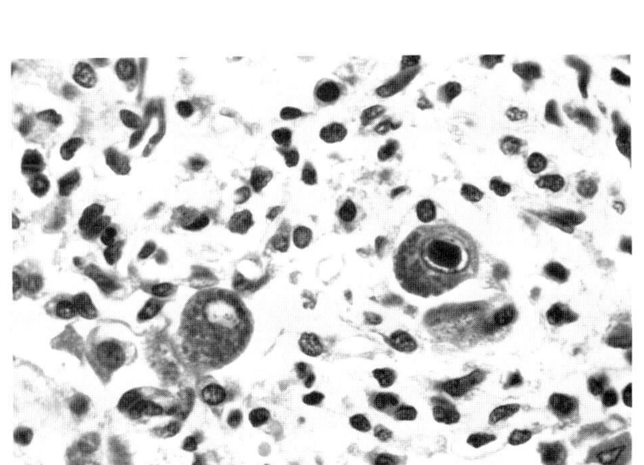

Figure 5–7   Two typical CMV-infected cells.

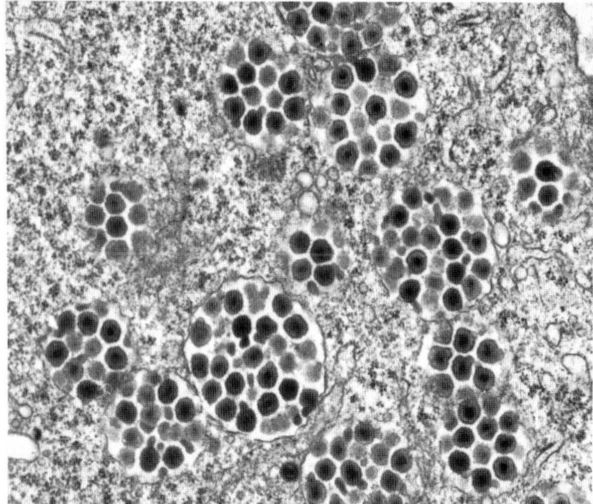

Figure 5–8   Electron microscopy of CMV shows the cytoplasmic virions to be included in membrane-bound vesicles.

The involved nucleus contains a prominent central inclusion surrounded by a halo and marginated chromatin. Cytoplasmic inclusions and perinuclear basophilic specks are also present (Fig. 5–7). By electron microscopy, the nucleus contains free uncoated virions, while the cytoplasm shows coated virions in membrane-bound vesicles (Fig. 5–8). These vesicles give rise to the speckled nature of the cytoplasmic inclusions.

BACTERIAL INFECTIONS

Immunocompromised patients are at increased risk for community-acquired and nosocomial bacterial pneumonia of various etiologies, including the more common agents such as *Hemophilus* and *Streptococcus*, as well as agents that seldom cause disease in normal hosts.

Pseudomonas aeruginosa

Pseudomonas aeruginosa is a gram-negative bacterium that causes necrotizing pneumonia with abscesses, hemorrhagic infarcts, and a characteristic proliferation of bacteria in vessel walls with minimal reaction, giving the impression of a "blue haze" (Fig. 5-9) (Soave et al, 1978).

Serratia marcescens

Serratia marcescens may cause lethal nosocomial pneumonia in seriously ill patients. The reaction pattern is acute bronchopneumonia with abscesses and neutrophilic vasculitis in non-neutropenic patients, and diffuse alveolar damage and hemorrhage in neutropenic patients (Goldstein et al, 1982).

Nocardia asteroides

Nocardia asteroides is a gram-positive bacterium that occasionally causes pulmonary disease in the normal host but more commonly in the immunocompromised host. It is seen most often in patients with pulmonary alveolar proteinosis, following organ

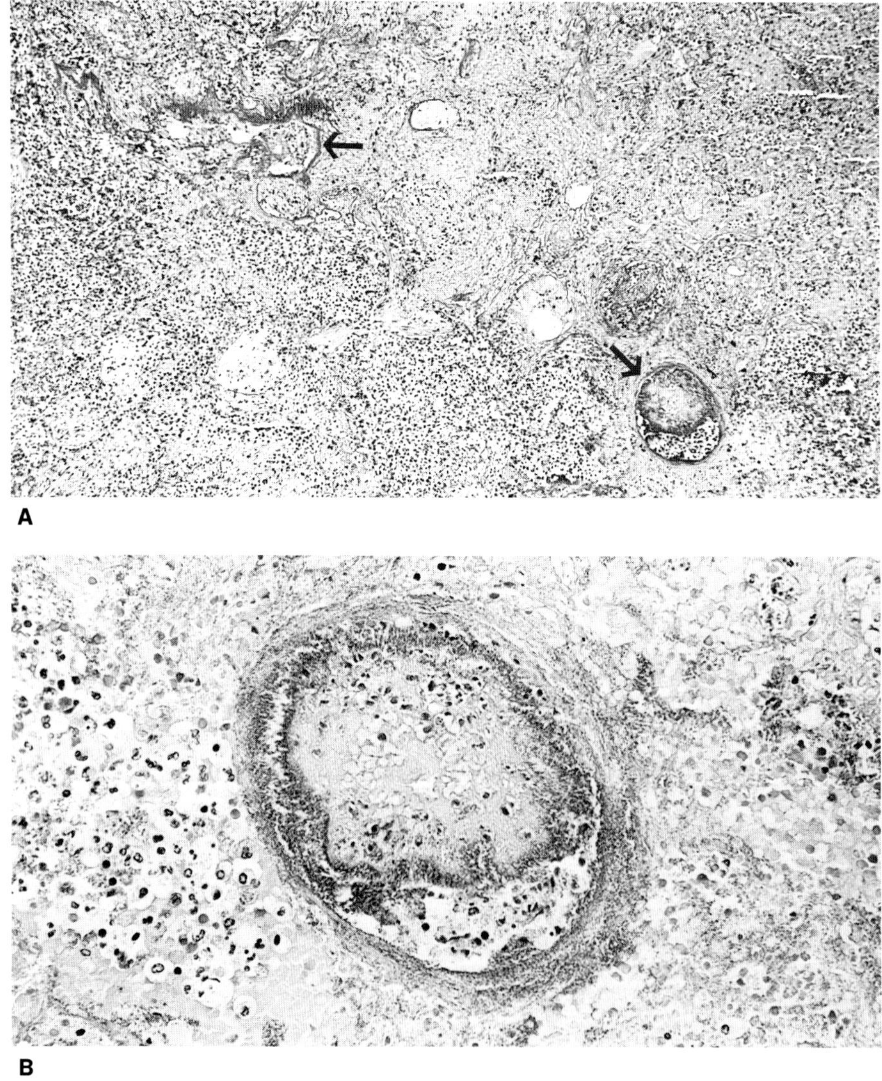

Figure 5-9   *A, Pseudomonas*-induced necrotizing pneumonia with vascular necrosis and thrombosis (*arrows*) (H&E). *B*, Circumferential proliferation of organisms in vessel wall (tissue Gram's stain).

transplantation, and in patients receiving immunosuppressive therapy (Williams et al, 1976a). Clinically, it may produce dry or productive cough, malaise, and fever. The radiologic manifestations are nonspecific. It may present with single or multiple nodules, lobar pneumonia, necrotizing bronchopneumonia, abscess formation, pleural extension with effusion, and chest wall invasion (Grossman et al, 1970). Diagnosis frequently requires lung aspiration or biopsy, since morphologic or culture proof of nocardiosis from sputum is not very accurate. The classic gross appearance of *Nocardia* pneumonia in the immunocompromised host is one of abscesses and/or cavities (Washington University CPC, 1982). The microscopic pattern is one of purulent inflammation. The organisms may be demonstrated in the inflammatory debris as branching, beaded, filamentous bacilli that are gram-positive, methenamine silver–positive, and weakly acid-fast (Fig. 5–10).

Legionella pneumophila

Legionella pneumophila is associated with pneumonia in immunocompromised patients, including renal transplant recipients, bone marrow transplant recipients (Kugler et al, 1983), and patients with AIDS (Murray et al, 1987). The pattern of reaction varies according to the ability of the host to respond. In these patients, *Legionella* pneumonia may be lethal in spite of appropriate therapy.

MYCOBACTERIAL INFECTIONS

Patients with various lymphoreticular and nonlymphoreticular malignancies are at higher risk for active tuberculosis than is the general population (Kaplan et al, 1974). However, the occurrence of both tuberculosis and nontuberculous mycobacteriosis in patients with AIDS is already extraordinarily common and is increasing in frequency.

Mycobacterium tuberculosis

M. tuberculosis is particularly frequent in Haitian patients with AIDS and drug-abuse risk factors and/or with a high risk of previous exposure to *M. tuberculosis* (Snider et al, 1987; Fournier et al, 1988). Without a high index of suspicion, the diagnosis may be elusive since the clinical, radiologic, and pathologic features are usually atypical. Fever, weight loss, and cough are the usual presenting symptoms. Radiologic infiltrates, when present, are often nonapical and noncavitary, and extrapulmonary disease is found in 60 to 70 percent of patients (compared with 16 percent for non-AIDS active tuberculosis patients) (Snider et al, 1987). Pathologically, granulomatous reaction is often very poorly developed, the organisms cannot be found by special stains, and definitive diagnosis is delayed until cultures become positive. Response to antituberculous therapy is usually good.

Mycobacterium avium-intracellulare

Of the nontuberculous mycobacterial infections, *M. avium-intracellulare* is the most common and is, in fact, more common overall than *M. tuberculosis* in patients with AIDS. As in the case of *M. tuberculosis*, the clinical findings are nonspecific and the symptoms are more often systemic than respiratory. Pathologically, the disease is ordinarily disseminated and granulomas are very poorly formed, but unlike tuberculosis, large numbers of organisms can usually be demonstrated (Klatt et al, 1987; Chaisson and Hopewell, 1989). There is some controversy over the significance of disseminated *M. avium* infection in patients with AIDS: Some investigators (Horsburgh and Selik, 1989) believe that it adversely affects survival, and some (Klatt et al, 1987; Chaisson and Hopewell 1989) view the infection as innocuous. Unlike *M. tuberculosis*, this infection responds very poorly to antimycobacterial drugs.

FUNGAL INFECTIONS

As mentioned in Chapter 4, a variety of fungal diseases occur in the nonimmunocompromised host,

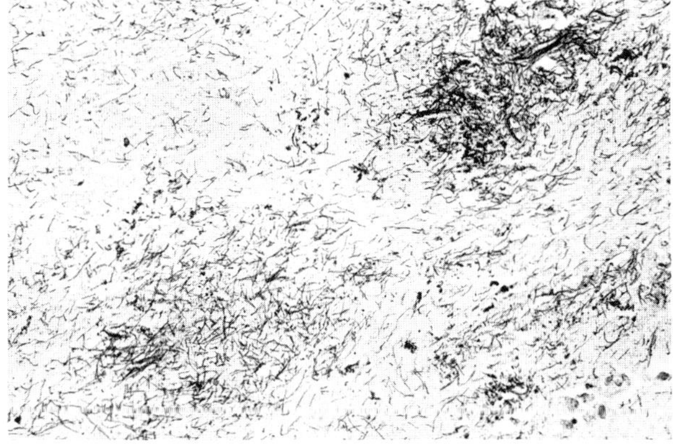

Figure 5–10   *Nocardia* (tissue Gram's stain).

but they are less commonly life-threatening than in the immunocompromised host.

Aspergillosis

Aspergillus is one of the most common organisms found in lung biopsies in the immunocompromised host (Orr et al, 1978). The organisms invade blood vessels, giving rise to infected infarcts that may cavitate (Fig. 5-11). The typical histologic appearance is one of septate hyphal thrombi, coagulative parenchymal necrosis, and hyphal proliferation in the dead tissue (see Fig. 5-11). Occasionally, particularly with large cavitated infarcts, the tissue temperature becomes sufficiently low (approaching 22°C) to support conidiospore formation (Fig. 5-12). Radiologically, invasive aspergillosis may present with subsegmental, segmental or lobar consolidation or with single or multiple nodules (Orr et al, 1978) (Fig. 5-13). When cavitation occurs, there is usually a rim of air surrounding the infarcted lung, causing an "air crescent sign" similar to that observed in mycetomas. In invasive aspergillosis, the air crescent represents air between retracted, infarcted lung and the

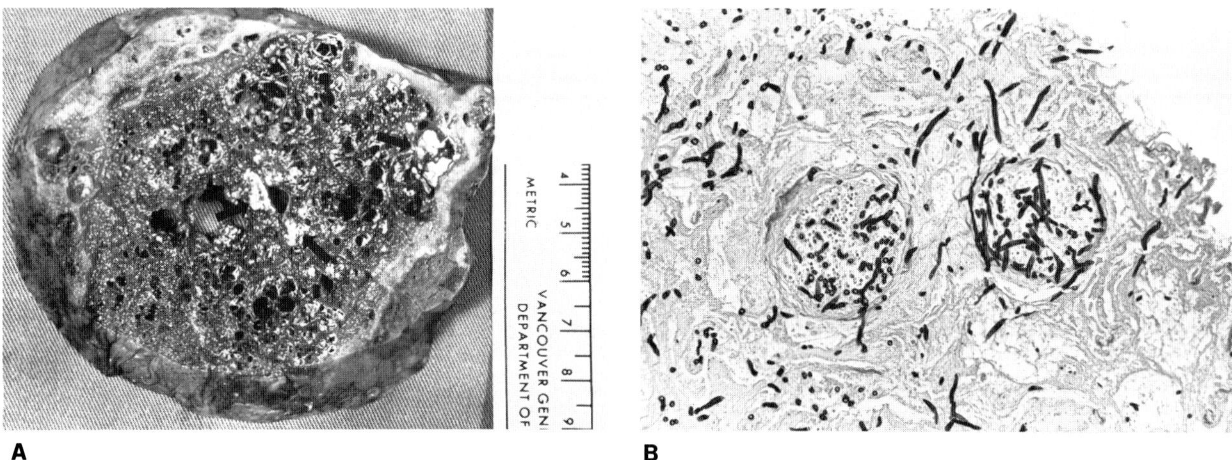

A   **B**

Figure 5-11   *A*, Massive *Aspergillus* infarct involving the apical segment of the upper lobe (cut in transverse plane). White flecks (*arrows*) are mold. *B*, Hyphal proliferation in vessels and adjacent tissue.

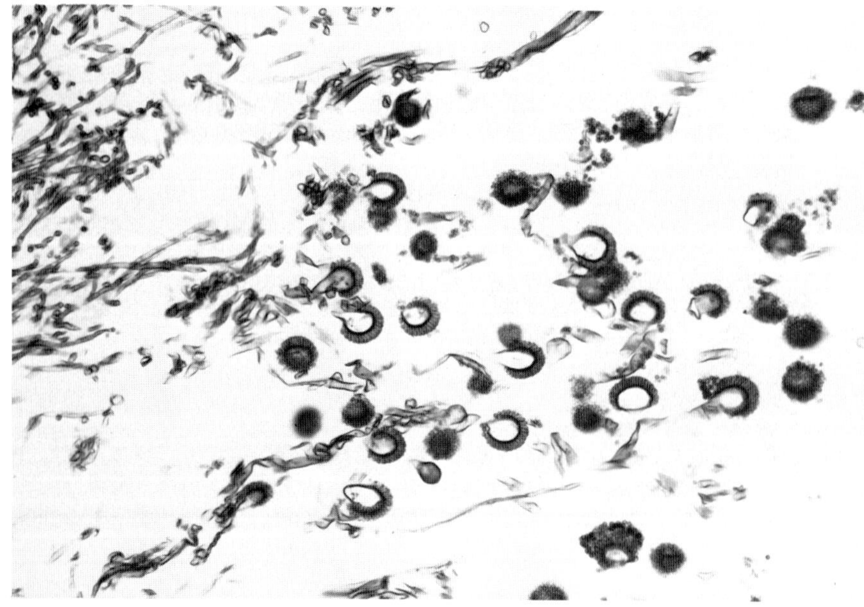

Figure 5-12   Conidiospores can form if tissue reaches a sufficiently low temperature.

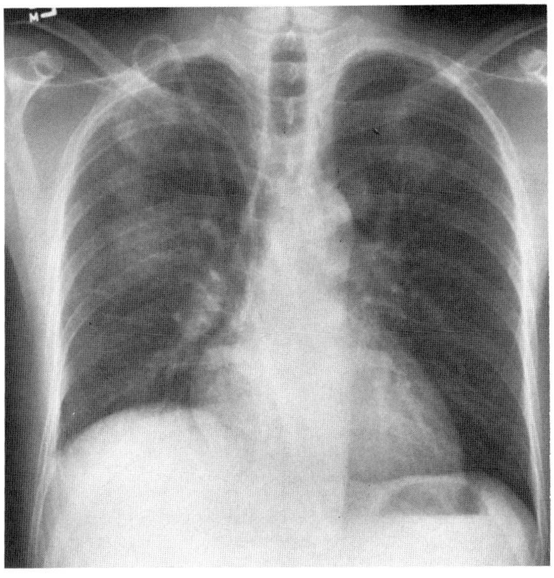

A

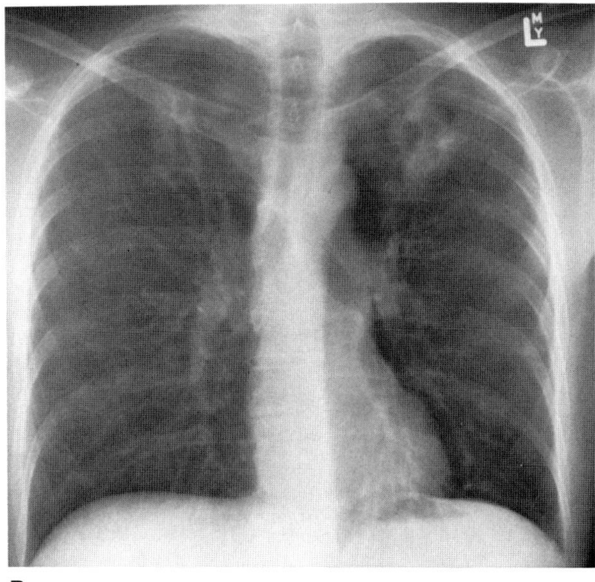

B

Figure 5–13 *A,* This 35-year-old man being treated for acute myelogenous leukemia developed invasive pulmonary aspergillosis. The chest radiograph shows bilateral upper lobe nodules. *B,* Chest radiograph in another patient with invasive pulmonary aspergillosis. A cavitating nodule is present in the left upper lobe. Ill-defined small areas of consolidation are present in the right upper lobe.

surrounding lung parenchyma (Curtis et al, 1979). Although in the appropriate clinical setting these findings may be highly suggestive, there is no single typical radiologic pattern of invasive aspergillosis. The radiograph is often normal or shows nonspecific infiltrates. The air crescent sign is also a late finding; diagnosis should have been made before the appearance of this sign. Recently, it has been suggested that CT might be helpful in the early diagnosis of invasive aspergillosis (Kuhlman et al, 1987). The findings on CT consisted of single peripheral mass-like infiltrates or multiple inflammatory nodules. A characteristic halo of low attenuation, seen surrounding the infiltrates, has been shown to be due to coagulative necrosis (Hruban et al, 1987).

Mucormycosis

Mucormycosis (Bigby et al, 1986) is less common and is nearly always seen in diabetic or immunocompromised patients. It gives rise to a pattern of lung injury similar to that of aspergillosis, specifically septic thrombi with infarction. The radiologic findings of mucormycosis are nonspecific, consisting of patchy airspace consolidation that may be uni- or bilateral and may cavitate (Barturm et al, 1975). Rarely, mucormycosis may present as a solitary nodule (Gale et al, 1972). Air crescent formation, similar to that seen in aspergillosis, may occur and may be

seen on CT before it is apparent on the radiograph (Silver et al, 1989).

Candidiasis

Candidiasis is a common infection in immunocompromised patients. The route of infection may be either aerogenous or hematogenous, these two patterns of infection being equally common in one large series (Dubois et al, 1977). In the event of aerogenous infection, bronchopneumonia is found with endobronchial yeast growth, peribronchial microabscesses, and predominantly lower lobe involvement. In the event of hematogenous infection, infected thrombi and diffuse microabscesses usually less than 5 mm in diameter are found (Fig. 5–14). The pattern of reaction of aerogenous *Candida* resembles bacterial bronchopneumonia, and that of hematogenous infection in some ways resembles aspergillosis and mucormycosis. We have also seen instances of granulomatous reaction to *Candida* simulating tuberculosis. Silver stains demonstrate budding yeast and/or hyphal fragments; the latter may be impossible to distinguish from *Aspergillus* morphologically. Culture is the only certain way of identification. The clinical and radiologic findings in *Candida albicans* pneumonia are nonspecific, and *Candida* infection is often seen in association with other pathogens. Buff et al, (1982) described the

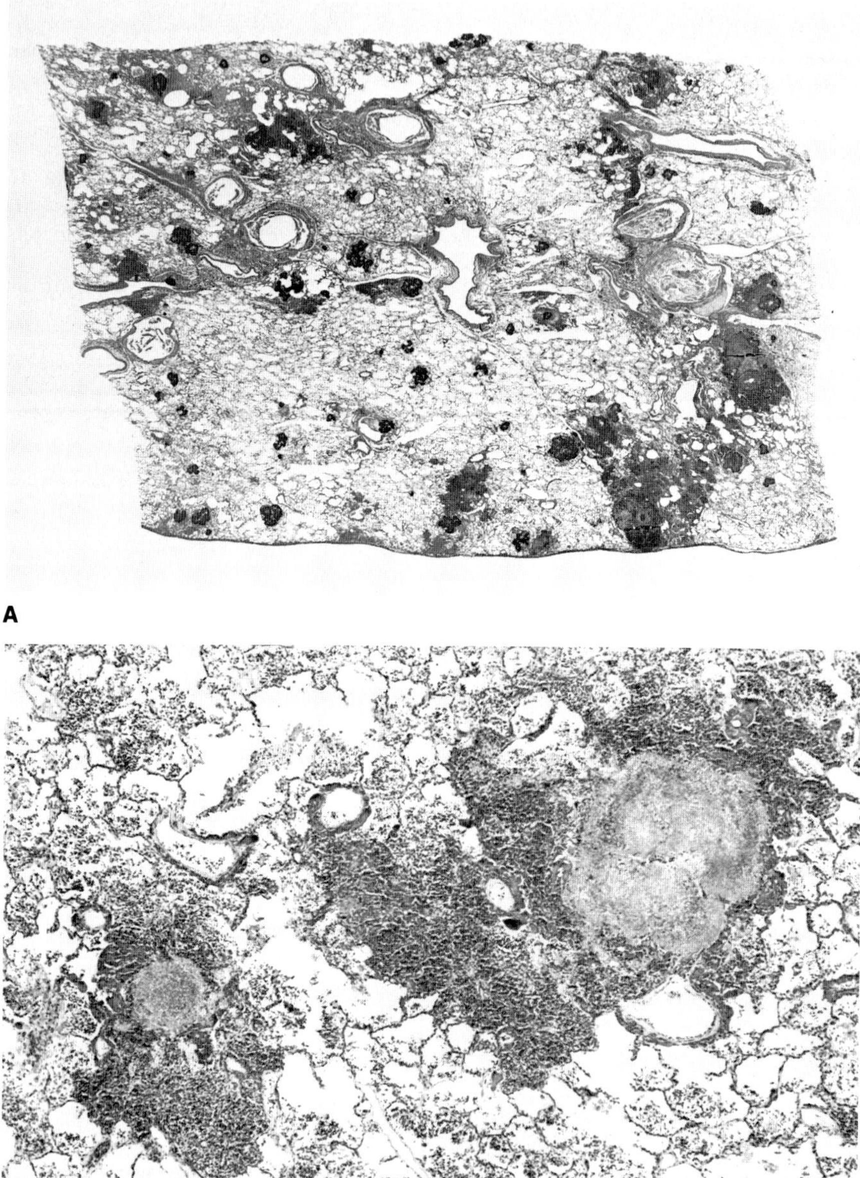

Figure 5–14   *A*, Scanning microscopic appearance of hematogenous *Candida*, with dozens of variably sized nodules, most surrounded by zone of hemorrhage. *B*, Colonies of *Candida* surrounded by hemorrhage with no inflammatory reaction in a profoundly neutropenic patient.

radiologic findings in patients with pure *Candida* pneumonia. All had airspace consolidation or mixed airspace and interstitial changes (Fig. 5-15). None developed cavitation. A miliary nodular pattern has been described by others (Pagani and Libshitz, 1981), presumably correlating with the hematogenous route of infection.

Cryptococcosis

Cryptococcosis (torulosis, European blastomycosis) is caused by the fungus *Cryptococcus neoformans.* Cryptococcosis is mainly a disease of the immunocompromised host or patients with underlying severe disease. In one series (McDonnell and Hutchins, 1985) 33 of 36 autopsied patients, most of whom would be classified as immunocompromised, had underlying debilitating disease. In these patients cryptococcosis was the major cause of death in 69 percent, and pulmonary cryptococcosis the cause of death in more than 25 percent. In 7 of the 36 patients one or more peripheral pulmonary granulomas were present, and these were variable in size. Granulomas are the most common reaction pattern encountered in the nonimmunocompromised host (see Fig. 4-11) and are usually an incidental finding in patients with cryptococcal meningitis. Occasionally the granulomas may be quite large, mimicking neoplasm, or may even cavitate. The most common form of involvement (53 percent) in the series referred to above was granulomatous pneumonia with intra-alveolar proliferation of organisms and varying degrees of

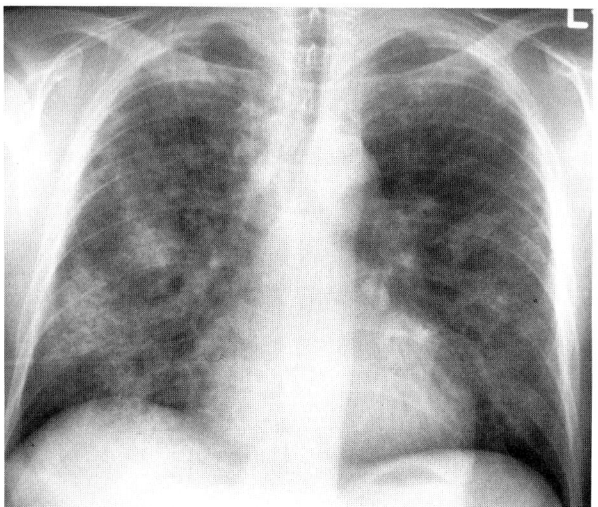

Figure 5-15   Chest radiograph in a 38-year-old patient with "pure" *Candida* pneumonia. The findings consist of patchy bilateral airspace consolidation.

inflammatory response. In 7 of the 36 patients, numerous organisms were present diffusely within alveolar capillaries and interstitial tissues, accompanied by either minimal inflammation or miliary granulomas. In a few patients, there were both intraalveolar and intravascular organisms with little inflammatory reaction. Recently it has become apparent that cryptococcosis is a common and serious complication of AIDS (Gal et al, 1986). It was found in about 10 percent of patients, and in them the cryptococcosis was characteristically interstitial and intravascular with minimal inflammation and no granuloma formation. The organisms are usually very abundant but may be hard to see with hematoxylin and eosin stains. They were seen lying free and also within giant cells. The characteristic feature is a large capsule that does not stain with hematoxylin and eosin but does stain with periodic acid–Schiff or mucicarmine (see Fig. 4-11). In patients with AIDS the capsule may be poorly formed and the organisms harder to identify with mucicarmine stains than with silver stains. Cryptococcosis in patients with AIDS typically becomes disseminated systemically and responds poorly to amphotericin (Wasser and Talavera, 1987).

Histoplasmosis

Histoplasma capsulatum causes lung disease in the immunocompromised host, usually as a component of disseminated infection (Kauffman et al, 1978; Goodwin et al, 1980, Salzman et al, 1988). In addition to lung disease, involvement of lymph nodes, bone marrow, liver, spleen, and oropharynx is common in these patients at the time of presentation. Patients who are immunocompromised on the basis of leukemia, lymphoma, steroid therapy, and AIDS are all susceptible (Fig. 5-16). The vast majority of infected patients live in or have lived in areas where histoplasmosis is endemic (Kauffman et al, 1978; Salzman et al, 1988). The phenomenon of histoplasmosis developing in a patient long after he has moved from an endemic area suggests the possibility of reactivation of infection. Unlike aspergillosis or candidiasis, in which infection is very common but virtually confined to the immunocompromised host, the prevalence of histoplasmosis is not dramatically increased in immunosuppressed individuals (Kauffman et al, 1978). However, in contrast to immunologically intact people in whom histoplasmosis usually causes pulmonary granulomas of little clinical significance, disseminated histoplasmosis in the immunocompromised host produces an interstitial histiocytic reaction with or without tuberculoid granulomas (Goodwin et al, 1980). The organisms

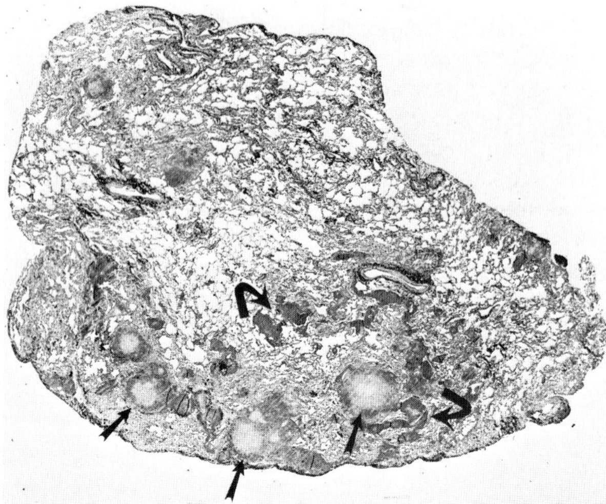

Figure 5–16 Patient with chronic lymphocytic leukemia (*curved arrows*) and granulomas due to histoplasmosis (*long arrows*).

are readily demonstrated by methenamine silver stains of tissue sections of biopsies of lung, bone marrow, or other involved sites. Bronchoalveolar lavage is insensitive in the diagnosis of histoplasmosis in the immunocompromised host (Salzman et al, 1988).

PROTOZOAL INFECTIONS

Pneumocystis carinii

Pneumocystis carinii is a protozoan that is nearly always encountered as a cause of pulmonary infiltrates in debilitated patients. *Pneumocystis carinii* pneumonia was at one time termed "plasma cell pneumonia", or "interstitial plasma cell pneumonitis." This terminology described the infantile form of the disease seen in malnourished babies living under conditions of profound deprivation. Currently, *Pneumocystis carinii* pneumonia is much more commonly seen in immunocompromised children and adults in general (Weber et al, 1977) and in patients with AIDS in particular (Murray et al, 1987). Extrapulmonary involvement also may occur (Grimes et al, 1987). Clinically, patients usually present with dry cough and progressive shortness of breath. They usually have severe hypoxemia (MacFarlane, 1985). In some patients, the diagnosis may be first suspected by radiologic abnormalities at the time when the patient is still asymptomatic (Engelberg et al, 1984). Radiologically, the first abnormality is often a bilateral perihilar linear process or perihilar haziness that progresses within 3 to 5 days to a more homogeneous

diffuse airspace consolidation (Forrest, 1972); Delorenzo et al, 1987) (Fig. 5–17). This pattern is characteristic but may be mimicked by a variety of other disease processes. Furthermore, *Pneumocystis carinii* infection may cause a variety of different radiographic patterns including uni- or bilateral, segmental or nonsegmental infiltrates (Fig. 5–18), or single or multiple nodules that may cavitate (Doppman et al, 1975; Barrio et al, 1986). It may have a striking upper-lobe predominance, mimicking tuberculosis (Milligan et al, 1985) (Fig. 5–19). In approximately 10 percent of patients, the radiograph at the time of diagnosis is normal. The diagnosis depends on demonstrating the organisms, which may be found by open lung biopsy or bronchoalveolar lavage. More recently, the ease with which the diagnosis can be made in patients with AIDS by sputum examination has been emphasized (Murray et al, 1987). *Pneumocystis carinii* is not well seen on hematoxylin and eosin–stained slides; methenamine silver stains show the cysts, which are approximately 6 μm in diameter and are folded or cup-shaped. The Giemsa's stain shows six to eight individual inner bodies within the cysts. The classic appearance of *Pneumocystis carinii* in the lung is a foamy eosinophilic intra-alveolar exudate (which contains the organisms), together with a mild mononuclear interstitial infiltrate. It is essential to recognize that many, if not most, cases of *Pneumocystis carinii* pneumonia do not have a classic histologic appearance. Absence of the foamy exudate,

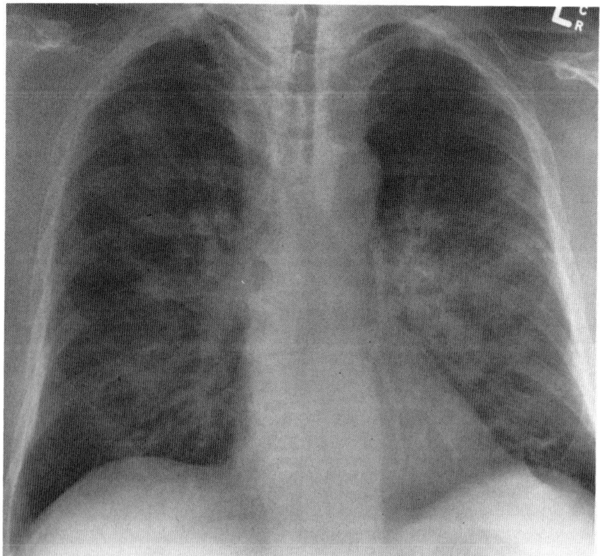

Figure 5–17 The patient is a 63-year-old man with *Pneumocystis carinii* pneumonia. The chest radiograph shows bilateral ground-glass densities predominantly in the perihilar region.

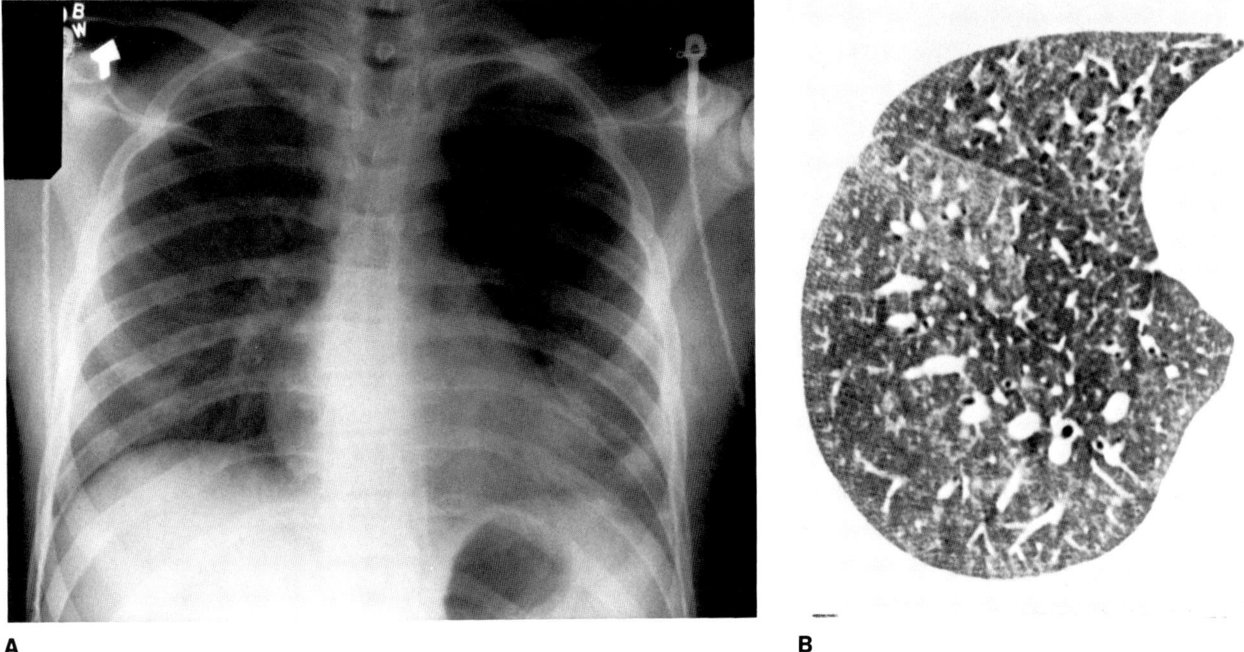

A   **B**

Figure 5–18 The patient is a 19-year-old male bone marrow transplant recipient. *A,* Chest radiograph shows ill-defined areas of ground-glass density bilaterally. The patient had previous open lung biopsy showing pneumocystic pneumonia. *B,* High-resolution CT through the right lower lung zone shows patchy distribution of ground-glass densities. These radiologic and CT findings are nonspecific.

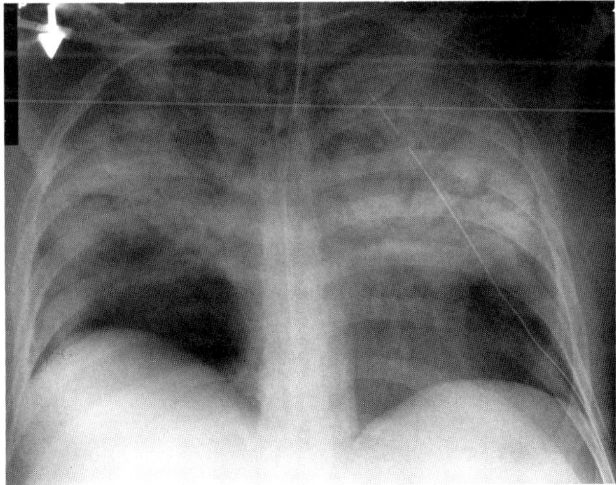

Figure 5–19 Chest radiograph of a 47-year-old man with severe pneumocystic pneumonia shows airspace consolidation with air bronchograms predominantly in the upper lobes. The left chest tube was inserted at the time of a recent open lung biopsy.

severe interstitial inflammation, fibrosis, marked intra-alveolar histiocytic reaction, and granulomatous inflammation have all been described in *Pneumocystis carinii* pneumonia (Weber et al, 1977; Bleiweiss et al, 1988; Luna and Cleary, 1989; Saldana and Mones, 1989) (Fig. 5–20). Since *Pneumocystis carinii* pneumonia is a treatable condition, it is imperative that it be suspected in all immunocompromised hosts and that silver stains be performed on all lung biopsies from these patients.

Toxoplasmosis

Toxoplasma gondii is a relatively uncommon pathogen in patients who are immunocompromised from malignancy, chemotherapy, or AIDS (Williams et al, 1976b; Vietzke et al, 1968; Catterall et al, 1986; Murray et al, 1987). Disseminated toxoplasmosis in this population appears to be due to reactivation of latent infection in most instances (Williams et al, 1976b). Pulmonary disease is usually overshadowed by central nervous system involvement, although radiologic pulmonary infiltrates are described in approximately half of patients with *Toxoplasma* encephalitis. The histologic changes of *Toxoplasma* pneumonitis are subtle. The reaction pattern varies

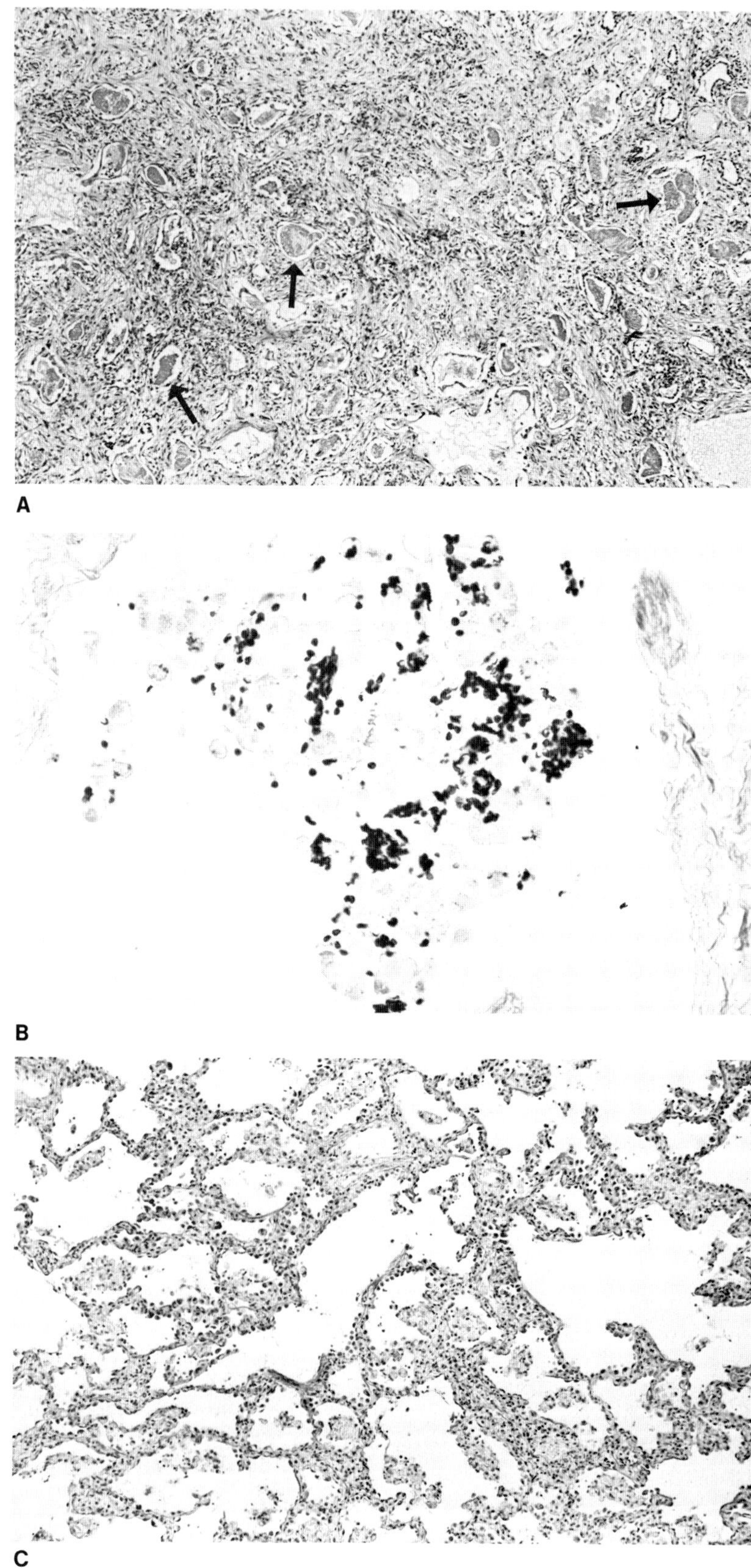

Figure 5–20   *A*, Severe fibrosing reaction to *Pneumocystis* with eosinophilic clusters of organisms in remnant alveoli (*arrows*). *B*, Intra-alveolar histiocytic reaction containing organisms (methenamine silver). *C*, Reaction to *Pneumocystis* simulating desquamative interstitial pneumonia, with mononuclear cell alveolitis, type-II cell hyperplasia, and intra-alveolar histiocytes.

from focal necrosis to diffuse interstitial pneumonitis with a fibrinopurulent alveolar exudate. The inflammatory reaction is variable, depending on the host's ability to respond. Identification of the trophozoites can sometimes be accomplished by hematoxylin and eosin, silver, or Giemsa's stains; immunohistochemical stains for toxoplasma antigen detection may prove to be more sensitive. Mixed pulmonary infections in patients with neurotoxoplasmosis, particularly viral pneumonitis due to CMV or HSV are described as being common (Vietzke et al, 1968); these viral agents may be responsible for the pulmonary infiltrates in patients with predominantly central nervous system disease and/or may mask minor degrees of pulmonary toxoplasmosis.

Strongyloidiasis

Strongyloides occasionally causes opportunistic infections including pneumonia in immunocompromised patients (Williams et al, 1976b; Genta et al, 1989). Patients who once lived in areas where *Strongyloides* is endemic seem to be at particular risk. Peripheral blood eosinophilia is seen in the majority of these patients. The diagnosis of pulmonary *Strongyloides* infection may be established by the identification of larvae in sputum or bronchoalveolar lavage fluid. In the immunocompromised host, the infection is often fatal in spite of appropriate treatment.

DRUG REACTIONS: CYTOTOXIC CHEMOTHERAPEUTIC DRUGS

The features of diffuse alveolar damage induced by antineoplastic therapeutic agents include type-II cell proliferation, interstitial fibrosis, and relative preservation of lung structure. Advanced honeycombing is not common, although the interstitial fibrosis may develop over a very short period of time. A characteristic feature of antineoplastic drug-induced lesions is the presence of large type-II cells that frequently have atypical, hyperchromatic nuclei with prominent nucleoli. Electron-microscopically, the nuclei often contain tubular structures thought to represent the products of altered nucleic acid metabolism brought about by the anticancer agents. A reasonably safe working assumption is that any antineoplastic drug may produce diffuse alveolar damage. However, from the clinical point of view there are some drugs—5-fluorouracil, adriamycin, thiotepa, azathioprine—that very rarely, if ever, produce pulmonary lesions. With the increasing number of agents available, the number of toxic agents will increase. Because a comprehensive list has recently been compiled (Colby and Carrington, 1988), only

two will be mentioned here: bleomycin, because it is commonly used and a useful example of diffuse alveolar damage; and methotrexate because it produces an unusual reaction.

Bleomycin

Bleomycin is a glycopeptide that is used in the treatment of epidermoid carcinoma, lymphoma, and malignant testicular tumors (Holoye et al, 1978). It is concentrated in skin, lungs, and lymph. Lung lesions are not related to pre-existing areas of disease, but the risk of lung toxicity is increased with increasing age, previous or concurrent radiotherapy, concurrent oxygen therapy, and/or concurrent additional cytotoxic drug therapy (Cooper et al, 1986a). Cumulative dose is an important factor in bleomycin toxicity. Toxicity appears at an average total dose of 100 to 150 units, with a significant increase at 450 units. Symptoms include a dry cough and progressive dyspnea. Rales, usually at the base of the lungs, are the earliest physical sign. Radiographic abnormalities typically lag behind the development of symptoms and function defects. Bleomycin may produce bilateral airspace, reticular, or reticulonodular changes that are usually predominantly in the lower lung zones. Functionally, restrictive lung disease occurs. In experimental studies the initial site of injury is the venous endothelial cell (Adamson and Bowden, 1974). The cell cytoplasm appears attenuated and vacuolated. The perivascular tissue is edematous, and an infiltrate of lymphocytes and plasma cells is seen. Type-I pneumonocytes become focally necrotic, and fibrin and other proteinaceous material leak into alveoli. Subsequently there is type-II cell hyperplasia, and bizarre type-II cells appear (Fig. 5–21). The intra-alveolar fibrin is organized by fibroblasts, and a characteristic intra-alveolar fibrosis occurs (De Lena et al, 1972). Interstitial fibroblasts also multiply, and septal widening results. Electron-microscopically, intranuclear inclusions of curious tubular structures have been seen in type-II cells (Gyorkey et al, 1980). Similar structures were also seen by these authors in patients who had been given busulfan. Hypersensitivity pneumonitis has been reported with bleomycin (Holoye et al, 1978).

Methotrexate

Methotrexate is toxic at least partly because of a hypersensitivity reaction (Clarysse et al, 1969). A dose relationship is not evident, although frequency of administration and concurrent other cytoxic drugs may increase toxicity and corticosteroids may be protective (Cooper et al, 1986a). The incidence of lung toxicity in methotrexate therapy is uncertain but is

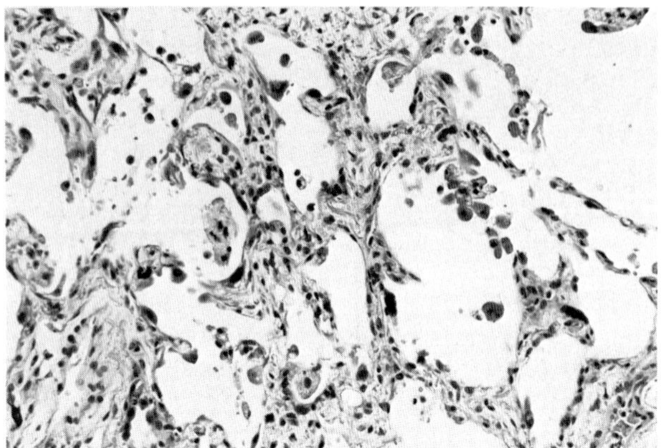

Figure 5–21   Interstitial fibrosis and bizarre type-II cells typical of cytotoxic drug reaction.

estimated to be less than 10 percent. A cough occurs anywhere from a few days to many months after administration, followed by malaise, raised temperature, and increasing dyspnea. About half of patients have peripheral eosinophilia. Radiographic manifestations include bilateral reticulonodular or irregular linear densities and, more commonly than with other drugs, bilateral airspace consolidation (Cooper and Matthay, 1987). Pleural effusions are common. Microscopically, an interstitial infiltrate of lymphocytes, plasma cells, and eosinophils is seen. Granulomas together with multinucleate giant cells are common. After 20 to 40 days of drug withdrawal, symptoms gradually subside in nearly all cases. Mortality is approximately 1 percent.

RADIATION PNEUMONITIS

Fajardo and Berthrong (1978) found that 5 to 20 percent of the patients treated for thoracic neoplasms by radiation developed clinical pneumonitis, and this resulted in the death of 8 percent of them. Damage was related to the amount of lung irradiated, the total dose, and the number of doses delivered, in addition to the treatment time. Concurrent infection (Bennett et al, 1969), chemotherapeutic agents (Phillips et al, 1975), or steroid withdrawal (Castellino et al, 1974) are known to increase radiation damage.

Signs and symptoms are often initially absent or mild. Cough, often harsh and nonproductive, results from bronchial epithelial damage. Progressive dyspnea may occur two to three months after irradiation. Functionally, a restrictive defect occurs. Radiologically, airspace consolidation is seen 1 to 6 months

after cessation of radiotherapy. The extent of radiation pneumonitis may vary from mild and patchy to complete consolidation of the entire irradiated zone. The pneumonitis is followed by progressive fibrosis, leading to loss of volume and bronchiectasis. Characteristically the changes are usually limited to the radiation port, but this is not invariably the case (Fennessy, 1987; Gibson et al, 1988). The fibrosis does not progress after 9 to 12 months (Libshitz and Southard, 1974).

In a recent prospective study, radiation pneumonitis could be detected on CT before the radiograph and was apparent on CT in patients in whom the radiograph remains normal (Ikezoe et al, 1988). Out of 17 patients, radiation pneumonitis was seen on CT within 4 weeks of completion of radiotherapy in 13 patients, by 8 weeks in one patient, and by 13 weeks in another patient. The pneumonitis on CT was seen as homogeneous, patchy, or discrete airspace consolidation. In four patients the radiation pneumonitis extended beyond the radiation portal. In three of the 15 patients with radiation pneumonitis, no abnormality was detected on the chest radiograph, whereas in three others it was seen much earlier on CT than on the radiograph.

Two phases of radiation damage are recognized (White, 1976; Gross, 1977). The *initial* phase starts in 1 to 2 hours and lasts for about 2 months. Clinically the differential diagnosis includes opportunistic infection and tumor infiltration. Histologically, diffuse alveolar damage is the predominant finding. Vascular changes may not be obvious, and special stains may be necessary to show fibrin in vessels. The interstitial space becomes widened, and alveoli become filled with necrotic type-I alveolar cells and exudate and prominent hyaline membranes. Macrophages accumulate in alveoli and mononuclear cells are present in the septa, but neutrophils are absent. Proliferating type-II cells classically appear large, with bizarre hyperchromatic nuclei. Although the cellular atypicality is similar to many forms of cytotoxic drug reaction, this feature is an important one in the differential diagnosis with infection, nonspecific diffuse alveolar damage, etc. Myointimal cells of small vessels proliferate, incorporate lipid, and produce intimal foam cells that are characteristic of radiation pneumonitis. As indicated, the differential diagnosis of acute radiation pneumonitis includes diffuse alveolar damage due to antineoplastic drugs (reviewed above) and coincident infections. All of these may mimic radiation pneumonitis, and the precise diagnosis may be extremely difficult.

The *chronic* manifestation of radiation is characterized by vascular sclerosis and repair. Hyaline membranes become phagocytosed or incorporated into intra-alveolar fibrous tissue. The interstitium is thickened, and there is broadening of the interlobular septa. The microvasculature is obliterated. Medium and small arteries have vascular sclerosis, which is present in an eccentric and discontinuous fashion along the vessel. Ischemia produces more fibrosis, and a vicious circle is established. Bronchioles may be distorted by the fibrosis so that bronchiolectasis with an obstructive pneumonitis may result.

Chronic radiation pneumonitis may histologically simulate usual interstitial pneumonia (UIP) on lung biopsy, although it tends to be confined to the radiation port, while UIP is usually most marked in the periphery of the lower lobes. The hyperplastic type-II cells and alveolar macrophages of UIP do not show the bizarre cellular features of radiation damage. Although there is sclerosis of the large to medium-sized vessels in UIP, the microvasculature is not involved. Radiation lesions in larger vessels, in contrast to the symmetric sclerosis of UIP, are eccentric and discontinuous.

Most histologic descriptions of radiation pneumonitis precede modern anticancer therapeutic agents and the considerable improvement in radiotherapeutic techniques. Expert opinion (Katzenstein and Askin, 1982) is that the lesions of antitumor drugs and radiation pneumonitis are in practice identical, except for foam cells within the intima and media associated with radiation. The practical problem is whether a pulmonary infiltrate in a previously radiated patient is due to tumor, infection, drug reaction, or radiation pneumonitis. It is usually possible to diagnose or exclude the first two; the other two are diagnosed on the basis of clinical information and morphologic changes that are consistent with the diagnosis.

GRAFT-VERSUS-HOST DISEASE

Graft-versus-host disease (GVHD) must be included in the differential diagnosis of pulmonary dysfunction in bone marrow transplant patients. This is a difficult and elusive diagnosis at the time of this writing. The diagnostic criteria are not so well delineated as for the more commonly recognized sites of GVHD such as skin, gut, and liver for several reasons. Bone marrow transplant patients are always immunocompromised and thus at high risk for various other acute lung diseases that may obscure the changes of GVHD. Systemic GVHD itself appears to predispose the patient for lung infection (Krowka et al, 1985), which would obscure the pulmonary GVHD component. Lung biopsy is not so innocuous as skin and gut biopsy, and thus the histologic evolu-

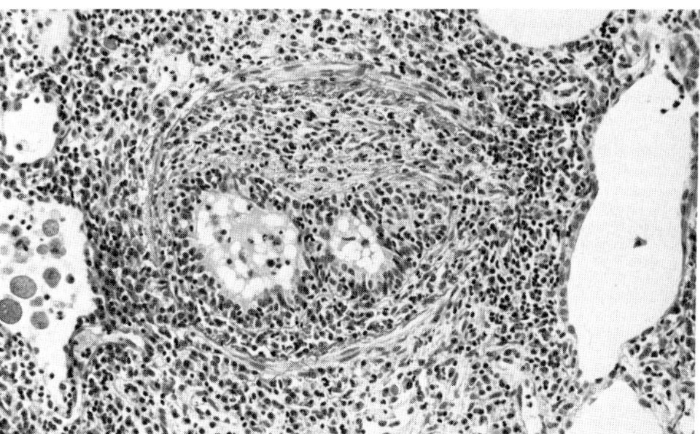

Figure 5–22 Mononuclear bronchiolitis with fibrous obliteration of the lumen in graft-versus-host disease.

tion of lung lesions cannot be as easily traced. Nevertheless, pulmonary GVHD is believed to exist, and its target is believed to be primarily the epithelium of the conducting airways. Beschorner et al, (1978) described a bronchial lesion that they believed represented GVHD, consisting of a relatively monomorphous, mature lymphocytic infiltrate in the bronchial walls and bronchial glands, associated with single-cell necrosis, analogous to the single-cell necrosis typical of acute GVHD in other sites (Snover, 1984). Most other investigators (Krowka et al, 1985; Snover 1984; Urbanski et al, 1987) view lymphocytic bronchitis as a nonspecific reaction. However, bronchiolitis obliterans is estimated to occur in 10 percent of patients with chronic GVHD and has been found to be responsible for severe obstructive lung disease in bone marrow transplant patients in the absence of infection. The histology of such cases is described (Ralph et al, 1984; Urbanski et al, 1987) as showing a cellular infiltrate in the walls of small bronchioles associated with variable degrees of peribronchiolitis, peribronchiolar alveolitis, and fibrous obliteration of the bronchiolar lumina (Fig. 5–22). Intrabronchiolar granulation tissue polyps are uncommon. The cellular infiltrate may be either mononuclear or polymorphonuclear (Urbanski et al, 1987). The proximal bronchi in three of four patients in the series of Ralph et al (1984) were described as showing acute inflammatory or purulent changes, although it was uncertain whether these changes were partly related to infection. We have seen one case of apparent pulmonary GVHD with conspicuous bronchiolar granulation polyps (Fig. 5–23) and one case with dramatic purulent bronchitis and proximal bronchiolitis (see Fig. 5–23). Treatment of pulmonary GVHD is immunosuppression; death occurs in approximately half of patients, and stable to slowly progressive obstructive lung disease occurs in the others.

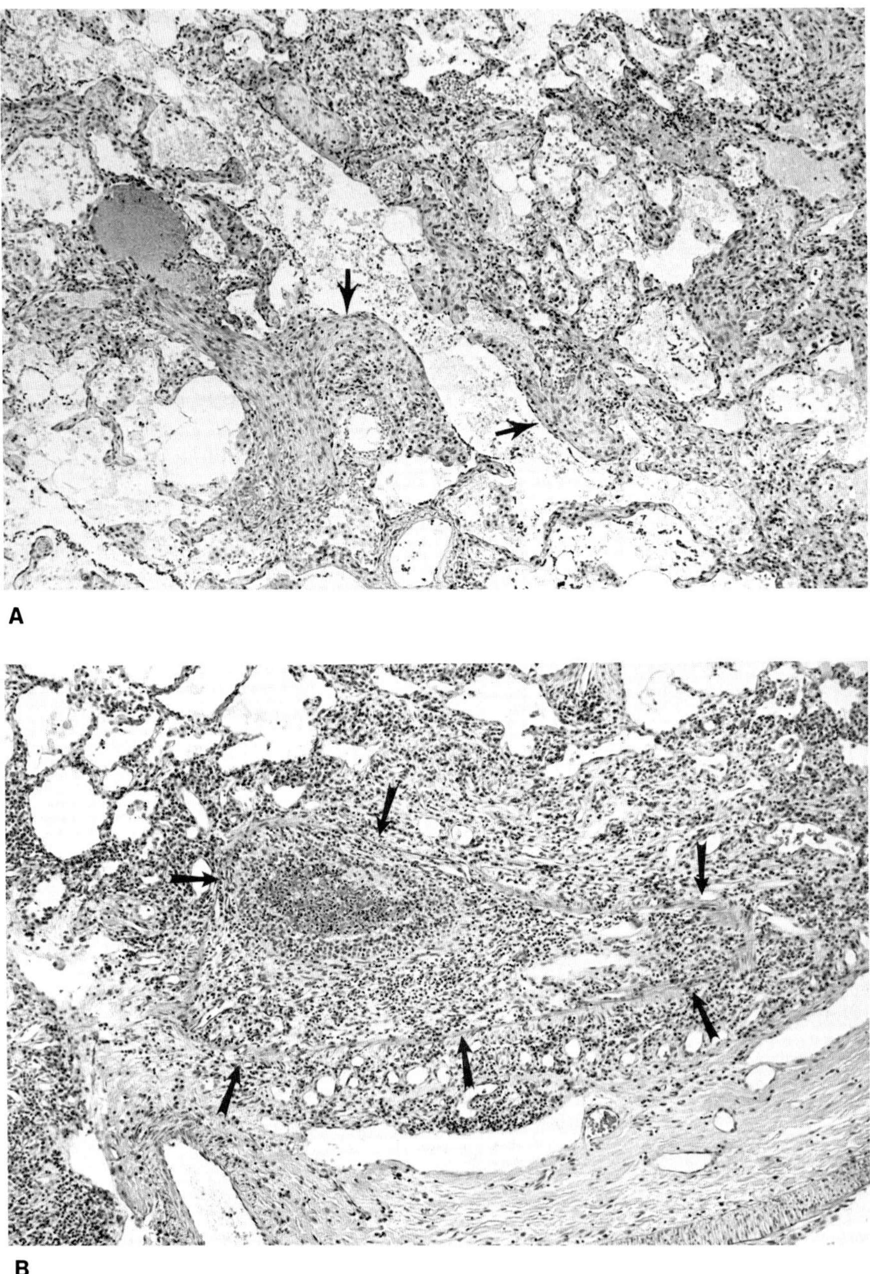

Figure 5–23 *A*, Clinical graft-versus-host disease with granulation tissue polyps in alveolar ducts (*arrow*) simulating bronchiolitis obliterans–organizing pneumonia. *B*, Purulent exudate in a bronchiole markedly narrowed by graft-versus-host disease (*arrows* at original bronchiolar submucosa).

OTHER

Pulmonary Alveolar Proteinosis

Pulmonary alveolar proteinosis is found in immunocompromised patients, particularly those with hematologic malignancies and myeloproliferative disorders. These patients very commonly have opportunistic lung infections including various fungal and mycobacterial infections as well as nocardiosis. Alveolar proteinosis in this setting is more fully discussed in Chapter 7.

Tumors

Tumors may present as acutely developing infiltrates in the immunocompromised host. The most common tumors to behave in this fashion are lymphomas, leukemias, and Kaposi's sarcoma in patients with AIDS. These lesions are discussed in Chapter 8.

Diffuse Pulmonary Hemorrhage

Diffuse pulmonary hemorrhage is an important cause of acute and rapidly developing infiltrates in immunocompromised patients. This may be due to infection with secondary hemorrhage (see Fig. 5–14), to primary hemorrhage due to thrombocytopenia or coagulopathies, or to Kaposi's sarcoma in patients with AIDS. Diffuse pulmonary hemorrhage is more fully discussed in Chapter 6.

REFERENCES

Abdallah PS, Mark JBD, Merigan TC. Diagnosis of cytomegalovirus pneumonia in compromised hosts. Am J Med 1976; 61:326–332.

Adamson IYR, Bowden DH. The pathogenesis of bleomycin-induced pulmonary fibrosis in mice. Am J Pathol 1974; 77:185–198.

Barrio JL, Svarez M, Rodrigues JL, et al. *Pneumocystis carinii* pneumonia presenting as cavitating and non-cavitating solitary pulmonary nodule in patients with the acquired immunodeficiency syndrome. Am Rev Respir Dis 1986; 134:1094–1096.

Barturm RJ, Watnick M, Herman PG. Roentgenographic findings in pulmonary mucormycosis. Am J Roentgenol Radium Ther Nucl Med 1975; 113:810–815.

Becroft DMO, Osborne DRS. The lungs in fatal measles infection in childhood: pathological, radiological and immunological correlations. Histopathology 1980; 4:401–412.

Bedrossian CWM, Luna MA, Conklin RH, Miller WC. Alveolar proteinosis as a consequence of immunosuppression: a hypothesis based on clinical and pathologic observations. Hum Pathol 1980; 11:527–535.

Bennett DE, Million RR, Ackerman LV. Bilateral radiation pneumonitis: a complication of the radiotherapy of bronchogenic carcinoma. (A report and analysis of seven cases with autopsy.) Cancer 1969; 23:1001–1018.

Beschorner WE, Saral R, Hutchins GM, et al. Lymphocytic bronchitis associated with graft-versus-host disease in recipients of bone-marrow transplants. N Engl J Med 1978; 299:1030–1036.

Bigby TD, Serota ML, Tierney LM Jr, Matthay MA. Clinical spectrum of pulmonary mucormycosis. Chest 1986; 89:435–439.

Bleiweiss IJ, Jagirdar JS, Klein MJ, et al. Granulomatous *Pneumocystis carinii* pneumonia in three patients with the acquired immune deficiency syndrome. Chest 1988; 94:580–583.

Blum RH, Carter SK, Agre K. A clinical review of bleomycin—a new antineoplastic agent. Cancer 1973; 31:903–914.

Buff SJ, McLelland R, Gallis HA, et al. *Candida albicans* pneumonia: radiographic appearance. AJR 1982; 138:645–648.

Castellino RA, Glatstein E, Turbow MM, et al. Latent radiation injury of lungs or heart activated by steroid withdrawal. Ann Intern Med 1974; 80:593–599.

Catterall JR, Hofflin JM, Remington JS. Pulmonary toxoplasmosis. Am Rev Respir Dis 1986; 133:704–705.

Catterall JR, McCabe RE, Brooks RG, Remington JS. Open lung biopsy in patients with Hodgkin's disease and pulmonary infiltrates. Am Rev Respir Dis 1989; 139:1274–1279.

Chaisson RE, Hopewell PC. Mycobacteria and AIDS mortality (editorial). Am Rev Respir Dis 1989; 139:1–3.

Clarysse AM, Cathey WJ, Cartwright GE, et al. Pulmonary disease complicating intermittent therapy with methotrexate. JAMA 1969; 209:1861–1864.

Colby TV, Carrington CB. Infiltrative lung disease. In Thurlbeck WM, ed. Pathology of the lung. New York: Thieme, 1988:425–517.

Cooper JAD Jr, Matthay RA. Drug-induced pulmonary disease. DM 1987; 33:61–120.

Cooper JAD Jr, White DA, Matthay RA. Drug-induced pulmonary disease, part I: cytotoxic drugs. Am Rev Respir Dis 1986a; 133:321–340.

Cooper JAD Jr, White DA, Matthay RA. Drug-induced pulmonary disease, part 2: noncytotoxic drugs. Am Rev Respir Dis 1986b; 133:488–505.

CPC 37-1978. N Engl J Med 1978; 299:644–650.

Curtis AM, Smith GJW, Ravin CE. Air crescent sign of invasive aspergillosis. Radiology 1979; 133:17–21.

DeLena M, Guzzon A, Monfardini S, Bonadonna G. Clinical, radiologic and histopathologic studies on pulmonary toxicity induced by treatment with bleomycin (NSC-125066). Cancer Chemother Rep 1972; 56:343–355.

Delorenzo LJ, Huang CT, Maguire UP, Stone DJ. Roentgenographic patterns of *Pneumocystis carinii* pneumonia in 104 patients with AIDS. Chest 1987; 91:323–327.

Devogelaer JP, Pirson Y, Vandenbroucke JM, et al. D-penicillamine induced crescentic glomerulonephritis: report and review of the literature. J Rheumatol 1987; 14:1036-1041.

Dickout WJ, Chan CK, Hyland RH, et al. Prevention of acute pulmonary edema after bone marrow transplantation. Chest 1987; 92:303-309.

Doppman JL, Glenn UW, DeVito VT. Atypical radiographic features in *Pneumocystis carinii* pneumonia. Radiology 1975; 114:39-44.

Douglas RG Jr, Anderson MS, Weg JG, et al. Herpes simplex virus pneumonia. JAMA 1969; 210:902-904.

Dubois PJ, Myerowitz RL, Allen CM. Pathoradiologic correlation of pulmonary candidiasis in immunosuppressed patients. Cancer 1977; 40:1026-1036.

Engelberg LA, Lerner CW, Tapper ML. Clinical features of *Pneumocystis carinii* in the acquired immune deficiency syndrome. Am Rev Respir Dis 1984; 130:689-694.

Fajardo LF, Berthrong M. Radiation injury in surgical pathology, part 1. Am J Surg Pathol 1978; 2:159-199.

Fennessy JJ. Irradiation damage to the lung. J Thorac Imag 1987; 2:68-79.

Forrest JV. Radiologic findings in *Pneumocystis carinii* pneumonia. Radiology 1972; 103:539-544.

Fournier AM, Dickinson GM, Erdfrocht IR, et al. Tuberculosis and nontuberculous mycobacteriosis in patients with AIDS. Chest 1988; 93:772-775.

Gal AA, Koss MN, Hawkins J, et al. The pathology of pulmonary cryptococcal infections in the acquired immunodeficiency syndrome. Arch Pathol Lab Med 1986; 110:502-507.

Gale AM, Kleitsch WP. Solitary pulmonary nodule due to phycomycosis (mucormycosis). Chest 1972; 62:752-755.

Genta RM, Miles P, Fields K. Opportunistic *Strongyloides stercoralis* infection in lymphoma patients. Cancer 1989; 63:1407-1411.

Gibson PG, Bryant DH, Morgan GW, et al. Radiation-induced lung injury: a hypersensitivity pneumonitis? Ann Intern Med 1988; 109:288-291.

Glenville AR, Baldwin JC, Burke CM, et al. Obliterative bronchiolitis after heart-lung transplantation: apparent arrest by augmented immunosuppression. Ann Intern Med 1987; 107:300-304.

Goldstein JD, Godleski JJ, Balikian JP, Herman PG. Pathologic patterns of *Serratia marcescens* pneumonia. Hum Pathol 1982; 13:479-484.

Goodwin RA Jr, Shapiro JL, Thurman GH, et al. Disseminated histoplasmosis: clinical and pathologic correlations. Medicine 1980; 59:1-33.

Greene R. Opportunistic pneumonias. Semin Roentgenol 1980; 15:50-72.

Greenman RL, Goodall PT, King D. Lung biopsy in immunocompromised hosts. Am J Med 1975; 59:488-496.

Grimes MM, LaPook JD, Bar MH, et al. Disseminated *Pneumocystis carinii* infection in a patient with acquired immunodeficiency syndrome. Hum Pathol 1987; 18:307-308.

Gross NJ: Pulmonary effects of radiation therapy. Ann Intern Med 1977; 86:81-92.

Grossman CB, Bragg DG, Armstrong D. Roentgen mani-

festations of pulmonary nocardiosis. Radiology 1970; 96:325-330.

Gyorkey F, Gyorkey P, Sinkovics JG. Origin and significance of intranuclear tubular inclusions in type II pulmonary epithelial cells of patients with bleomycin and busulfan toxicity. Ultrastruct Pathol 1980; 1:211-221.

Handwerger S, Mildvan D, Senie R, McKinley FW. Tuberculosis and the acquired immunodeficiency syndrome at a New York City hospital: 1978-1985. Chest 1987; 91:176-180.

Hanson PJ, Harcourt-Webster JN, Gazzard BG, Collins JV. Fiberoptic bronchoscopy in diagnosis of bronchopulmonary Kaposi's sarcoma. Thorax 1987; 42:269-271.

Holoye PY, Luna MA, MacKay B, Bedrossian CWM. Bleomycin hypersensitivity pneumonitis. Ann Intern Med 1978; 88:47-49.

Horsburgh CR Jr, Selik RM. The epidemiology of disseminated non-tuberculous mycobacterial infection in the acquired immunodeficiency syndrome (AIDS). Am Rev Respir Dis 1989; 139:4-7.

Hruban RH, Meziane MA, Zerhouni EA, et al. Radiologic-pathologic correlation of the CT halo sign in invasive pulmonary aspergillosis. J Comput Assist Tomogr 1987; 11:534-536.

Ikezoe J, Takashima S, Morimoto S, et al. CT appearance of acute radiation-induced injury in the lung. AJR 1988; 150:765-770.

Jehn U, Göldel N, Reinmüller R, Wilmanns W. Noncardiogenic pulmonary edema complicating intermediate and high-dose Ara C treatment for relapsed acute leukemia. Med Oncol Tumor Pharmacother 1988; 5:41-47.

Kaplan MH, Armstrong D, Rosen P. Tuberculosis complicating neoplastic disease. Cancer 1974; 33:850-858.

Katzenstein A-LA, Askin FB. Surgical pathology of non-neoplastic lung disease. Philadelphia: WB Saunders, 1982:37.

Kauffman CA, Israel KS, Smith JW, et al. Histoplasmosis in immunosuppressed patients. Am J Med 1978; 64:923-932.

Klatt EC, Jensen DF, Meyer PR. Pathology of *Mycobacterium avium-intracellulare* infection in acquired immunodeficiency syndrome. Hum Pathol 1987; 18:709-714.

Krowka MJ, Rosenow EC III, Hoagland HC. Pulmonary complications of bone marrow transplantation. Chest 1985; 87:237-246.

Kugler JW, Armitage JO, Helms CM, et al. Nosocomial Legionnaires' disease. Am J Med 1983; 74:281-288.

Kuhlman JE, Fishman EK, Burch PA, et al. Invasive pulmonary aspergillosis in acute leukemia: the contribution of CT to early diagnosis and aggressive management. Chest 1987; 92:95-99.

Libshitz HI, Southard ME. Complications of radiation therapy: the thorax. Semin Roentgenol 1974; 9:41-49.

Lombard CM, Churg A, Winokur S. Pulmonary veno-occlusive disease following therapy for malignant neoplasms. Chest 1987; 92:871-876.

Luna MA, Cleary KR. Spectrum of pathologic manifestations of *Pneumocystis carinii* pneumonia in patients with neoplastic diseases. Semin Diagn Pathol 1989; 6: 262-272.

McDonnell JN, Hutchins GM. Pulmonary cryptococcosis. Hum Pathol 1985; 16:121-128.

MacFarlane JT. *Pneumocystis carinii* pneumonia (editorial). Thorax 1985; 40:561-570.

Meduri GU, Stover DE, Lee M, et al. Pulmonary Kaposi's sarcoma in the acquired immune deficiency syndrome: clinical, radiographic, and pathologic manifestations. Am J Med 1986; 81:11-18.

Miliauskas JR, Webber BL. Disseminated varicella at autopsy in children with cancer. Cancer 1984; 53: 1518-1525.

Milligan SA, Stulbarg MS, Hamyu H, Holden JA. *Pneumocystis carinii* pneumonia radiographically simulating tuberculosis. Am Rev Respir Dis 1985; 132: 1124-1126.

Murray JF, Garay SM, Hopewell PC, et al. Pulmonary complications of the acquired immunodeficiency syndrome: an update. Am Rev Respir Dis 1987; 137:504-509.

Nash G. Necrotizing tracheobronchitis and bronchopneumonia consistent with herpetic infection. Hum Pathol 1972; 3:283-291.

Nash G. Pathologic features of the lung in the immunocompromised host. Hum Pathol 1982; 13:841-858.

Ognibene FP, Shelhamer JH. Kaposi's sarcoma. Clin Chest Med 1988; 9:459-465.

Orr DP, Myerowitz RL, Dubois PJ. Pathoradiologic correlation of invasive pulmonary aspergillosis in the compromised host. Cancer 1978; 41:2028-2039.

Pagani JJ, Libshitz HI. Opportunistic fungal pneumonias in cancer patients. AJR 1981; 137:1033-1039.

Phillips TL, Wharam MD, Margolis LW. Modification of radiation injury to normal tissues by chemotherapeutic agents. Cancer 1975; 35:1678-1684.

Ralph DD, Springmeyer SC, Sullivan KM, et al. Rapidly progressive air-flow obstruction in marrow transplant recipients. Am Rev Respir Dis 1984; 129:641-644.

Rosenow EC III. Drug-induced lung diseases. In Kelley WN, ed. Textbook of internal medicine. Vol. 2. Philadelphia: JB Lippincott, 1989:1939-1943.

Rosenow EC III, Wilson WR, Cockerill FR III. Pulmonary disease in the immunocompromised host, part I. Mayo Clin Proc 1985; 60:473-487.

Saldana MJ, Mones JM. Cavitation and other atypical manifestations of *Pneumocystis carinii* pneumonia. Semin Diagn Pathol 1989; 6:273-286.

Salzman SH, Smith RL, Aranda CP. Histoplasmosis in patients at risk for the acquired immunodeficiency syndrome in a non-endemic setting. Chest 1988; 93:916-921.

Samuels ML, Johnson DE, Holoye PY, et al. Large-dose bleomycin therapy and pulmonary toxicity: a possible role of prior radiotherapy. JAMA 1976; 235:1117-1120.

Schulman LL. Cytomegalovirus pneumonitis and lobar consolidation. Chest 1987; 91:558-561.

Silver SF, Torymalashi M, Boshnen CH, et al. Pulmonary consolidation with an air crescent sign in an immunocompromised woman. J Can Assoc Radiol 1989; 40:167-169.

Singer C, Armstrong D, Rosen PP, et al. Diffuse pulmonary infiltrates in immunosuppressed patients: prospective study of 80 cases. Am J Med 1979; 66:110-120.

Snider DE Jr, Hopewell PC, Mills J, Reichman LB. Mycobacterioses and the acquired immunodeficiency syndrome. Am Rev Respir Dis 1987; 136:492-496.

Snover DC. Acute and chronic graft-versus-host disease. Hum Pathol 1984; 15:202-205.

Soave R, Murray HW, Litrenta MM. Bacterial invasion of pulmonary vessels. Am J Med 1978; 65:864-867.

Sobonya RE, Hiller C, Pingleton W, Watanabe I. Fatal measles (rubeola) pneumonia in adults. Arch Pathol Lab Med 1978; 102:366-371.

Triebwasser JH, Harris RE, Bryant RE, Rhoades ER. Varicella pneumonia in adults. Medicine 1967; 46:409-423.

Tucker MA, Coleman CN, Cox RS, et al. Risk of second cancers after treatment for Hodgkin's disease. N Engl J Med 1988; 318:76-81.

Tuxen DV, Cade JF, McDonald MI, et al. Herpes simplex virus from the lower respiratory tract in adult respiratory distress syndrome. Am Rev Respir Dis 1982; 126:416-419.

Urbanski SJ, Kossakowska AE, Curtis J, et al. Idiopathic small airways pathology in patients with graft-versus-host disease following allogeneic bone marrow transplantation. Am J Surg Pathol 1987; 11: 965-971.

Vernon SE. Cytologic features of nonfatal herpes virus tracheobronchitis. Acta Cytol 1982; 26:237-242.

Verweij J, van Zanten T, Souren T, et al. Prospective study on the dose relationship of mitomycin C–induced interstitial pneumonitis. Cancer 1987; 60:756-761.

Vietzke WM, Gelderman AH, Grimley PM, Valsamis MP. Toxoplasmosis complicating malignancy. Cancer 1968; 21:816-827.

Washington University CPC. Cavitary lung disease following renal transplantation. Am J Med 1982; 72: 145-155.

Wasser L, Talavera W. Pulmonary cryptococcosis in AIDS. Chest 1987; 92:692-695.

Weber WR, Askin FB, Dehner LP. Lung biopsy in *Pneumocystis carinii* pneumonia: a histopathologic study of typical and atypical features. Am J Clin Pathol 1977; 67:11-19.

Weiner RS, Bortin MM, Gale RP, et al. Interstitial pneumonitis after bone marrow transplantation: assessment of risk factors. Ann Intern Med 1986; 104:168-175.

White DC: The histopathologic basis for functional decrements in late radiation injury in diverse organs. Cancer 1976; 37:1126-1143.

Williams DM, Krick JA, Remington JS. Pulmonary infection in the compromised host, part I. Am Rev Respir Dis 1976a; 114:359-394.

Williams DM, Krick JA, Remington JS. Pulmonary infection in the compromised host, part II. Am Rev Respir Dis 1976b; 114:593-627.

Wilson WR, Cockerill FR III, Rosenow EC III. Pulmonary disease in the immunocompromised host, part II. Mayo Clinic Proc 1985; 60:610-631.

CHAPTER 6

DIFFUSE PULMONARY HEMORRHAGE

Diffuse pulmonary hemorrhage (DPH) is a syndrome that consists of hemoptysis, iron-deficiency anemia and, radiologically, airspace infiltrates, which rapidly worsen and clear (Albelda et al, 1984). The DPH syndrome implies bilateral, diffuse, widespread hemorrhage from the microvasculature without localized or endobronchial sources. Many cases of DPH are related to autoimmunity, and in these cases, the hemorrhage is thought to be primarily at the alveolar capillary level. There are, however, other cases of the DPH syndrome in which autoimmunity is not involved and the precise level(s) of hemorrhage cannot be specified. The presence of hemosiderin-laden macrophages is characteristic but not diagnostic of DPH (Hay and Turner-Warwick, 1988); these cells indicate that bleeding into the lung has occurred primarily at the alveolar capillary level, but this finding cannot be used to ascertain whether the bleeding is diffuse or localized, immune or nonimmune (Leatherman, 1987).

The acute stage of DPH is characterized radiologically by the presence of nodular or confluent airspace infiltrates. The nodular densities measure 2 to 10 mm in diameter and have ill-defined borders (Sybers et al, 1965; Bowley et al, 1979). These presumably represent blood-filled pulmonary acini. Confluent airspace consolidation may be patchy, diffuse, or predominantly perihilar (Fig. 6–1). The lung periphery and the lung apices are often spared

(Bowley et al, 1979; Proskey et al, 1970). The infiltrates are usually bilateral, although they may be asymmetric; air bronchograms are common. Two to three days after the acute episode, as the blood is being absorbed into the interstitium, the fluffy airspace infiltrates are gradually replaced by a reticular pattern. Unless bleeding recurs, the radiograph returns to normal within 1 to 2 weeks (Bowley et al, 1979). If the patient experiences repeated episodes of hemorrhage and develops progressive interstitial fibrosis, the reticular pattern persists (Bruwer et al, 1956; Sybers et al, 1965). The radiologic appearance of DPH is nonspecific and cannot be distinguished from that of pulmonary infection or edema. Patients may also have extensive pulmonary hemorrhage and a normal chest radiograph and in these instances, pulmonary hemorrhage may be detected by carbon monoxide uptake (Bowley et al, 1979; Ewan et al, 1976). With bleeding at the alveolar capillary level the diffusing capacity for carbon monoxide increases due to uptake of carbon monoxide by the intra-alveolar blood cells and has been found to be an effective way to assess active bleeding (Addleman et al, 1985)

Many classification schemes for DPH have been offered (Albelda et al, 1984; Leatherman, 1987; Hay and Turner-Warwick, 1988; Wilson, 1988; Miller, 1988) and no one scheme is universally accepted. Figure 6–2 suggests a diagnostic algorithm for the

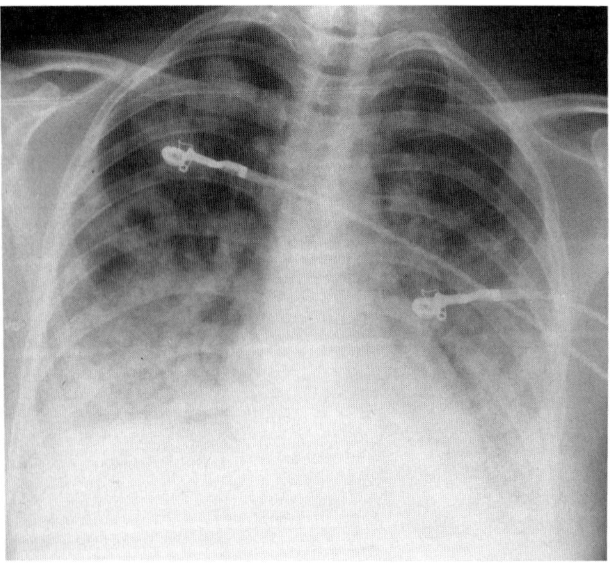

A

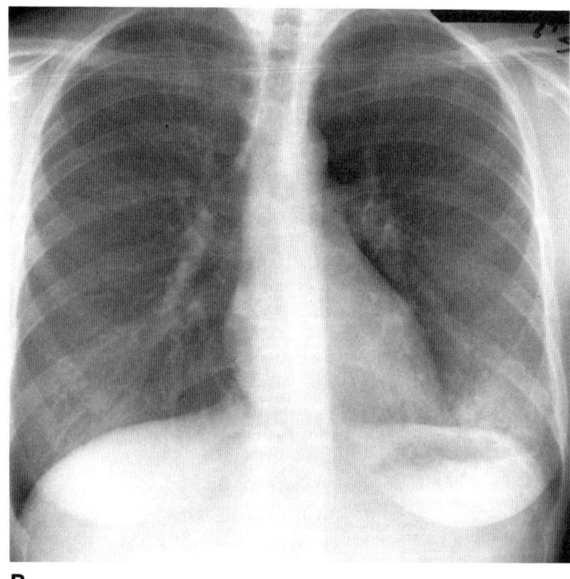

B

Figure 6–1   Young woman with repeated episodes of pulmonary hemorrhage related to mixed collagen vascular disease. *A,* Some of the episodes of DPH were associated with extensive bilateral airspace consolidation. *B,* Other episodes were associated with mild, patchy areas of consolidation predominantly in the lower lung zones.

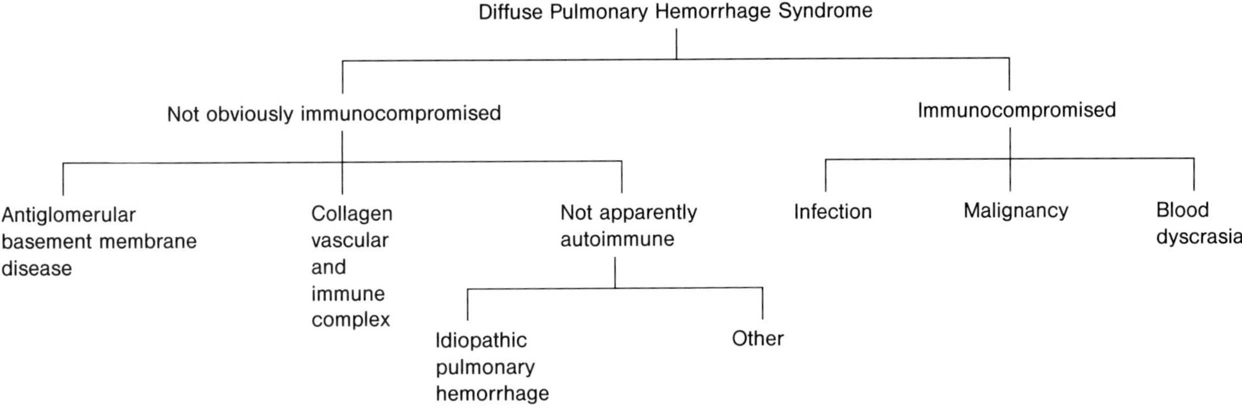

Figure 6–2 Etiologies of diffuse pulmonary hemorrhage syndrome.

classification of DPH. According to this scheme, the first major branch point is whether the patient is immunocompromised (at the time of presentation) from malignancy, acquired immunodeficiency syndrome (AIDS), cytotoxic therapy, and so on. If the patient is not immunocompromised, the major differential diagnoses include antiglomerular basement membrane disease, immune complex disease, idiopathic pulmonary hemosiderosis, and a variety of miscellaneous not obviously immune-related causes and associations. If the patient is immunocompromised, the major differential diagnostic considerations include infection, malignancy, and blood dyscrasia. Each of these categories are considered separately below.

DIFFUSE PULMONARY HEMORRHAGE IN THE NONIMMUNOCOMPROMISED HOST

Antiglomerular Basement Membrane Disease

Often referred to (incorrectly) as Goodpasture's syndrome (Goodpasture, 1919), antiglomerular basement membrane disease (AGBMD) consists of the triad of circulating anti-GBM antibody, DPH, and glomerulonephritis. It usually occurs in young adult males, although the age range is wide; we have seen an 80-year-old patient with this disease, but it is rare before age 16 years. Presenting symptoms are generally respiratory rather than renal. The usual lesion in the kidney is diffuse crescentic glomerulonephritis, but occasionally the glomeruli are normal by standard light microscopy. Renal immunofluorescence studies show linear deposits (versus "lumpy bumpy"

in membranous glomerulonephritis) of IgG on glomerular basement membranes, although this finding is not considered absolutely diagnostic since non-immunologic nonspecific linear fluorescence may occasionally be found in normal and diabetic patients (Wilson, 1988). The diagnosis must be established by specific elution from tissue or by detecting anti-GBM antibody in the serum, with radioimmunoassay or enzyme-linked immunosorbent assay, either of which has sensitivity and specificity rates in excess of 95 percent (Leatherman, 1987). There is a small group of patients with DPH and circulating anti-GBM who never develop overt renal failure. Some of these patients can be demonstrated to have linear IgG glomerular deposits and some cannot (Albelda et al, 1984). Lung biopsy is rarely, if ever, necessary (Leatherman, 1987). The findings are nonspecific, consisting of hemorrhage, hemosiderin deposition, and variable interstitial inflammation and fibrosis; immunofluorescence is not as reliable in the lung as it is in the kidney. In some instances, AGBMD may be associated with diffuse alveolar damage or with a neutrophilic capillaritis (Soergel and Sommers, 1962, Lombard et al, 1989). Capillaritis, however, is a well-recognized feature of Wegener's granulomatosis and systemic lupus erythematosus (SLE), complicated by DPH.

The clinical association of glomerulonephritis and DPH of whatever cause(s) is referred by some as "Goodpasture's syndrome" (Wilson, 1988), although it is not our policy to use this terminology. An interesting association between DPH and rapidly progressive glomerulonephritis that is AGBM antibody-negative has been detailed by Leatherman et al (1984). Life-threatening DPH and immune complex-negative rapidly progressive glomerulonephritis occurred in five of their patients, the association closely simulating AGBMD clinically. The DPH in these patients responded to corticosteroids, although its precise pathogenesis remains obscure so far. Treatment consists of corticosteroids and possibly other immunosuppressants such as azathioprine or cyclophosphamide. Plasmapheresis to remove AGBM antibodies has also been used.

DPH associated with Collagen Vascular Disease and/or Immune Complex Disease

DPH occurs in a variety of immune-complex–related collagen vascular diseases and systemic vasculitides, including SLE, Wegener's granulomatosis, polyarteritis nodosa (Goodpasture's case [1919] had necrotizing angiitis), cryoglobulinemia, rheumatoid arthritis, and scleroderma. An underlying acute capillaritis with or without larger vessel vasculitis is usually found in the lung; these patients may or may not have concurrent renal lesions. DPH in SLE and DPH in Wegener's granulomatosis deserve specific mention.

DPH in SLE typically occurs in patients with an established diagnosis of lupus and active extrapulmonary disease (Albelda et al, 1984; Leatherman, 1987; Hay and Turner-Warwick, 1988), although on occasion DPH may be the presenting symptom (Myers and Katzenstein, 1986). This complication of SLE is frequently fatal but can be successfully treated in some cases with high-dose immunosuppressive agents (Myers and Katzenstein, 1986; Churg et al, 1980). In addition to recent hemorrhage, fibrin, and hemosiderin, SLE-associated DPH is characterized by mild to severe degrees of acute capillaritis with accentuation of alveolar walls by a neutrophil infiltrate, areas of alveolar wall necrosis, and a patchy neutrophilic small-vessel arteritis. A nonspecific mononuclear infiltrate with type-II cell hyperplasia may accompany the vasculitis. Immunofluorescence usually shows granular deposits of IgG and C3 along alveolar septa; these deposits may also be seen ultrastructurally (Myers and Katzenstein, 1986).

Wegener's granulomatosis is occasionally associated with DPH, either as the presenting symptom or in a patient with an established diagnosis of Wegener's granulomatosis (Leatherman, 1987; Myers and Katzenstein, 1987; Travis et al, 1987). In such patients, the classic findings of necrotizing granulomas and larger-vessel vasculitis are focally present but are overshadowed by hemorrhage and acute capillaritis similar to that described above for SLE. Immune complexes cannot be documented.

Goldstein et al (1986) reported a case of immune complex proliferative glomerulonephritis with DPH. In this case, immune complexes were not found in the lung, no antiglomerular basement membrane antibodies were detected and the patient completely recovered with short-term steroid therapy.

Idiopathic Pulmonary Hemosiderosis

Idiopathic pulmonary hemosiderosis (IPH) is characterized by iron-deficiency anemia and radiologic infiltrates, but there are no associated renal abnormalities and, by definition, no demonstrable immunologic abnormalities. IPH most commonly occurs in either children under 10 years of age or in young adults. The pathologic and radiologic features are similar between these two populations, but some of the clinical features are dissimilar. Emphasis on this dissimilarity is given particularly by Hay and Turner-Warwick (1988), who view childhood and adult pulmonary hemosiderosis as two different clinical variants of the disease. In childhood cases, sex incidence is equal. Systemic symptoms such as fever and weight loss may be much more dramatic than the chest findings. Since children frequently swallow their expectorations, "hemoptysis" is sometimes not a feature, which adds further diagnostic difficulty. Hilar, and rarely mediastinal, adenopathy are also seen in the childhood variant (CPC 30–1988). While the radiologic findings of diffuse airspace disease together with chronic cough, dyspnea, and iron-deficiency anemia in a child are suggestive of IPH, open lung biopsy is usually required for a definitive diagnosis (Cutz, 1987). Recently, Rubin et al, (1989) described the magnetic resonance imaging (MRI) findings in a 2½-year-old boy. The pulmonary parenchymal hemosiderin causes a T2 shortening due to the presence of paramagnetic ferric iron. Thus, while the T1-weighted MRI image showed diffusely increased signal intensity, the T2-weighted MRI image showed a markedly reduced signal intensity. The MRI diagnosis allowed initiation of therapy and stabilization of the patient before the diagnosis was confirmed by open lung biopsy. MRI, therefore, has the potential of confirming the clinical suspicion of repeated diffuse pulmonary hemorrhage in patients in whom the clinical findings are equivocal.

Adult patients are usually males in their 20s or 30s, although cases in elderly patients are also described (Hay and Turner-Warwick, 1988). The disease in adults is usually milder than in children. Occasional patients have an acute episode of massive life-threatening hemoptysis, but this occurs less often than in AGBMD. Both childhood and adult cases of IPH may progress to fibrosis after repeated episodes of hemorrhage. Both also have a peculiar and poorly understood association with either morphologic villous atrophy of the small bowel or overt celiac disease (Hay and Turner-Warwick, 1988).

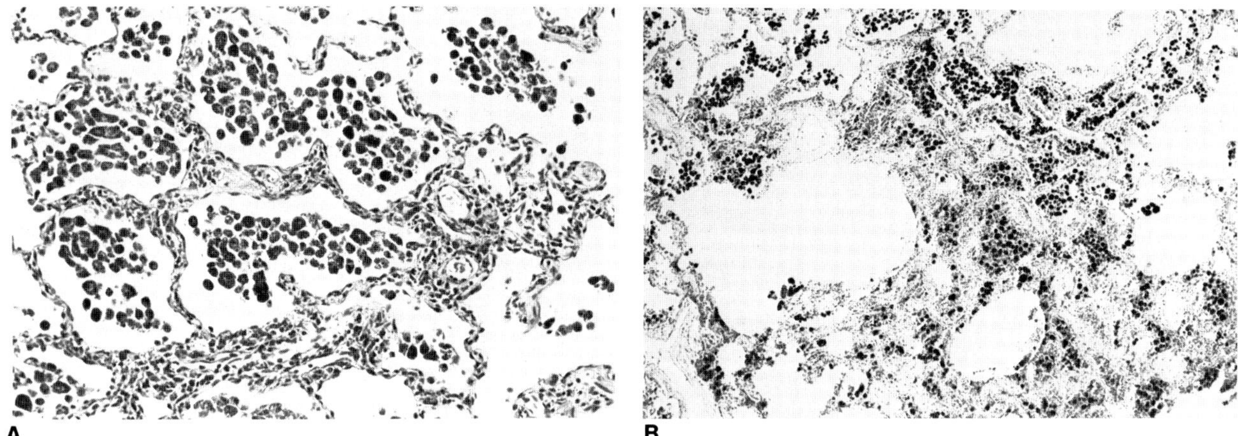

Figure 6-3 Open lung biopsy from a 12-year-old female with hemoptysis. *A*, H&E stain shows intra-alveolar hemosidero-phages and mild mononuclear alveolitis. (× 265). *B*, Iron stain highlights the hemosiderosis. (× 96).

Immunosuppressive therapy has been tried, although the results have not been spectacular. Spontaneous remissions and exacerbations commonly occur in both childhood and adult variants. In some long-term survivors, interstitial fibrosis seems to progress slowly in the absence of clinically obvious continuing bleeding.

By light microscopy, the appearance of IPH is similar to that of AGBMD (Fig. 6-3*A*). Hemorrhage, hemosiderin-laden intra-alveolar macrophages, variable interstitial fibrosis, and variable type-II cell reaction are seen. The amount of hemosiderin present may be accentuated by histochemical stains (see Fig. 6-3*B*). Vasculitis is not present. By definition, immu-

nofluorescent stains are noncontributory. Ultrastructural studies describe rupture, splitting, and reduplication of alveolar basal lamina (Hay and Turner-Warwick, 1988), but these findings are not particularly useful in separating IPH from the other DPH syndromes.

Other Causes of DPH in the Nonimmunocompromised Host

There are numerous causes of DPH in this category, some of which are obvious clinically and some of which are elusive. These causes should always be kept in mind in the differential diagnosis of DPH,

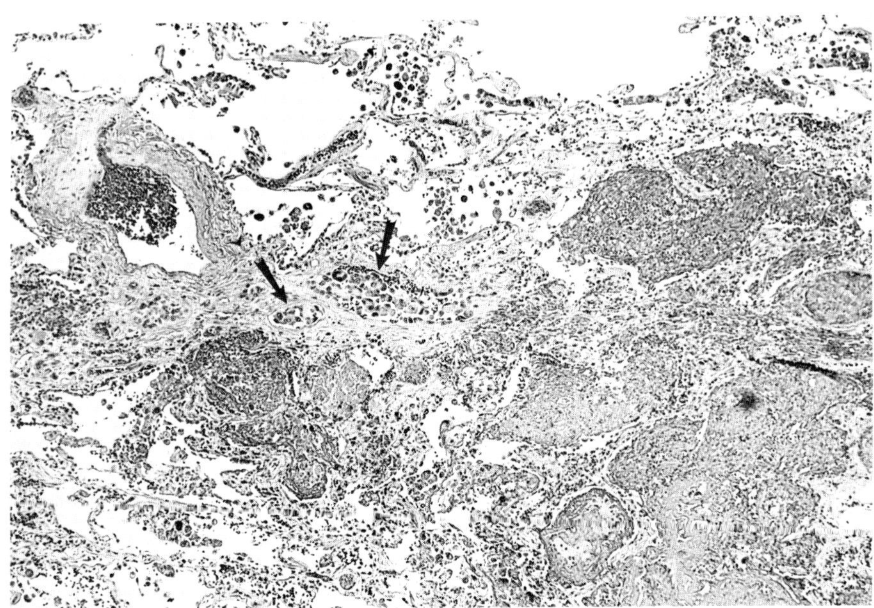

Figure 6-4 Metastatic angiosarcoma occupying pulmonary vein (*arrows*) associated with marked intra-alveolar hemorrhage. (H&E, × 96).

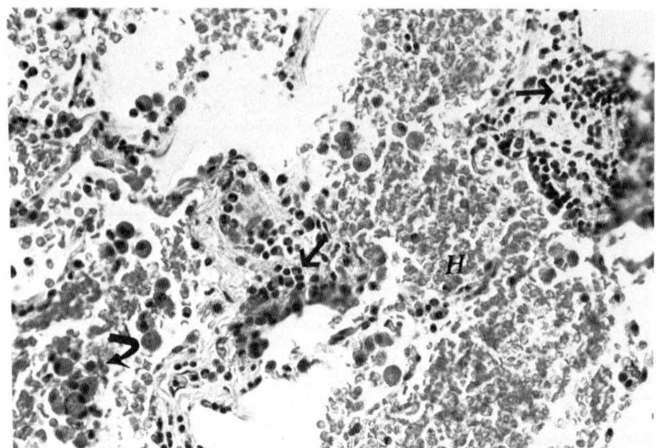

Figure 6–5   Chronic eosinophilic pneumonia presenting as DPH. Note interstitial eosinophils (*straight arrows*), hemosiderophages (*curved arrow*), and recent hemorrhage (H).

particularly in cases that are unusual clinically and pathologically. *Drug reaction* to penicillamine, trimetallic anhydride, and lymphangiography have been described as causing DPH (Miller, 1988). Murray et al (1988) reported an intriguing case of DPH with peripheral blood eosinophilia that appeared to be due to the use of freebase cocaine. *Cardiovascular disorders* such as mitral stenosis, pulmonary venoocclusive disease, severe pulmonary edema (Albelda et al, 1984), and even amyloidosis (Road et al, 1985) may cause DPH. Lymphangioleiomyomatosis, further discussed in Chapter 7, may present with or be complicated by DPH, presumably due to occlusive smooth muscle proliferation in the pulmonary veins (Hay and Turner-Warwick, 1988). A *generalized bleeding tendency* such as anticoagulation therapy, disseminated intravascular coagulation, and drug-induced (Albelda et al, 1984) or immune thrombocytopenia (Martinez et al, 1983) may be complicated by DPH. Systemic bleeding is a well recognized complication of bleeding disorders; it is surprising that it is so uncommon in the lung. *Lung damage*, either traumatic, inhalation, or from necrotizing pneumonia, may result in DPH. *Primary and metastatic malignancies*, particularly angiosarcomas, may present as DPH (Spragg et al, 1983; Miller, 1988; Segal et al, 1988; Yousem, 1986) (Fig. 6–4). *Chronic eosinophilic pneumonia* may be complicated by hemoptysis due to DPH (Carrington et al, 1969) (Fig. 6–5).

DIFFUSE PULMONARY HEMORRHAGE IN THE IMMUNOCOMPROMISED HOST

Clinically obvious DPH is relatively uncommon in the immunocompromised host, but is well recog-

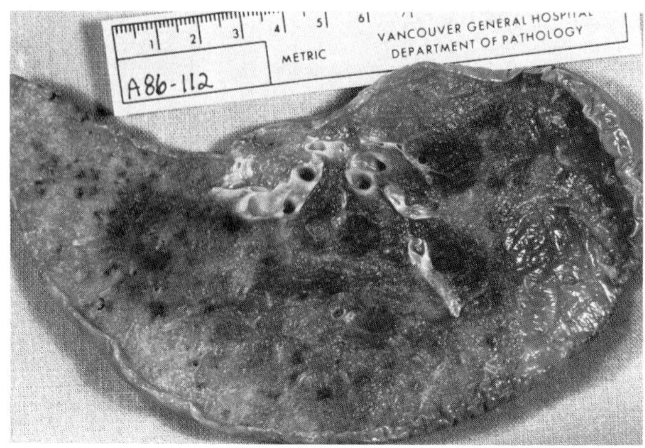

A

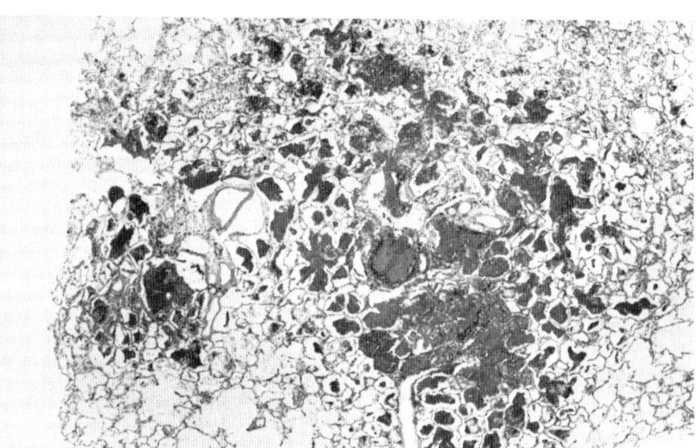

B

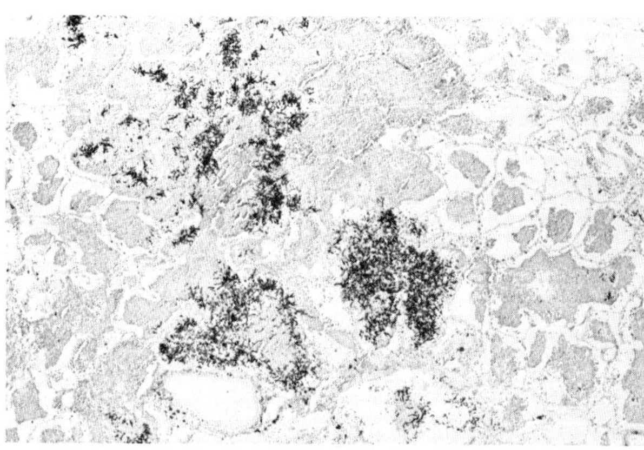

C

Figure 6–6   Leukemic patient with DPH due to pulmonary candidiasis. *A*, Hemorrhage occupies most of the central parenchyma. *B*, H&E stain shows vaguely nodular intra-alveolar hemorrhage with little reaction ($\times$ 25). *C*, Methanamine silver stains show a large number of *Candida* organisms ($\times$ 63).

nized (Tenholder and Hooper, 1980; Smith and Katzenstein, 1982; Dutcher et al, 1984; Kahn et al, 1987). The etiology in the great majority of cases is either infection, malignancy, or blood dyscrasia. The most common fungal *infections* that cause DPH are aspergillosis and candidiasis (Tenholder and Hooper, 1980). In most instances, hemorrhage due to aspergillosis is probably related to multiple infarcts (see Chapter 5) and thus cannot be strictly viewed as DPH. In hematogenous candidiasis, the pattern of involvement is one of bilateral diffuse miliary abscesses surrounded by hemorrhage, and thus intrapulmonary hemorrhage is frequently a serious complication of candidiasis (Rosen, 1976) (Fig. 6-6). Necrotizing gram-negative bacterial pneumonia and viral infection, particularly cytomegalovirus, are also occasionally complicated by DPH.

Of the *malignancies* associated with DPH in the immunocompromised host, by far the most common are Kaposi's sarcoma in patients with AIDS (see Chapter 9) and leukemic infiltrates (Tenholder and Hooper, 1980).

The occurrence of DPH due to uncomplicated *thrombocytopenia* is somewhat controversial, since it has been suggested (Smith and Katzenstein, 1982) that some degree of diffuse alveolar damage must be present for DPH to occur. Other investigators (Dutcher et al, 1984; Kahn et al, 1987) have shown that DPH does occur, albeit uncommonly, as the result of apparently uncomplicated thrombocytopenia of less than 50,000 platelets per cubic millimeter.

The histologic criteria for the diagnosis of DPH in the immunocompromised host are similar to those in immunologically intact patients—namely hemorrhage and hemosiderophages diffusely in the alveolar spaces with variable degrees of organization and reaction. The diagnosis of DPH in the immunocompromised host can sometimes alternatively be made by finding hemosiderin-laden macrophages in bronchoalveolar lavage fluid (Cordonnier et al, 1986; Kahn et al, 1987). Obviously, cultures and a variety of histochemical stains are also necessary to detect concurrent infection.

REFERENCES

Addleman W, Wagan AS, Grossman RF. Monitoring intrapulmonary hemorrhage in Goodpasture's Syndrome. Chest 1985; 87:119-120.

Albelda SM, Gefter WB, Epstein DM, Miller WT. Diffuse pulmonary hemorrhage: a review and classification. Radiology 1984; 154:289-297.

Bowley NB, Steiner RE, Chin WS. The chest x-ray in antiglomerular basement membrane antibody disease (Goodpasture's syndrome). Clin Radiol 1979; 30:419-429.

Bruwer AJ, Kennedy RLJ, Edwards JE. Recurrent pulmonary hemorrhage with hemosiderosis: so-called idiopathic pulmonary hemosiderosis. AJR 1956; 76:98-107.

Carrington CB, Addington WW, Goff AM, et al. Chronic eosinophilic pneumonia. N Engl J Med 1969; 280:788-798.

Churg A, Franklin W, Chan KL, et al. Pulmonary hemorrhage and immune complex deposition in the lung: complications in a patient with systemic lupus erythematosus. Arch Pathol Lab Med 1980; 104:388-391.

Cordonnier C, Bernaudin JF, Bierling P, et al. Pulmonary complications occurring after allogeneic bone marrow transplantation: a study of 130 consecutive transplanted patients. Cancer 1986; 58:1047-1054.

CPC 30-1988. N Engl J Med 1988; 319:227-237.

Cutz E. Idiopathic pulmonary hemosiderosis and related disorders in infancy and childhood. Perspect Pediatr Pathol 1987; 11:47-81.

Dutcher JP, Schiffer CA, Aisner J, et al. Incidence of thrombocytopenia and serious hemorrhage among patients with solid tumors. Cancer 1984; 53:557-562.

Ewan PW, Jones HA, Rhodes CG, Hughes JMB. Detection of intrapulmonary hemorrhage with carbon monoxide uptake. N Engl J Med 1976; 259:1391-1396.

Goldstein J, Weil J, Liel Y. Intrapulmonary hemorrhages and immune complex glomerulonephritis masquerading as Goodpasture's syndrome. Hum Pathol 1986; 17:754-757.

Goodpasture EW. The significance of certain pulmonary lesions in relation to the etiology of influenza. Am J Med Sci 1919; 158:863-870.

Hay JG, Turner-Warwick M. Pulmonary hemosiderosis, hemorrhagic syndromes and other rare infiltrative disorders. In Murray JF, Nadel JA, eds. Textbook of respiratory medicine. Philadelphia: WB Saunders, 1988.

Kahn FW, Jones JM, England DM. Diagnosis of pulmonary hemorrhage in the immunocompromised host. Am Rev Respir Dis 1987; 136:155-160.

Leatherman JW. Immune alveolar hemorrhage. Chest 1987; 91:891-897.

Leatherman JW, Davies SF, Hoidal JR. Alveolar hemorrhage syndromes: diffuse microvascular lung hemorrhage in immune and idiopathic disorders. Medicine 1984; 63:343-361.

Lombard CM, Colby TV, Elliott CG. Surgical pathology of the lung in anti-basement membrane antibody-associated Goodpasture's syndrome. Hum Pathol 1989; 20:445-451.

Martinez AJ, Maltby JD, Hurst DJ. Thrombotic thrombocytopenic purpura seen as pulmonary hemorrhage. Arch Intern Med 1983; 143:1818-1820.

Miller RR. Diffuse pulmonary hemorrhage. In Thurlbeck WM, ed. Pathology of the lung. New York: Thieme, 1988:303-310.

Murray RJ, Albin RJ, Mergner W, Criner GJ. Diffuse alveolar hemorrhage temporally related to cocaine smoking. Chest 1988; 93:427-429.

Myers JL, Katzenstein A-LA. Microangiitis in lupus-induced pulmonary hemorrhage. Am J Clin Pathol 1986; 85:552-556.

Myers JL, Katzenstein A-LA. Wegener's granulomatosis

presenting with massive pulmonary hemorrhage and capillaritis. Am J Surg Pathol 1987; 11:895-898.

Proskey AJ, Weatherbee L, Easterlung RE, et al. Goodpasture's syndrome: a report of five cases and review of the literature. Am J Med 1970; 48:162-173.

Road J, Jacques J, Sparling JR. Diffuse alveolar septal amyloidosis presenting with recurrent hemoptysis and medial dissection of pulmonary arteries. Am Rev Respir Dis 1985; 132:1368-1370.

Rosen PP. Opportunistic fungal infections in patients with neoplastic diseases. Path Annu 1976; 11:255-315.

Rubin GD, Edwards DK, Reicher MA, et al. Diagnosis of pulmonary hemosiderosis by MR imaging. AJR 1989; 152:573-574.

Segal SL, Lenchner GS, Cichelli AV, et al. Angiosarcoma presenting as diffuse alveolar hemorrhage. Chest 1988; 94:214-216.

Smith LJ, Katzenstein A-L. Pathogenesis of massive pulmonary hemorrhage in acute leukemia. Arch Intern Med 1982; 142:2149-2152.

Soergel KH, Sommers SC. Idiopathic pulmonary hemosiderosis and related syndromes. Am J Med 1962; 39:499-511.

Spragg RG, Wolf PL, Haghighi P, et al. Angiosarcoma of the lung with fatal pulmonary hemorrhage. Am J Med 1983; 74:1072-1076.

Sybers RG, Sybers JL, Dickie HA, Paul LW. Roentgenographic aspects of hemorrhagic pulmonary-renal disease (Goodpasture's syndrome). AJR 1965; 94:674-680.

Tenholder MF, Hooper RG. Pulmonary hemorrhage in the immunocompromised host—an elusive reality [abstract]. Am Rev Respir Dis 1980; 121 [suppl]:198.

Travis WD, Carpenter HA, Lie JT. Diffuse pulmonary hemorrhage: An uncommon manifestation of Wegener's granulomatosis. Am J Surg Pathol 1987; 11:702-708.

Wilson CB. Immunologic diseases of the lung and kidney (Goodpasture's syndrome). In Fishman AP, ed. Pulmonary diseases and disorders. 2nd ed. New York: McGraw-Hill, 1988.

Yousem SA. Angiosarcoma presenting in the lung. Arch Pathol Lab Med 1986; 110:112-115.

Chapter 7

Chronic Infiltrative Lung Disease

Lung biopsy is most commonly performed in patients with chronic infiltrative lung disease. Numerous diseases may produce the syndrome. The common causes are listed in Table 7–1 according to the largest series (490 cases) of open lung biopsies that has been analyzed (Carrington and Gaensler, 1978). It is meant as an indication of the frequency of diagnoses in chronic infiltrative lung disease. One feature of this series is the high percentage of pneumoconiosis, especially asbestosis. This represents Gaensler's interest in occupational lung disease. The other oddity is the 4:3 ratio of usual interstitial pneumonia (UIP) compared with desquamative interstitial pneumonia (DIP); a more realistic figure is 10:1 or higher.

USUAL INTERSTITIAL PNEUMONIA (FIBROSING ALVEOLITIS)

Many terms—Hamman-Rich syndrome, fibrosing alveolitis, cryptogenic fibrosing alveolitis, idiopathic pulmonary fibrosis, idiopathic interstitial fibrosis of the lung, usual interstitial pneumonia—have been used to designate this condition, reflecting the fact that no one term describes the condition

precisely. We prefer the term "usual interstitial pneumonia" (UIP). Hamman and Rich (1944) described a small group of patients who had diffuse, rapidly progressive fibrosis of the lungs and evidence of subacute inflammation. In retrospect, it is hard to decide exactly what they described, but these cases probably correspond to what is now known as acute interstitial pneumonia, or rapidly progressive pulmonary fibrosis (see p. 111). Most commonly, patients with usual interstitial pneumonia have an insidious onset of breathlessness; 25 to 40 percent date the onset of their symptoms to a flu-like illness. However, prospective studies have not shown evidence that well-documented viral pneumonia progresses to UIP. No age is exempt, but most patients are between 40 and 70 years old, and men are slightly more commonly affected than women. Physical findings characteristically include clubbing (but not pulmonary osteoarthropathy) and late fine inspiratory crackles ("Velcro crackles") at the bases of lungs. Pulmonary hypertension and right ventricular hypertrophy and failure occur only terminally. A high erythrocyte sedimentation rate is common, but polycythemia is rare. Most patients die of respiratory failure, often precipitated by pulmonary infection. The average duration of symptoms in one series was 3 years (Crystal et al, 1976), and the mean survival from time of diagnosis was 4 years, with a range of 0.4 to 20 years, in another series (Stack et al, 1972).

The radiologic features include reticular, reticulonodular, ground-glass, and ill-defined densities. The reticulonodular and ground-glass densities are generally equally frequent, and the bases are more severely involved than the apices. Terminal stages show coarse reticulation, often associated with cystic lesions, which are usually seen in the lower zones of the lung and decreased lung volumes (Genereux, 1975). Computed tomography (CT) has led to a more precise diagnosis prior to biopsy. On CT, UIP is characterized by the presence of reticular densities and small cystic airspaces predominantly in the periphery (subpleural regions) of the lower lung zones (Müller et al, 1986). This peripheral predominance is present in the vast majority of patients whether they have mild or severe disease (Fig. 7–1). The pattern and distribution of abnormalities in UIP usually allow for a confident diagnosis to be made on CT even when the radiographic findings are nonspecific (Mathieson et al, 1989). CT may also be used to assess disease activity in UIP (Müller et al, 1987a). The increased interstitial and airspace cellularity associated with disease activity result in areas of ground-glass density on CT (Fig. 7–2). Radiologic disease activity as well as areas of fibrosis are usually most marked in the subpleural lung regions. Because different lung regions show varying degrees of alveolar

---

TABLE 7–1

BIOPSIES IN CHRONIC DIFFUSE INFILTRATIVE LUNG DISEASE*

Interstitial pneumonias	24.9%
UIP 12.5%	
DIP 9.2%	
LIP 0.9%	
Environmental lung disease	21.6%
Asbestosis 11.8%	
Silicosis, coal, graphite 4.3%	
Allergic alveolitis 1.0%	
Sarcoidosis	13.2%
Nonspecific	13.1%
Unusual specific disorders	9.4%
Eosinophilic granuloma 3.1%	
Alveolar proteinosis 2.7%	
Diffuse pulmonary hemorrhage 1.6%	
"Allergic" reactions	4.5%
Eosinophilic pneumonia 4.3%	
Infections	3.8%
Pulmonary vascular disease	3.5%
Malignant neoplasm	2.9%
Chronic passive congestion	1.4%
No diagnosis	1.0%

*Modified from Carrington CB, Gaensler EA. Clinical-pathologic approach to diffuse infiltrative lung disease. In Thurlbeck WM, Abell MR, eds. The lung: structure, function and disease. Baltimore: Williams & Wilkins, 1978:58–87. This table describes the diagnosis in 490 lung biopsies. The percentage of major categories is shown and, within them, the percentage of subcategories, all expressed as a percentage of the 490 biopsies.

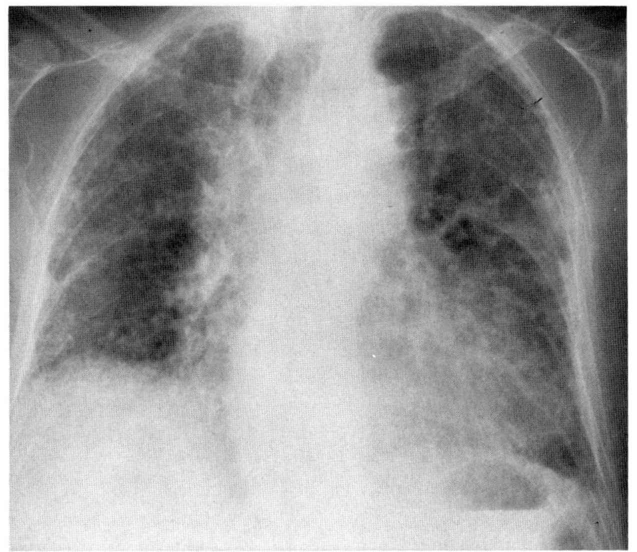

A

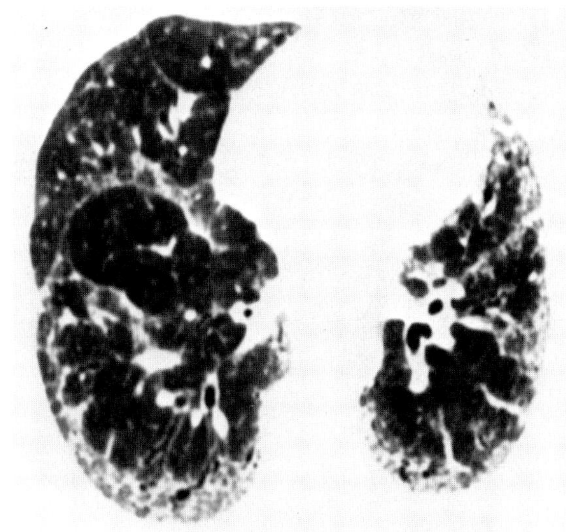

B

C

Figure 7–1   *A*, Chest radiograph of a 77-year-old patient with severe usual interstitial pneumonia (UIP), showing extensive bilateral coarse irregular linear opacities and low lung volumes. *B*, CT scan in a patient with early, mild UIP. Irregular linear densities are present predominantly in the subpleural lung regions. The fibrosis can be seen to extend also along the right major fissure. The asymmetric distribution of the disease is evident with more severe involvement of the left lung and relative sparing of the right middle lobe. The ground-glass increased density seen posterolaterally, particularly on the right side, is due to filling of airspaces with histiocytes. The presence of ground-glass density on CT in a patient with UIP has been shown to represent evidence of disease activity. *C*, Patient with end-stage lung due to UIP. Extensive "honeycombing" is present in the lower lobes and is associated with traction bronchiectasis. The subpleural predominance of the changes is still evident in the right middle lobe and, to a lesser extent, in the lingula.

wall inflammation, intra-alveolar cellularity, and fibrosis, CT allows a much better assessment of the overall parenchymal changes than any other method. CT also correlates better than the radiograph with the clinical and functional impairment in UIP (Staples et al, 1987). In a review of 23 patients, Staples et al demonstrated a significant correlation between extent of disease on CT and the severity of dyspnea as well as the impairment in gas transfer as assessed by the carbon monoxide diffusing capacity. As previously demonstrated by others, there was poor correlation between the chest radiographic findings and

the clinical and functional parameters. Except in scleroderma, pulmonary artery pressures are out of proportion to the changes seen on chest radiograph.

Classification

Identical clinical, radiologic, and morphologic changes may be seen in the lungs of patients with systemic sclerosis (scleroderma), systemic lupus erythematosus, dermatomyositis, and rheumatoid arthritis (see Chapter 8). Also, a substantial number of patients have some of the serologic features of the

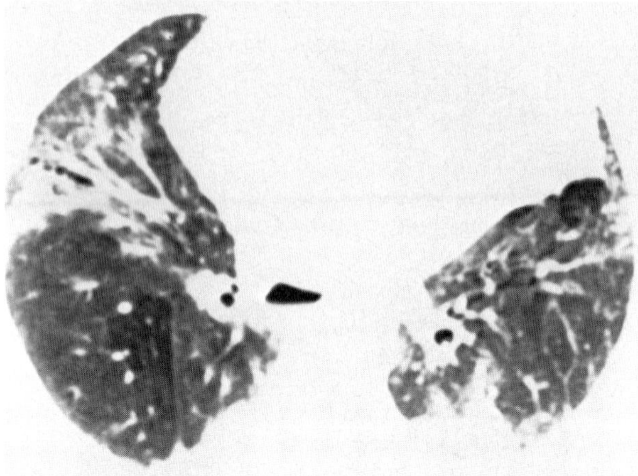

Figure 7–2 CT scan in a patient with marked disease activity in UIP. The areas of disease activity are seen on CT as ground-glass densities. Areas of disease activity, as areas of fibrosis, in UIP often have a patchy distribution although they still are predominantly subpleural. In this patient the areas of fibrosis and disease activity are predominantly in the posterior basal segments and near the right major fissure. The image also illustrates the need to use CT to guide the surgeon to the appropriate biopsy site.

collagen vascular diseases without the clinical syndrome. Patients were frequently found to have non-organ-specific autoantibodies in one series, including 27 percent with rheumatoid factor and 40 percent with antinuclear antibodies (Turner-Warwick et al, 1971). Others (Crystal et al, (1976) found that the proportion of these antibodies was lower, but elevated cryoglobulins occurred in 41 percent and elevated IgA was present in 39 percent. It has therefore been suggested that patients with UIP should be classified into three categories: (1) patients with clinical features of collagen vascular disease, (2) patients without clinical features of collagen vascular disease but with immunologic serum abnormalities and (3) patients with neither clinical features of collagen vascular disease nor immunologic serum abnormalities. The proportion of patients falling into each of the categories is uncertain because no series has a sufficiently large number of randomly acquired cases to determine the figures precisely. Referral patterns would likely affect certain series, and accumulation of case reports in the literature is unsatisfactory since cases are likely to be preferentially reported. UIP has also been reported in association with other diseases such as tubular acidosis (Mason et al, 1970; Zalin et al, 1970) and celiac disease (Smith et al, 1971).

Etiology and Pathogenesis

The association of UIP with the collagen vascular diseases suggests that immunologic mechanisms may be involved. Turner-Warwick and colleagues (1971) found complement and immunoglobulins in the lung parenchyma in some patients, and Dreisin et al, (1978) noted circulating immune complexes together with deposition of immunoglobulins in lung tissue.

Bronchoalveolar lavage (BAL) has shown an increased number of inflammatory cells, and neutrophils constitute an average of 33 percent of the cells obtained (Reynolds et al, 1977). Eosinophils were invariably present and remained after corticosteroid treatment. In contrast to allergic alveolitis, the number of lymphocytes was not increased. The significance of BAL findings is at present controversial, and the interpretation of BAL is awaiting the definitive National Institutes of Health Idiopathic Pulmonary Fibrosis study. Of patients with UIP 95 percent have been found to have circulating lymphocytes that produce migration inhibitory factor when exposed to type-I collagen (Kravis et al, 1976). These findings suggest that pulmonary fibrosis results from continued injury to the alveolar interstitium, brought about by mediators from cells that congregate at the site of collagen-induced, cell-mediated immunologic phenomena.

Familial fibrosing alveolitis is well documented, and it has been suggested that familial cases may constitute as much as 20 percent of cases of fibrosing alveolitis in children (Donohue et al, 1959). While the true figure is likely to be much lower, even in children, this may indicate that particular HLA antigens may be involved (Solliday et al, 1973). Bitterman et al (1986) have made the interesting observation that approximately half of clinically well people from families with familial fibrosing alveolitis have BAL evidence of interstitial inflammation, the natural history of which is as yet uncertain.

Morphologic and Diagnostic Features

The lung at the time of autopsy usually has a characteristic hobnailed external surface, and this appearance can also be recognized in lung biopsies. The lung is firm and the cut surface gray-white, often with a multicystic appearance (Fig. 7–3). The condition is usually more chronic and advanced (end-stage lung or honeycombing) in the lower zones of the lung, especially subpleurally. It has been stated that in about 35 percent of the cases, fibrosis is focal, and most of the lung is normal; in another 25 percent,

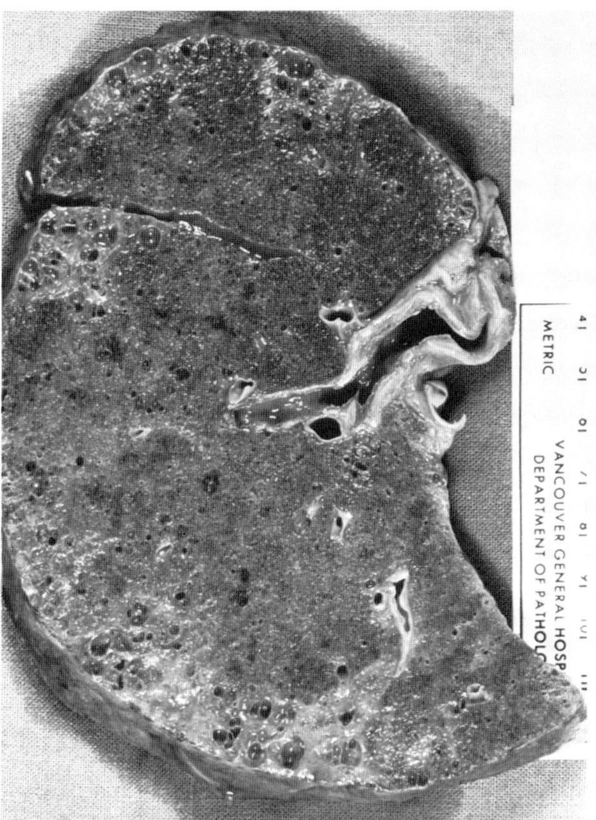

Figure 7–3   Gross appearance of upper lobe and superior segment of lower lobe in a patient dying of idiopathic UIP, cut horizontally in the plane of a CT scan. Note the multicystic architectural abnormality in the subpleural zones.

there is more fibrous than normal tissue; and in the remainder, most of the lung tissue is abnormal (Crystal et al, 1976). However, the extent of fibrosis was probably overestimated. The appearance of extensive fibrosis is clearly not compatible with life; it represents a nonrepresentative biopsy, which by the nature of the procedure, preferentially samples subpleural lung tissue. Increased collagen, by definition, is always present, although original biochemical studies did not show an increased amount of collagen per unit weight of lung. This may be due in part to the change in the denominator as well as in the numerator, and in part it may represent a shift from type-III collagen (which does not stain histologically) to type-I collagen (typical histologic collagen), so the total amount of collagen as assayed biochemically may be little altered (Fulmer and Crystal, 1976). More recent studies, however, have indicated that there is an increase in collagen (Murray and Laurent, 1988). In addition, Gadek et al (1979) detected increased collagenase activity in the lavage fluid of

patients with UIP, and hypothesized a sequence of collagen lysis followed by disordered resynthesis and interstitial remodeling.

The basic abnormalities in UIP include a combination of mononuclear cell alveolar wall inflammation, intra-alveolar histiocytes, young granulation tissue being incorporated into the interstitium, alveolar wall fibrosis, and end-stage lung. Carrington and Gaensler (1978) stressed that the most characteristic feature of the lung biopsy specimen grossly and microscopically is a heterogeneity of lesions, and the appearance is variable even within a given biopsy specimen or slide. Thus, depending on the biopsy site, one histologic section may contain normal lung, active inflammation, and honeycombed areas distributed among each other in a patchy fashion (Fig. 7–4). Interstitial inflammation is always observed, but its severity is variable. Crystal et al (1976) reported that in 13 percent of cases, it was heavy; in 54 percent, moderate; and in 33 percent, only scattered inflammatory cells were apparent. The majority of the cells are lymphocytes, macrophages, and plasma cells. Nodular collections of lymphocytes are present in many cases. Neutrophils and occasional eosinophils can usually be found, although they are not very obvious and are often found in the cystic spaces. Nonspecific type-II cell hyperplasia is often found in inflamed areas (Fig. 7–5). Interstitial granulomas and tissue eosinophilia are not features of UIP. Macrophages in the airspaces are also invariably present but, when present in large numbers, are characteristic of DIP. The presence of interstitial granulation tissue presents a problem with differential diagnosis of bronchiolitis obliterans–organizing pneumonia or cryptogenic organizing pneumonia (BOOP and COP, respectively). In general, in UIP the new granulation tissue is not extensive and is obviously limited to the airspace walls. In COP, the granulation tissue is within airspaces, often not in continuity with their walls, and the alveolar walls are relatively normal. These features of interstitial inflammation, intra-alveolar histiocytes, and young granulation tissue are considered signs of active and potentially reversible disease with probable steroid responsiveness (Watters et al, 1986; Müller et al, 1987a).

Alveolar wall fibrosis and honeycombing are considered to be irreversible. A less well-recognized and probably irreversible feature is the distortion and narrowing of bronchioles together with peribronchiolar fibrosis and inflammation. This observation may account for the functional evidence of small airway obstruction that is found in some patients with UIP (Ostrow and Cherniack, 1973). An interesting finding is the presence of cholesterol-ester clefts within airspaces. These clefts are said to be associated with more severe pulmonary fibrosis and

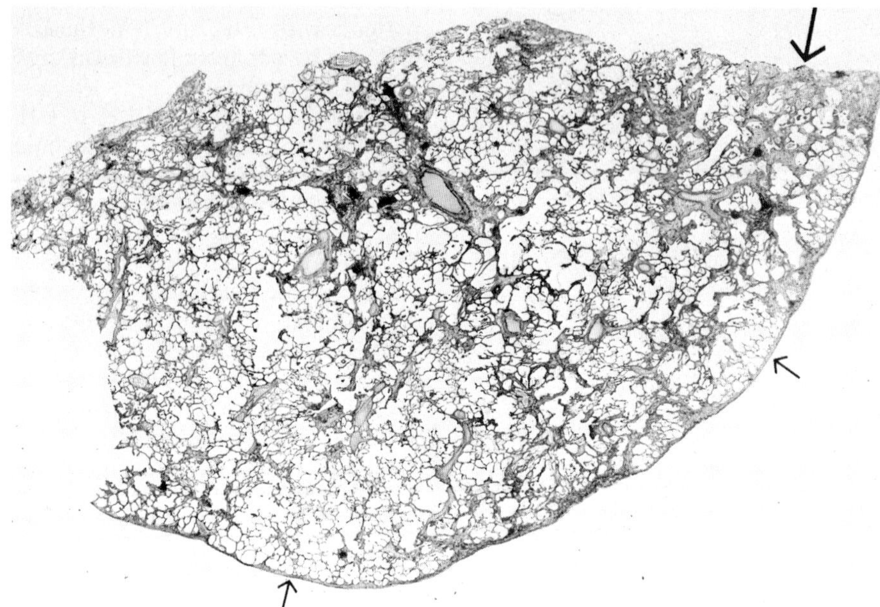

Figure 7–4   Scanning microscopic appearance of open lung biopsy from a patient with active UIP showing normal areas (*short arrow*) and honeycombed areas (*long arrow*) interspersed with areas of cellular interstitial widening.

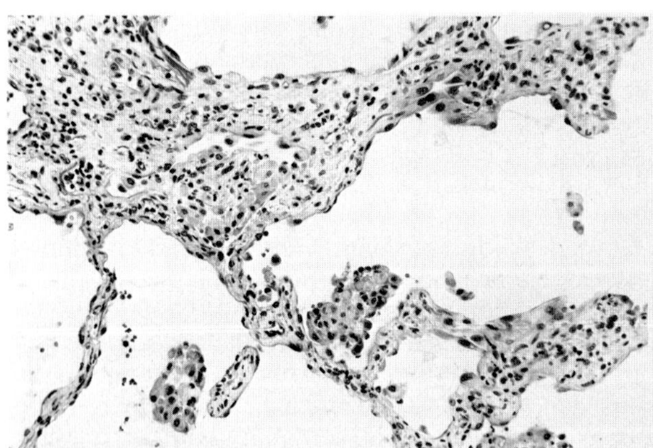

Figure 7–5   Typical area of active UIP showing mononuclear alveolitis with a modest degree of type-II cell hyperplasia and intra-alveolar histiocytes.

pulmonary hypertension (Crystal et al, 1976). The pulmonary vessels may have thickened walls due to increased intimal and medial thickness, and these changes occur in areas of pronounced interstitial fibrosis. Smooth muscle hyperplasia may also occur in the fibrotic areas of UIP due to muscularization of scars.

Ideally, quantitative assessment of the reversible versus irreversible components in an open lung biopsy might correlate with response to therapy and prognosis (Watters et al, 1986; Müller et al, 1987a). However, this assessment is highly dependent on biopsy site selection. We believe that biopsy site selection is best guided by CT, but it must be realized that a biopsy cannot necessarily be assumed to be "representative" in UIP.

It is critical to recognize that UIP and end-stage lung (Genereux, 1975) or honeycomb lung are not synonymous. UIP often has significant honeycombing in its later stages, particularly in a subpleural distribution (Fig. 7-6). However, all causes of chronic infiltrative lung disease may end up as end-stage lung. Thus, it is important to search carefully for any specific lesions in patients with honeycomb lung and to make quite certain that there are no clues to the etiology from the clinical history or radiographs. Asbestosis may be a problem, although it is usually easily recognized by the presence of obvious asbestos bodies and by the pattern of fibrosis. However, cases are seen where the lesions appear typical of UIP but only an occasional asbestos body may be found. Sometimes asbestos bodies may not be found although the patient has been exposed to asbestos. Under these circumstances, the diagnosis of idiopathic fibrosing alveolitis (UIP) seems unreasonable. As indicated, all cases of pulmonary fibrosis should be examined using polarized light, and it may be wise to include a stain for iron since the occasional asbestos body may be hard to recognize with hemotoxylin and eosin staining, and asbestos bodies are not doubly refractile.

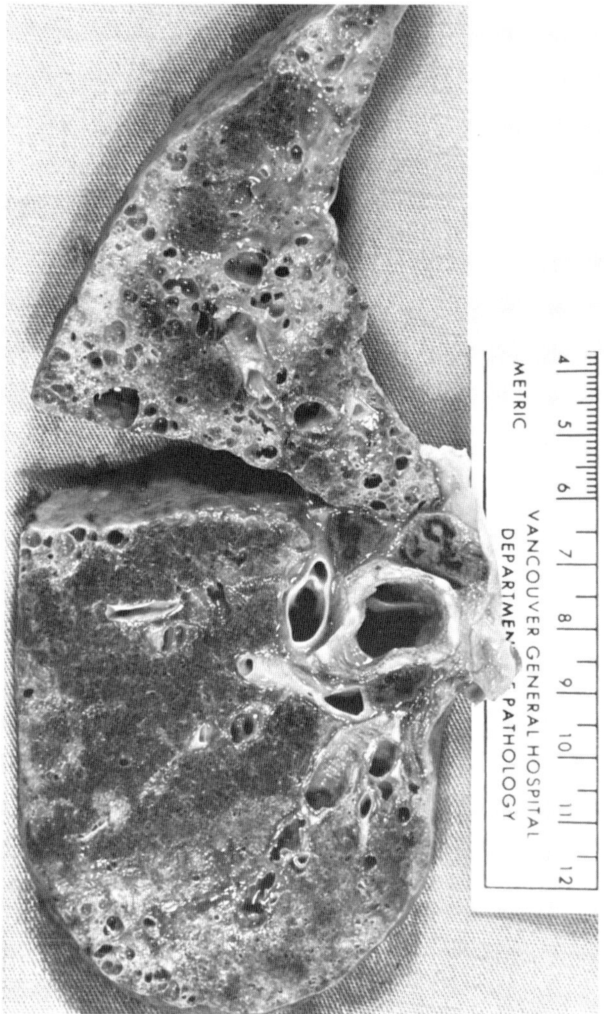

Figure 7–6 End-stage honeycombing in a subpleural distribution. This patient had had an open lung biopsy showing active UIP 5 years before.

Desquamative Interstitial Pneumonia

In 1965 Liebow et al described 18 patients with infiltrative lung disease that differed in many ways from UIP. They were slightly younger, symptoms were usually milder (Table 7–2), clubbing was not a characteristic feature, and radiologically the patients usually had ground-glass opacities, particularly at the bases and at the costophrenic angles. There was less evidence of restrictive lung disease and, in many, lung volumes were relatively normal (Carrington et al, 1978). The diagnostic histologic feature that Liebow and coworkers believed distinguished these patients from those with UIP was the presence of numerous large histiocytes cells filling the airspaces. Initially it was thought that the cells were chiefly

TABLE 7–2

DESQUAMATIVE AND USUAL INTERSTITIAL PNEUMONIAS*

	DIP	UIP
Average age at diagnosis (yrs)	42.3	50.9
Duration of symptom (yrs)	0.9	2.5
Survival (yrs)	12.2	5.6
Improved	61.5%	11.5%
Worse	27.0%	69.2%
Mortality	27.5%	66.0%

*From Carrington CB, Gaensler EA. Clinical-pathologic approach to diffuse infiltrative lung disease. In Thurlbeck WM, Abell MR, eds. The lung: structure, function and disease. Baltimore: Williams & Wilkins, 1978:58–87.

desquamated alveolar lining cells, hence the term "desquamative interstitial pneumonia." It is now known that the cells within the airspaces are macrophages, whereas the cells that line the involved alveoli are mainly type-II epithelial cells (Farr et al, 1970). The original description emphasized the presence of green-brown pigment in the cytoplasm of cells in the airspaces. The pigment stained strongly with periodic acid–Schiff stain and was diastase-resistant; only occasional iron-staining granules were present. Liebow et al (1965) also recognized intracytoplasmic "blue bodies" that occurred in the cells in the airspaces in about 10 percent of their patients. They are 15 to 25 μm in diameter, stain deeply with hematoxylin, and have a central round or oval core surrounded by a clear space, with an outer rim of granular brown material. Electron-microscopically, the central core consists of radially arranged fibrillar material. It is thought that this material may be connective tissue mucin and that the outer rim stains for iron (Gardiner and Uff, 1978). Eosinophilic intranuclear inclusions occur in the cells lining the air spaces and the cells lying free in airspaces in 5 to 80 percent of cases. These were originally described as "virus-like," but electron-microscopically they consist of myelin figures (Tubbs et al, 1978). The significance of the pigment, blue bodies, and intranuclear inclusions in the etiology and diagnosis of DIP is unknown.

Additional features of DIP include the relative preservation of lung architecture, with mild thickening of alveolar walls and absence of severe fibrosis or honeycombing. An interstitial mononuclear inflammatory infiltrate is present, sometimes with the formation of lymphoid follicles (Fig. 7–7).

Liebow et al (1965) and Carrington et al (1978) regarded DIP as a distinct entity, but this has been challenged by several investigators. The histologic

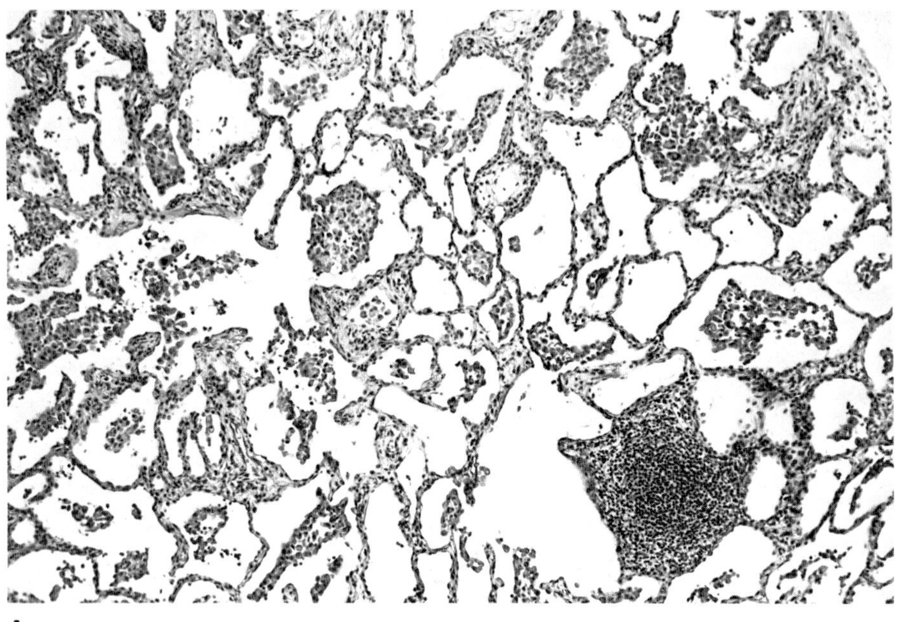

A

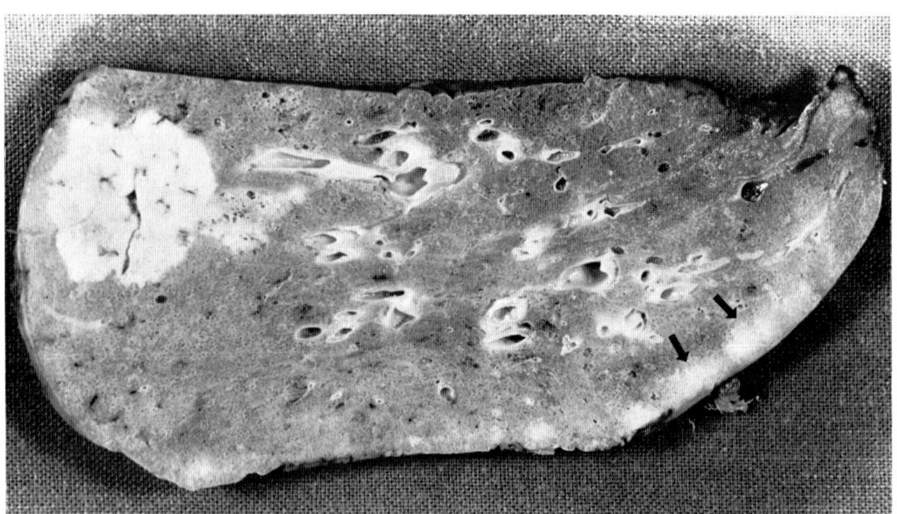

B

Figure 7–7 *A*, Typical histologic appearance of DIP, with prominent intra-alveolar histiocytes, alveolar wall inflammation with minimal fibrosis, and a lymphoid center. *B*, DIP reaction (*arrows*) in a patient with bronchoalveolar carcinoma. The histiocytic infiltrate is in the characteristic peripheral distribution of DIP and is not spatially related to the tumor. However, this patient had no clinical or radiologic evidence of idiopathic infiltrative lung disease.

appearance of DIP is not specific. A DIP-like reaction has been reported in asbestosis (Corrin and Price, 1977) and other dust-caused diseases (Coates and Watson, 1971) following nitrofurantoin therapy (Bone et al, 1976), is characteristically found in airspaces adjacent to the nodules of eosinophilic granuloma, and is occasionally found in association with tumors (Fig. 7–7). Foci of DIP morphology are commonly present in otherwise typical cases of UIP, and cases have been reported in which classic DIP "progressed to fibrosing alveolitis" (McCann and Brewer, 1974; Patchefsky et al, 1973). The notion that DIP is different from early UIP was primarily based on histopathologic differences in appearance. This basis is theoretically imperfect since, in biologic systems, age quite often changes morphology considerably (Color Plate). Thus DIP may represent an idiopathic disease with unique characteristics, a nonspecific reaction to injury, or an early stage in the development of UIP. Figure 7–8 is a schematic view of the

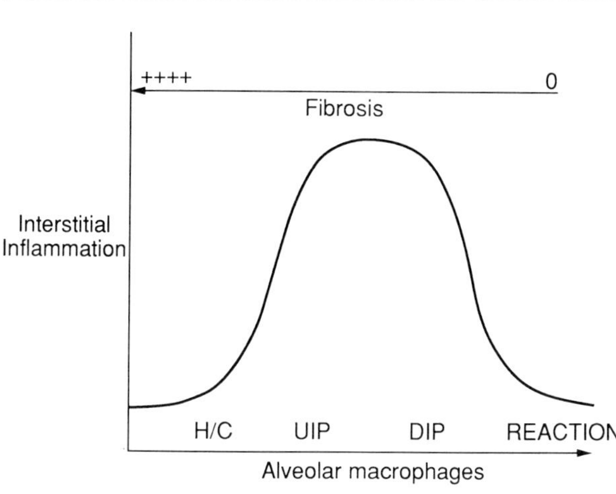

Figure 7–8 Schematic bell-shaped curve illustrating hypothetical relationship between DIP reaction, DIP, UIP, and honeycombing (H/C).

hypothetical interrelationship of honeycomb lung, UIP, DIP, and a DIP-like histiocytic reaction. According to this view, the morphologic separation of these entities is not always clearcut but rather is based on the relative degrees of intra-alveolar histiocytic collections (greatest in reaction and DIP), active interstitial inflammation (greatest in DIP and UIP), and irreversible fibrosis (greatest in honeycomb lung and UIP). The prognosis generally deteriorates with increasing fibrosis.

Regardless of the theoretical relationship between UIP and DIP, it is important to distinguish between the two since, even if they are related conditions, it has been shown that the clinical features are different, the prognosis is much better in DIP, and the response to steroids is greater in DIP (Carrington et al, 1978) (see Table 7–2). In classical instances, the distinction between DIP and fibrosing alveolitis is easy, but in many cases it is not. Radiologically and grossly, both UIP and DIP have a peripheral distribution but DIP tends to be less fibrotic (Vedal et al, 1988). The main distinguishing features of DIP histologically are the massive collection of macrophages in the airspaces and the greater uniformity of morphology from field to field in DIP. In addition, there is usually maintenance of alveolar architecture and only a mild degree of fibrosis. However, if there are massive intra-alveolar collections of cells, the diagnosis can be made even in the presence of distortion of lung parenchyma, pulmonary fibrosis, or areas of end-stage lung.

LYMPHOID INTERSTITIAL PNEUMONIA

In this interesting but as yet poorly understood condition, there is an exquisitely interstitial infiltrate of lymphocytes, plasma cells, and large mononuclear cells. There is a distinct clinical overlap between it, "pseudolymphoma of the lung," Sjögren's syndrome, Waldenström's macroglobulinemia, and involvement of the lung by lymphoma. Spencer (1977) has grouped the conditions together as "prelymphomatous states," and Gibbs and Seal (1978) have referred to them as "primary lymphoproliferative conditions of the lung."

In 1966 Liebow and Carrington briefly presented a group of cases and used the term "lymphoid interstitial pneumonia" (LIP) to describe them, later amplifying this description (Liebow and Carrington, 1969a). In 1973 they described 18 cases of LIP associated with dysproteinemia. The proportion of patients with LIP who have dysproteinemia is not completely certain; it is likely that it is the majority since 10 of 13 patients in the only other large series reported had dysproteinemia (Strimlan et al, 1978). LIP is uncommon, and in one series was 10 times less frequent than DIP (Carrington and Gaensler, 1978). It is the most common between 40 and 70 years of age, but it may occur at all ages, including children. Cough and insidious dyspnea are the most common complaints, but pneumonia was the initial symptom in a significant proportion of the cases. Arthralgia, arthritis, and positive rheumatoid factor occurred only rarely. Radiologically, bilateral reticular or reticulonodular infiltrates are most common, but a coarsely nodular pattern has been seen in patients with raised IgG levels (Liebow and Carrington, 1973). These authors also found that pleural effusion, in each instance on the right side, occurred in three of 18 patients. Functionally, a restrictive defect is present. The overall clinical pattern of LIP is likely to change in the future since LIP has now been described as a feature of the acquired immunodeficiency syndrome (AIDS). Originally reported in children (Joshi et al, 1985, 1986), it is now well documented in adults (Solal-Celigny et al, 1985; Griecho and Chinoy-Acharya, 1985; Morris et al, 1987). This is further evidence that it is a manifestation of immunologically mediated disease.

The characteristic histologic lesion is a diffuse infiltrate limited to the interstitium of the lung, consisting of lymphocytes, plasma cells, large mononuclear and "reticuloendothelial cells," and lymphoid centers (Fig. 7–9). The infiltrates are typically polymorphous, and either lymphocytes or plasma cells predominate. The general characteristics of the infiltrate are similar to those described by Saltzstein

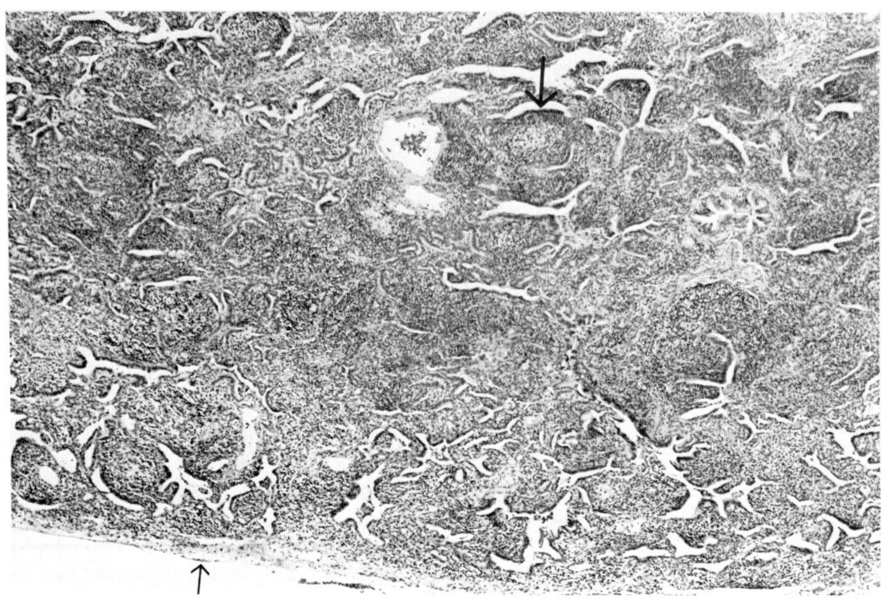

Figure 7–9 Lymphoid interstitial pneumonitis: open lung biopsy from a 9-year-old girl with hypogammaglobulinemia and bilateral interstitial infiltrates. Dense cellularity with lymphoid center (*long arrow*) and relative pleural sparing (*short arrow*).

(1963) in his description of "pseudolymphoma of the lung," but the two conditions differ in that pseudolymphoma of the lung is generally a localized disease. Poorly formed granulomas consisting of localized accumulations of large reticuloendothelial cells, mononuclear cells, epithelioid cells, and Touton giant cells were seen in four of 18 cases (Liebow and Carrington, 1973). The granulomas were not so compact as in sarcoidosis, and hyalinization was not seen. Similar granulomas were seen in the lymph nodes in one instance.

LIP can be regarded as the pulmonary analog of Sjögren's syndrome. In addition, it is very difficult in the lung, just as in other organs in Sjögren's syndrome, to distinguish benign from malignant infiltrations, and a spectrum exists (Anderson and Talal, 1972). It may also be that LIP may "transform" into lymphoma, as illustrated by Weisbrodt (1976) in his report of a patient with LIP and Sjögren's syndrome who developed lymphomatoid granulomatosis. LIP has also been described in association with diphenylhydantoin use (Chamberlain et al, 1986), pernicious anemia, the autoerythrocyte sensitization syndrome, chronic active hepatitis, and chronic graft-versus-host disease (Perreault et al, 1985). We have seen a case associated with polymyositis.

The main histologic differential diagnosis is between a benign infiltrate of the lung (LIP) or a malignant infiltration. The distinction between benignancy and malignancy is made on the characteristics of the infiltrate, the nature of the involvement of the lung, and evidence of extrapulmonary disease. In LIP, the infiltrate is classically polymorphous, and the more purely lymphocytic the infiltrate, the more likely it is to be malignant. Involvement of the pleura is also used as a distinguishing feature. While LIP may involve the deep layers (i.e., toward the airspaces) of the pleura, extension through all layers of the pleura is suggestive of malignancy. Involvement of the parietal pleura and adjacent fat is diagnostic of malignancy. Extensive involvement of airways with ulceration of the epithelium and destruction of cartilage indicates malignancy. Lymphoma is said to "track" along lymphatic channels (Colby and Carrington, 1983) (see Chapter 9). Definitive criteria of malignancy include involvement of extrapulmonary sites, usually intrathoracic lymph nodes, extrathoracic nodes, or the spleen. Clinical evidence of splenic enlargement is inadequate; histologic evidence of malignancy is required. Extrinsic allergic alveolitis should be included in the differential diagnosis and is usually excluded by the extent of the infiltration, which is more extensive and severe in LIP. Furthermore, the characteristic bronchiolitis and granulomas with foreign bodies of extrinsic allergic alveolitis are absent in LIP. Lymphomatoid granulomatosis may sometimes also be included in the differential diagnosis but differs in that the infiltrate is often, indeed characteristically, cytologically atypical with angioinvasion and angiodestruction. Large areas of necrosis may result from the angioinvasive infiltrate. The exact status of "benign lymphocytic angiitis and granulomatosis" (Israel et al, 1977) is uncertain. It may be the same condition as LIP with a conspicuous vasocentric component.

GIANT CELL INTERSTITIAL PNEUMONIA

Giant cell interstitial pneumonia (GIP) is the least common variant of chronic interstitial pneumonia (Ohori et al, 1989). The clinical manifestations are similar to those of UIP or DIP: progressive dyspnea, cough, chest pain, fatigue, and weight loss, with clubbing and fine basal rales on physical examination. The chest film usually shows bilateral, patchy, reticulonodular infiltrates involving the mid-lung zones with sparing of the apices and costophrenic angles. In other cases, flame-shaped opacities have been described, while in others the radiograph has resembled that seen in DIP (Sokolowski et al, 1972). In their review of GIP, Ohori et al (1989) emphasized that most cases of GIP are related to hard-metal exposure. Histologically, GIP is characterized by a nonuniform distribution of disease, with great variability of appearance from field to field within the same biopsy wedge (Fig. 7-10). There are many macrophages in the alveolar spaces, including bizarre multinucleate histiocytes, which are the diagnostic feature of this disease. These cells are characteristically cannibalistic, engulfing other cells (see Fig. 7-10). Unlike UIP, DIP, or LIP, the disease process is bronchiolocentric, presumably reflecting its possible inhalation origin (see Fig. 7-10). There is also an interstitial infiltrate of mononuclear cells, mostly lymphocytes. Steroid treatment has been the therapeutic mainstay suggested in the literature, but the majority of patients ultimately die of the disease.

ACUTE INTERSTITIAL PNEUMONIA

This condition is difficult to fit into our somewhat arbitrary definition of "acute" and "chronic" infiltrative lung disease. It is acute compared to our description of the other interstitial pneumonias but

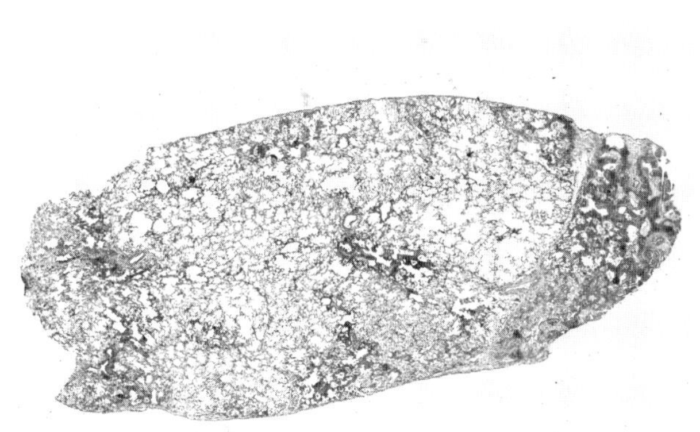

A

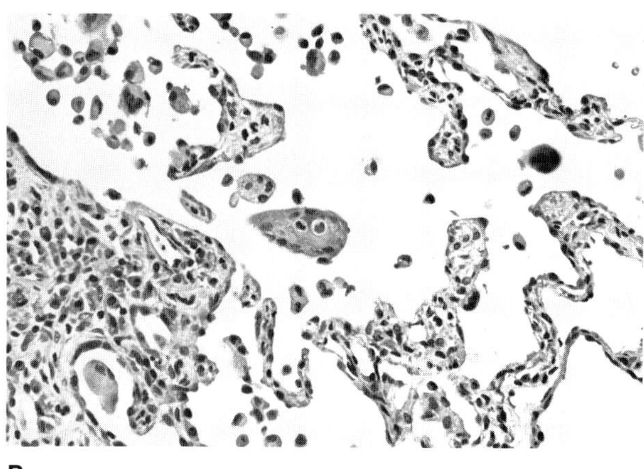

B

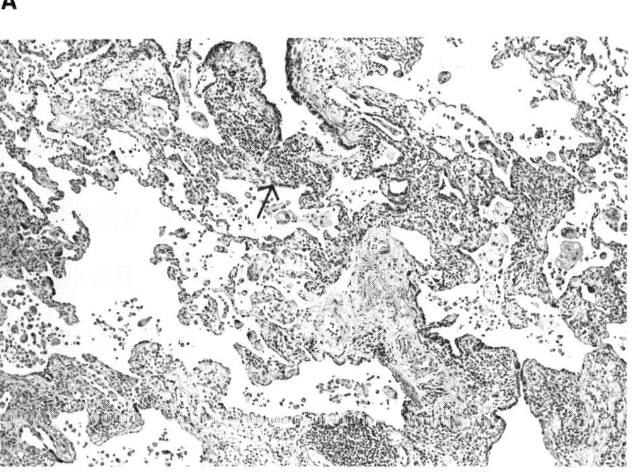

C

Figure 7–10   Giant cell interstitial pneumonitis: *A*, scanning microscopic view of biopsy showing nonuniformity of involvement; *B*, multinucleated histiocyte with engulfed cell fragment; *C*, bronchiolocentric accentuation of disease process with accompanying mononuclear bronchiolitis (*arrow*).

may be a variant of UIP and could be what Hamman and Rich described in 1944. It may also be a variant of diffuse alveolar damage in which catastrophic lung injury of unknown etiology occurs in previously healthy, relatively young people. The only thing clear at the present time is that it is a poorly defined entity, but this will undoubtedly change.

Katzenstein et al (1986a) coined the term to describe eight cases that had a sudden onset and a rapid course measured in days or weeks to institution of ventilatory therapy. The patients were young (13 to 50 years old, average age, 28 years), a pre-existing viral-like illness occurred in six, and two were pregnant women. The course was rapid, and death occurred in seven of the eight patients within 6 months of institution of therapy, and in five within 2 months. The radiology appears to be nonspecific, with a combination of diffuse reticulonodular and alveolar filling opacities. The histologic appearance was different from that of UIP in that the lesions were uniform in appearance and cellular fibroblastic proliferation was dominant, with an edematous stroma and little collagen. There was severe type-II cell metaplasia, and the cells often showed hyperchromaticity and prominent nucleoli. Remnants of hyaline membranes were seen in six. Squamous metaplasia of bronchioles with extension to adjacent airspaces was seen.

Pratt et al (1979) had previously described 12 patients with rapidly progressive infiltrative lung disease and used the term "rapidly fatal pulmonary fibrosis." However, their patients were in general older, with an average age of 62 years, and the course was rather more protracted (average, 4.2 months; maximum, 18 months). In addition, there was a male predominance of 3 to 1, five had collagen-vascular disease, and four had other diseases including syphilis, chronic eosinophilia, hypersensitivity reactions, and allergic disorders. Minimal pathology was presented in their paper, but they believed that their cases represented "the accelerated variant of interstitial pneumonitis" and resembled the cases reported by Hamman and Rich in 1944. In their review of the literature they found several similar previously reported cases.

CRYPTOGENIC ORGANIZING PNEUMONITIS *OR* BRONCHIOLITIS OBLITERANS-ORGANIZING PNEUMONIA

The term "bronchiolitis obliterans" has been used in so many different ways that it has become so ambiguous to be almost valueless. Probably three types of bronchiolar lesions fall under this heading:

the presence of loose granulation tissue within the lumens of bronchioles, partially or totally occluding them with preservation of the wall, as in rheumatoid bronchiolitis or measles (see Chapter 12); peribronchiolar fibrosis; and total obliteration of bronchioles with disappearance of the airways. The paradox is that once the airway is totally obliterated it cannot be seen; perhaps the best example of this sort of bronchiolar obliteration is in bronchiectasis, where loss of airways is well documented (Reid, 1950). It should also be borne in mind that classic bronchiolitis obliterans, defined as the presence of loose granulation tissue within bronchioles, may be seen in extrinsic allergic alveolitis, rheumatoid arthritis, and eosinophilic pneumonia.

The issue is further confused by the description of bronchiolitis obliterans and interstitial pneumonia ("BIP")(Liebow and Carrington, 1969a) in relation to other forms of interstitial pneumonia (UIP, DIP, LIP, and GIP). Precisely what was originally meant by this term is not clear. Our interpretation is that while active young connective tissue is commonly seen in UIP, it is seldom the dominant lesion; when it is dominant, then perhaps this was the condition referred to as BIP. A further complication is that the review of cases of "bronchiolitis obliterans" from the late Dr. Liebow's file clearly showed a concatenation of various diseases (Gosink et al, 1973).

Fortunately, Davison et al (1983) in Britain, and Epler et al (1985) in the United States produced clinical series that have led to much clarification. The Davison group termed their cases "cryptogenic organizing pneumonia" (COP), and the Epler group, "bronchiolitis obliterans and organizing pneumonia" (BOOP). COP is probably a more accurate description because (1) the dominant lesion is an organizing pneumonia, (2) true bronchiolitis obliterans, i.e. involving membranous bronchioles, is absent in one-third of cases, and (3) the term "bronchiolitis obliterans" is confusing insofar as patients with COP usually have a restrictive rather than an obstructive defect such as might be expected with bronchiolitis. The problem of bronchiolitis obliterans is further discussed in Chapter 12. Cryptogenic organizing pneumonia (COP) is an important part of the differential diagnosis of clinical infiltrative lung disease in general, and of UIP in particular.

Clinically the average age of patients with COP is about 60 years; the previous history is short (weeks to months) and frequently follows an apparent respiratory infection, sometimes in the immunocompromised host. Dyspnea is present in only half the patients, and fever is present in a small minority; clubbing is rare. In one study, restrictive lung disease was present in 40 percent of cases, but this was less common than in UIP, and the diffusing capacity

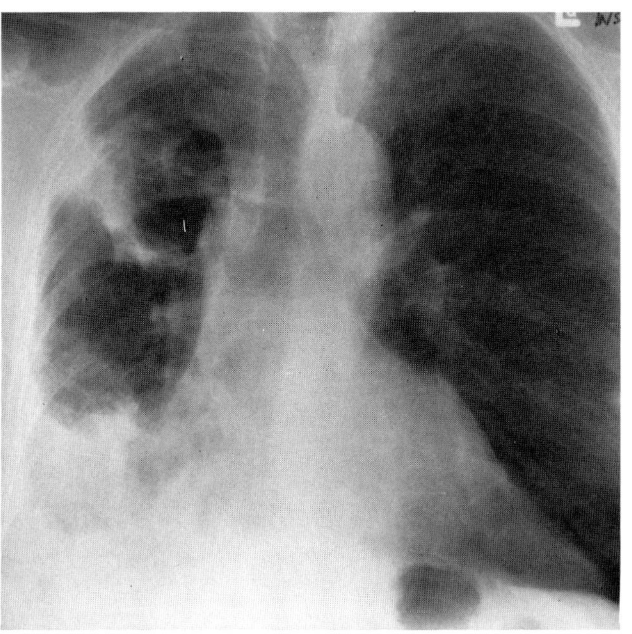
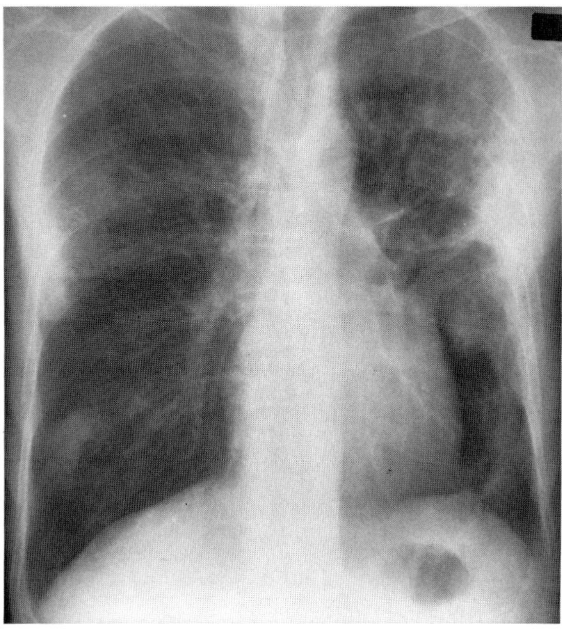

A   **B**

Figure 7–11   *A,* Cryptogenic organizing pneumonia (COP) or bronchiolitis obliterans–organizing pneumonia (BOOP) in a 70-year-old man. Chest radiograph shows extensive airspace consolidation in the right lung with associated loss of volume. The patient also had a small right pleural effusion. *B,* COP/BOOP in a 61-year-old male. Chest radiograph shows bilateral changes in a predominant subpleural distribution mimicking chronic eosinophilic pneumonia.

($D_L CO$) was reduced in only one-half (Katzenstein et al, 1986b). However, a subsequent study showed that evidence of lung restriction was about the same in UIP and BOOP, and $D_L CO$ was not significantly different between the groups (Guerry-Force et al, 1987). The radiologic findings usually consist of patchy bilateral nonsegmental areas of airspace consolidation (Müller et al, 1987b). Small, round, and irregular opacities may also be present. While these radiologic findings themselves are nonspecific, they often allow a confident diagnosis when seen in the appropriate clinical setting (Fig. 7-11). The importance of distinguishing UIP from COP is that the latter has a relatively good prognosis: about 50 percent resolve, mainly as a response to steroids, and 12.5 to 25 percent of patients die, usually in about 3 months. The clinical features of UIP and BOOP are compared in Table 7-3.

Morphologically, the major feature is organizing pneumonia mainly in alveoli, alveolar ducts, and respiratory bronchioles, and this is patchy and peribronchiolar (Fig. 7-12). All the lesions appear to be recent and of about the same age. Granulation tissue is often not present in membranous bronchioles, and at times may not even be seen in respiratory bronchioles (Davison et al, 1983), and this should not be a deterrent to the diagnosis of BOOP. Interstitial pneu-

TABLE 7–3

BRONCHIOLITIS OBLITERANS–ORGANIZING PNEUMONIA AND USUAL INTERSTITIAL PNEUMONIA*

	BOOP	UIP
Average age (yr)	57	55
Duration of symptoms	3 mo	2 yr
Dyspnea	50%	100%
Fever	58%	13%
Respiratory infection	21%	0%
Clubbing	15%	60%
Restrictive lung disease	50%	100%
Decreased diffusing capacity	50%	100%
Chest radiograph		
Airspace opacities	70%	0%
Interstitial opacities	38%	100%
Outcome		
Resolution	40%	0%
Residual disease	33%	31%
Death of disease	12.5%	62.5%
Mean survival to death	2.7 mo.	15 mo.

*Modified with permission from Davison AG, Heard BE, McAllister WC, Turner-Warwick MEH. Cryptogenic organizing pneumonitis. Q J Med 1983; 52(new series), No. 207:382–393. Epler GR, Colby TV, McLoud TC, et al. Bronchiolitis obliterans-organizing pneumonia. N Engl J Med 1985; 312:152–158; and Katzenstein A-LA, Myers JL, Prophet WD, et al. Bronchiolitis obliterans and usual interstitial pneumonia: a comparative clinicopathologic study. Am J Surg Pathol 1986b; 10:373–381.

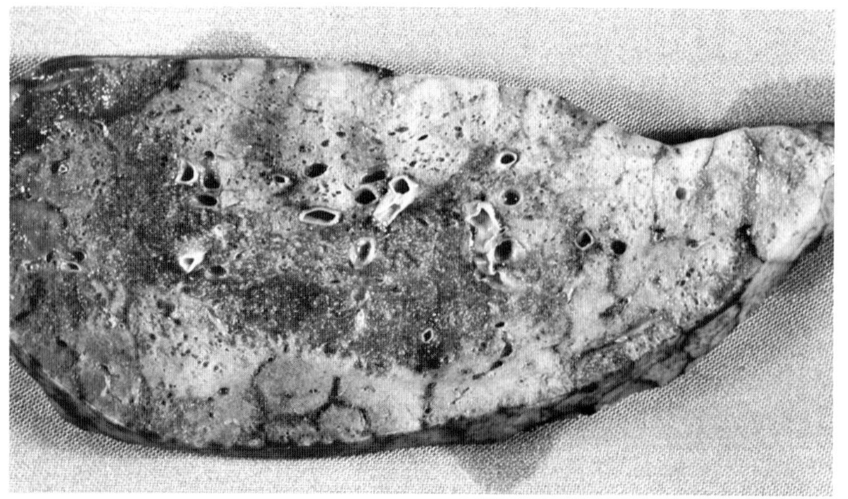

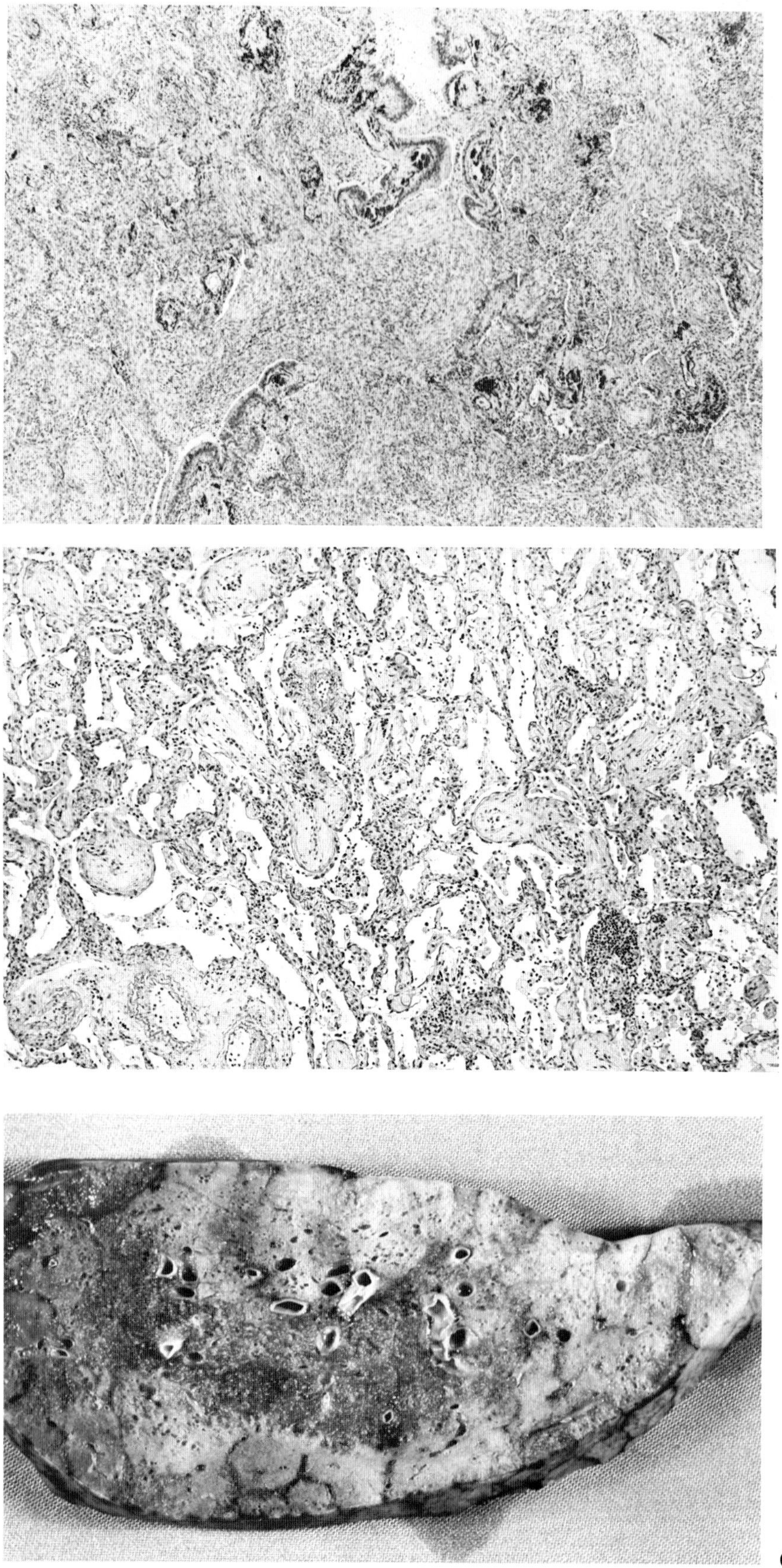

Figure 7–12 COP/BOOP: *A*, involving level of proximal respiratory bronchiole with branching of granulation tissue; *B*, involving level of alveolar ducts; and *C*, gross appearance showing peripheral distribution of fleshy infiltrates with minimal fibrosis.

TABLE 7–4

BRONCHIOLITIS OBLITERANS–ORGANIZING PNEUMONIA AND USUAL INTERSTITIAL PNEUMONIA*

	BOOP	UIP
Distribution of Lesions	Patchy, peribronchiolar	Diffuse, random
Location of Lesion	Dominantly airspaces	Predominantly interstitial
Temporal Appearance	Uniform, recent	Varying ages
Type of Fibrosis	Fibroblastic	Mainly collagen
Honeycombing	Unusual	Common
Foamy Macrophages	Common	Unusual

*Modified with permission from Katzenstein A-LA, Myers JL, Prophet WD, et al. Bronchiolitis obliterans and usual interstitial pneumonia: a comparative clinicopathologic study. Am J Surg Pathol 1986b; 10:373–381.

monia and type-II cell metaplasia are common, but extensive interstitial fibrosis is uncommon, and honeycombing is quite unusual. Obstruction of bronchioles may produce endogenous lipid ("golden or cholesterol") pneumonia. Vascular changes are slight.

Pathologically, the differential diagnosis is primarily with UIP. The distinction is generally easy, but discrepancies may occur even between expert pathologists, such as in the NIH Interstitial Lung Disease clinical trial. The difficulty arises when there is exuberant granulation tissue present, but it is not clear whether this is within the airspaces or in alveolar walls. As indicated previously, we suspect the latter were the cases originally described under the title BIP. Distinguishing morphologic features between UIP and BOOP are listed in Table 7-4.

The etiology is unknown. The histology suggests an infectious process, but infectious agents are usually not found. One case of COP and *Nocardia asteroides* infection has been reported (Camp et al, 1987). COP has also been found in patients treated with acebutolol and amiodarone (Camus et al, 1989) and with gold (Fort et al, 1988). COP has also been reported in patients with ulcerative colitis (Swinburn et al, 1988; Williams et al, 1982); this may have been due to medication as the patients were treated with either sulfasalazine or mesalazine. COP has also been described in association with free-base cocaine use (Patel et al, 1987). Thus, it may be that COP is a response to a variety of injuries to the lung.

NEUROFIBROMATOSIS (VON RECKLINGHAUSEN'S DISEASE)

Diffuse lung disease is seen in about 10 percent of all patients with neurofibromatosis and in about 20 percent of those who are over the age of 30. At least 31 cases have been reported in some detail (Webb and Goodman, 1977). Pulmonary involvement appears to be radiologically characteristic, with the presence of a mixture of linear or nodular opacities, particularly in the lower zones of the lung, and large bullae in the upper zones of the lungs. Diffuse interstitial fibrosis was present radiologically in 21 of the 31 reported cases, and bullae were present in 26. Bullae may rupture with consequent spontaneous pneumothorax. The functional pattern is of either restrictive or obstructive lung disease, depending on whether the bullous process or interstitial fibrotic lung disease dominates. The morphologic features of the lung lesions have not been described in detail but appear not to differ from those of classic UIP, although hyperplasia of the neurilemmal cells of intrapulmonary nerves and formation of glomus-like structures in small branches of the pulmonary arteries are described. Patients with bullae, but without radiologic evidence of interstitial fibrosis, may have histologic evidence of UIP (Massaro et al, 1966). Webb and Goodman (1977) described adenocarcinoma arising in fibrosing alveolitis and neurofibromatosis, presumably as a reflection of the increased frequency of carcinoma in pulmonary fibrosis.

SARCOIDOSIS

Sarcoidosis is a systemic disorder with both intrathoracic and extrathoracic granulomatous inflammation which is typically noncaseating. The etiology of the disease is unknown. It is much more common in black populations than most white populations (Hunninghake, 1986). Familial cases are described (Thomas and Hunninghake, 1987). Infection by acid-fast organisms and viruses and various environmentally encountered substances have been postulated as the etiology. A sarcoid-like reaction to malignancy is well known, and a few patients with malignancy seem to develop sarcoidosis following successful treatment (Abdi et al, 1987). Hunninghake

(1986) and Thomas and Hunninghake (1987) have reviewed the considerable amount of research concerning the immunology of sarcoid, and the interrelationships of the participating cells are complex. It has been suggested that the tissue reaction begins with an accumulation of helper T lymphocytes and monocytes in the alveolar wall. Subsequently, suppressor T cells and an appreciable number of B lymphocytes may be found in less active lesions (Daniele, 1986). Since over 90 percent of patients have intrathoracic involvement, the staging of the disease is based on radiologic involvement. Type-I sarcoidosis is defined as radiologic hilar/mediastinal adenopathy only, type-II as hilar/mediastinal and parenchymal involvement, and type-III by parenchymal involvement only. In general, the disease usually either resolves or improves, and only 5 to 10 percent of patients develop life threatening pulmonary fibrosis. Type-I patients are most likely to have a favorable outcome, type-III patients are most likely to progress, and type-II patients are intermediate. Acute onset and erythema nodosum are associated with favorable prognosis, independent of each other.

Sarcoidosis in the lung is characterized by the presence of noncaseating granulomas distributed in the lymphatics of the bronchovascular bundles, interlobular septa, and pleura (Fig. 7–13). The alveolitis that is postulated etiologically is not characteristic histologically; rather, the alveoli not involved by the granulomas are relatively normal. Occasional foci of necrosis within the granulomas are seen, and asteroid and Schaumann bodies within giant cells are common but not diagnostic. In spite of the presence of granulomas around pleural lymphatics, radiologically evident pleural effusion or pleural thickening is seen in less than 10 percent of cases (Wilen et al, 1974). Involvement of arteries and veins, separately or together is seen in the majority of cases.

The plain chest radiograph in 60 to 70 percent of patients with sarcoidosis has a typical appearance, showing enlarged bilateral hilar and paratracheal lymph nodes with or without concomitant parenchymal changes (Scadding and Mitchell, 1985). In 25 to

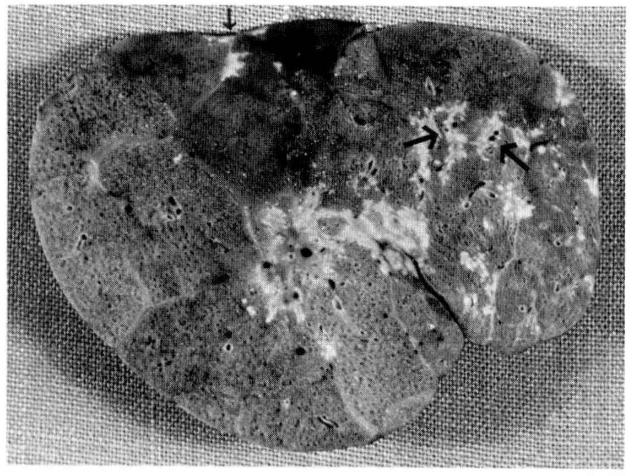

A

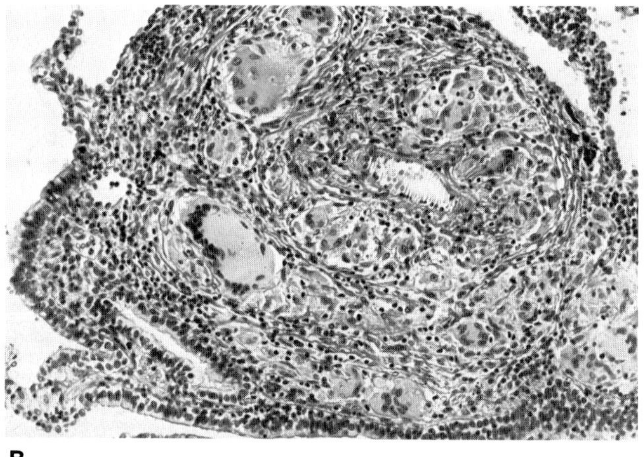

B

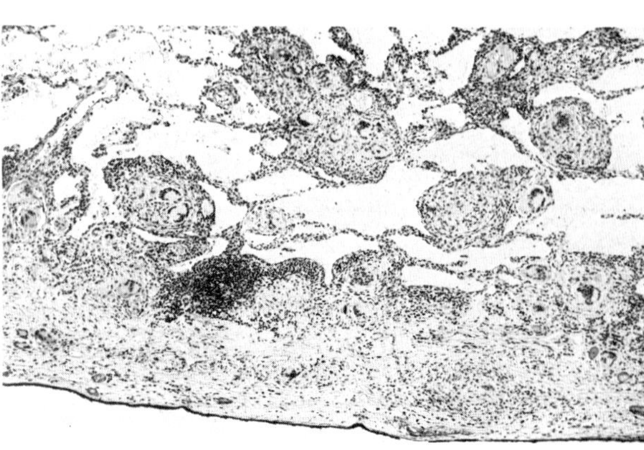

C

Figure 7–13 Sarcoidosis. *A,* Grossly characterized by nodules and linear infiltrates following bronchovascular bundles (*long arrows*), pleural and interlobular septa (*short arrows*). Well-formed noncaseating granulomas in bronchiolar mucosa (*B*) and pleura (*C*).

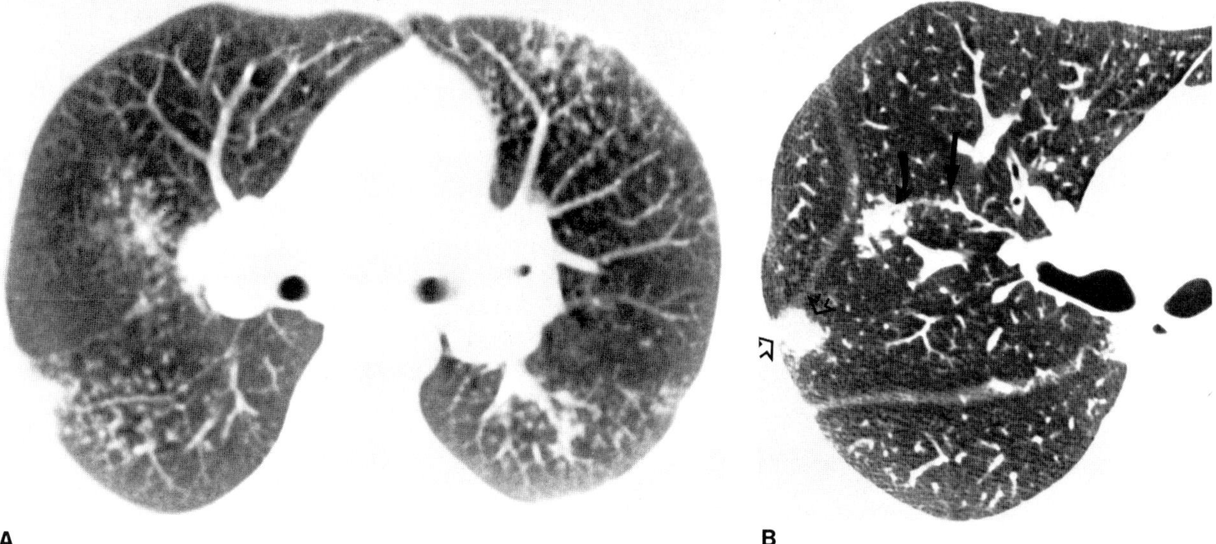

A   **B**

Figure 7–14   *A*, 10-mm collimation CT in a patient with sarcoidosis. The sarcoid granulomas are seen as small nodules situated predominantly along the bronchovascular bundles resembling leaves on a tree. A conglomerate of subpleural granulomas is present in the right lower lobe. Also noted is marked bilateral hilar and subcarinal lymphadenopathy. *B*, High-resolution CT at the level of the right minor fissure in a patient with mild, localized parenchymal changes due to sarcoidosis. A few localized granulomas can be seen closely associated with a pulmonary artery, giving it a beaded appearance (*arrow*). Several granulomas can be seen near branches of the same vessel (*curved arrow*). An irregular nodule, presumably representing a conglomerate of small granulomas, is present subpleurally (*open arrows*).

30 percent of cases, however, the radiologic findings are nonspecific, and in 5 to 10 percent of patients the radiograph is normal. The characteristic juxtalymphatic distribution of disease is usually difficult to appreciate on the radiograph but can be seen on CT (Müller et al, 1989) (Fig. 7–14). CT scan often allows a confident diagnosis even when the radiographic findings are nonspecific (Mathieson et al, 1989). As would be expected from the distribution of granulomas, pulmonary fibrosis due to sarcoidosis also has a predominantly peribronchovascular distribution (Fig. 7–15). In severe cases the chest radiograph shows a characteristic appearance of dense areas of fibrosis extending from the hila to the upper and mid lung zones (Fig. 7–16). Because of the tendency for peribronchial involvement, sarcoidosis is one of the few types of diffuse infiltrative lung diseases in which the presumptive diagnosis can be confirmed by transbronchial biopsy with a high degree of success (Carrington and Gaensler, 1978). Roethe et al (1980) took five biopsies from the upper lobe and five from the lower lobe in 37 patients and made a positive diagnosis in 36 of 37 patients and in all of ten patients with stage-1 disease (i.e., without radiologic evidence of parenchymal involvement).

In 1973 Liebow described a disease he termed "necrotizing sarcoid granulomatosis." The histologic criteria included granulomatosis or giant cell vascu-

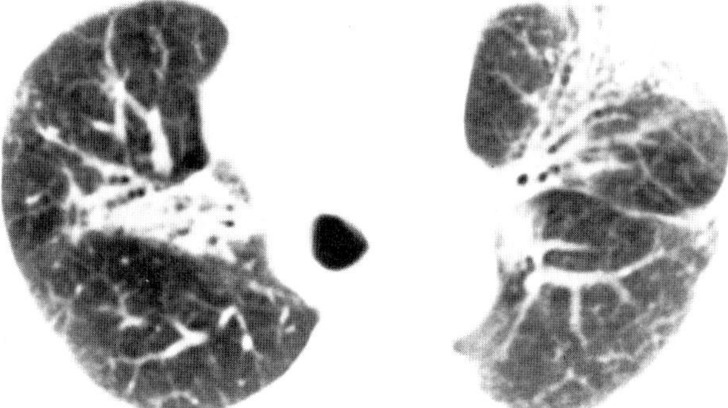

Figure 7–15   Patient with pulmonary fibrosis due to sarcoidosis. CT scan shows the fibrosis to be situated predominantly along the bronchovascular bundles. It can also be seen that the distribution of the fibrosis is patchy: while some areas have extensive fibrosis, others appear normal.

litis, variable parenchymal necrosis with or without cavitation, and sarcoid-like granulomas that often show central necrosis. He emphasized that various types of angiitis occurred, including extensive granulomatous inflammation with occlusion of vessels, granulomas around the external elastic lamella, simulating temporal arteritis, and a mononuclear infiltrative and occlusive vasculitis. The clinical presentation and radiologic findings were variable; hilar adenopathy and extrathoracic involvement were unu-

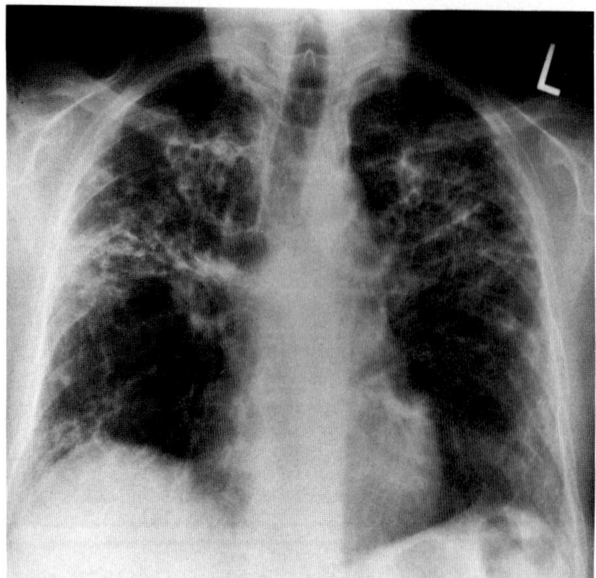

Figure 7–16 Chest radiograph in a patient with severe pulmonary fibrosis shows linear bands radiating from the hila to the upper and mid lung zones. This distribution is characteristic of end-stage sarcoidosis and reflects the distribution of disease predominantly along the bronchovascular bundles.

sual. In contrast to other forms of pulmonary angiitis, the patients tend to do well with surgical, steroid, or even no therapy (Koss et al, 1980; Singh et al, 1981; Leavitt et al, 1986). One report suggested that necrotizing sarcoid granulomatosis may be a hypersensitivity reaction to *Aspergillus* (Koss et al, 1980), but Churg (1983), Singh et al (1981), and Leavitt et al, (1986) viewed it as a variant of sarcoidosis. It is described in further detail on p. 176, where the case is made for the retention of the name in at least some cases.

EXTRINSIC ALLERGIC ALVEOLITIS

Lung disease can result from inhalation of various vegetable and animal dusts, but the lesions and the clinical syndromes may not be identical. In the majority, the disease is immunologically mediated, although the immunologic mechanisms have not been well documented in all conditions (Salvaggio and Karr, 1979). Cell-mediated (type IV) hypersensitivity reactions and possibly immune complex (type III) reactions are pathogenetically important (Fink, 1986; Salvaggio and deShazo, 1986). The prototypical example is "farmer's lung," which is the best studied. It is more common in Britain and Europe than in North America and is caused by hypersensitivity to

thermophilic actinomycetes (*Micromonospora vulgaris* and *Thermophylliae polyspora*) that grow in moldy hay. In North America, *Micropolyspora faeni* is the most common. Farmer's lung is most prevalent when the summers are wet. Cut hay is not gathered until it is dry, and thus there may be considerable multiplication of the organisms in the hay in the intervening period. The farmer is then exposed to the moldy hay, usually during winter feeding in an enclosed space. Symptoms appear a few hours later and consist of fever, malaise, cough, and dyspnea. Wheezing is uncommon. The symptoms disappear and then may reappear when the patient is exposed again.

Radiologically, acute heavy exposure to the antigen causes diffuse airspace consolidation. This resolves within a few days, after which a characteristic fine nodular appearance can often be seen (Cook et al, 1988). The nodules measure up to 3 mm in diameter and tend to spare the lung bases. On CT, small, poorly defined nodules are seen at this stage as well as areas of ground-glass increased density (Fig. 7–17). Repeated exposure to the antigen may lead to the chronic stage of interstitial fibrosis, which is often more severe in the upper lobes. The radiographic features are nonspecific, but occasionally the correct diagnosis can be suggested on CT (Silver et al, 1989).

The acute symptoms may be minimal or not be recognized in some patients and the patients develop progressive dyspnea. Functionally, restrictive lung disease occurs. Precipitating antibodies to the organic dust antigen are found in a higher proportion of subjects compared with nonaffected workers in the same environment (Fink, 1986).

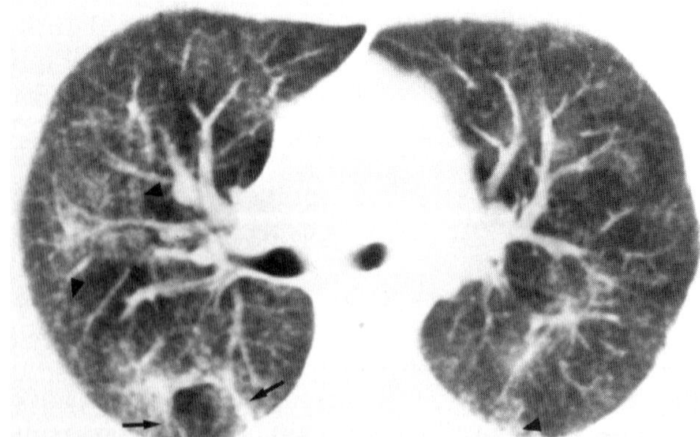

Figure 7–17 Extrinsic allergic alveolitis in a 31-year-old man. Ground-glass areas of increased density are present bilaterally, as well as numerous small, ill-defined nodules (*arrowheads*). The linear densities posteriorly on the right side (*arrows*) presumably represent fibrosis.

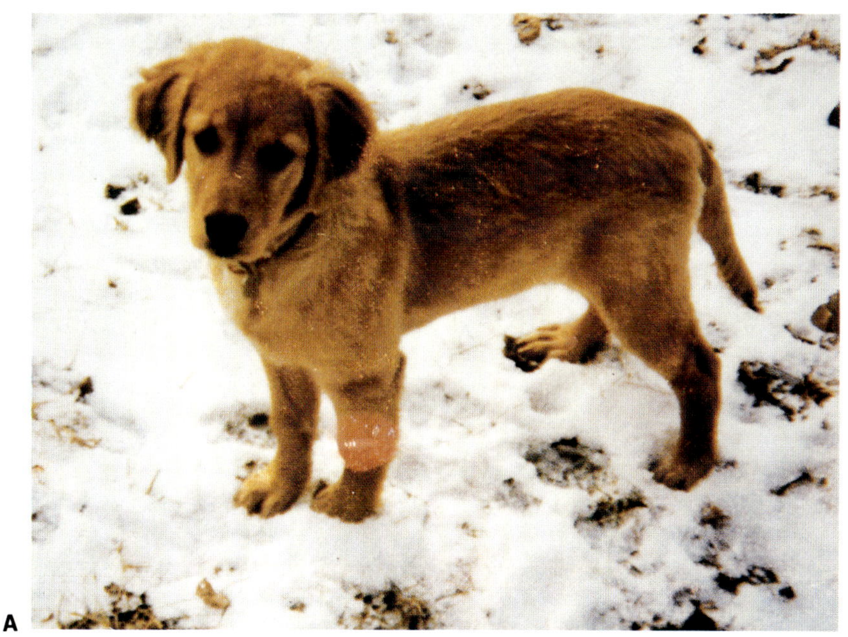

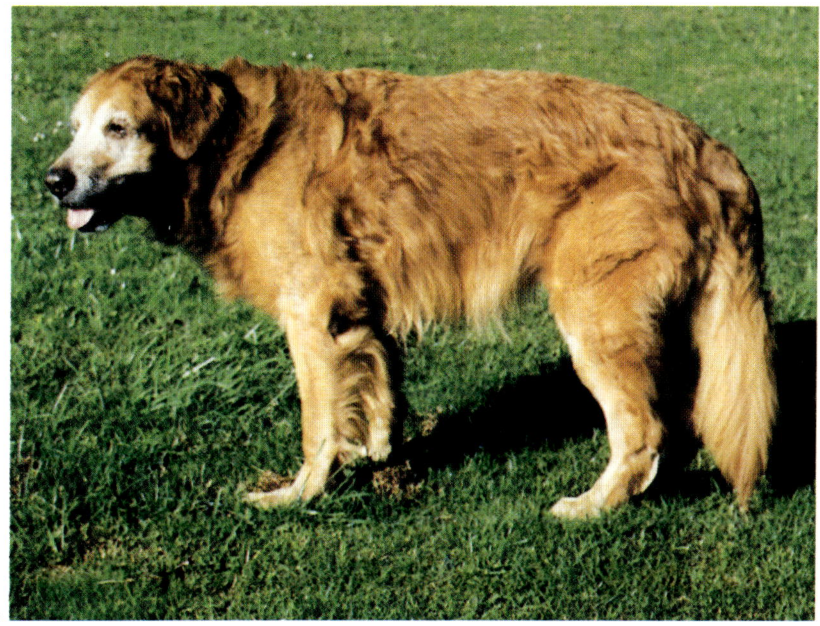

Color Plate   Biologic system ("Christie") showing dramatic morphologic changes over time (3 months [*A*] compared with 12 years [*B*] of age). Perhaps the morphologic differences between DIP and UIP are analogous to this phenomenon.

The histologic features of extrinsic allergic alveolitis (EAA) are similar, regardless of the organic dust responsible, but vary according to the stage at which the disease is seen. Most biopsies are taken in the subacute phase, and it is this stage that is best described histologically (Coleman and Colby, 1988). Lung structure is generally intact, so that alveoli can usually be distinguished. The dominant lesion is chronic interstitial pneumonia with lymphocytes and plasma cells in alveolar walls. Scattered, poorly formed granulomas are seen in the interstitium, which are noncaseating but more ill defined than sarcoid granulomas. The epithelioid cells are loosely arranged and mixed with lymphocytes. Very characteristically, the granulomas contain some giant cells of the foreign-body type and may contain cleft-like spaces or small doubly refractile particles, the exact nature of which is not known (Fig. 7–18). The third component of the histologic reaction is a cellular bronchiolitis of bronchioles, respiratory bronchioles, and sometimes alveolar ducts. The bronchiolitis is

also mononuclear in type. Lipid-laden macrophages may be found in alveolar spaces in the event of bronchiolar obstruction. In the series of Coleman and Colby (1988), each component of this triad was found in all 41 cases to a variable degree. Reyes et al (1982) described an interstitial infiltrate in all of their cases, granulomas in 70 percent, bronchiolitis obliterans in 50 percent, and lipid laden macrophages in 65 percent.

Few cases of EAA in the acute stages have been examined histologically. One patient has been described who died 10 to 12 days after the onset of symptoms (Barrowcliff and Arblaster, 1968). There was an acute respiratory bronchiolitis with destruction of the bronchiolar walls, fibrin thrombi in adjacent alveolar walls, and an infiltrate of neutrophils, eosinophils, and mononuclear cells. As EAA becomes chronic, fibrosis occurs with distortion of lung architecture, varying degrees of end-stage lung, and occasionally extensive pleural fibrosis. At this stage, the lesions may not be distinguishable from those of

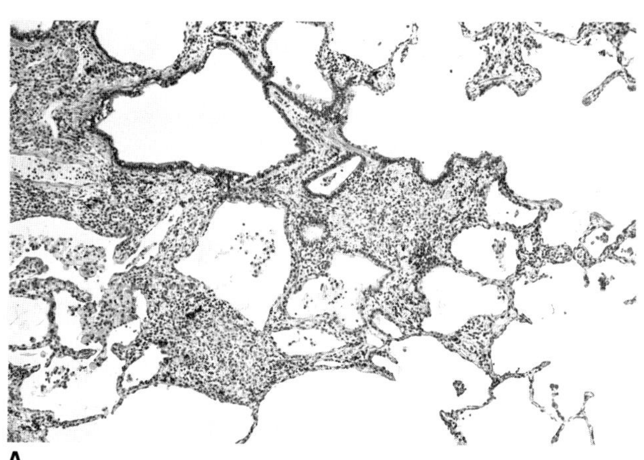

A

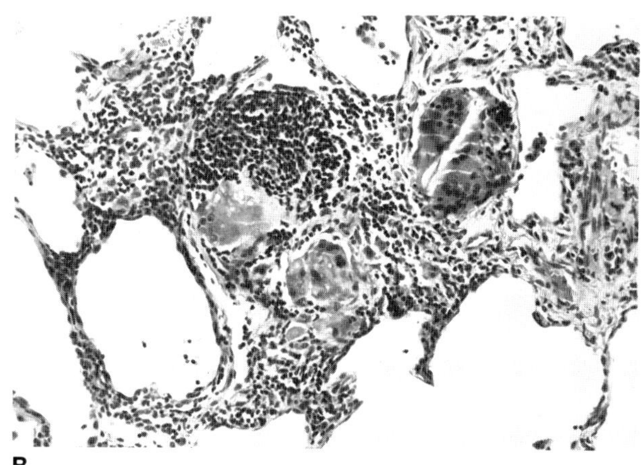

B

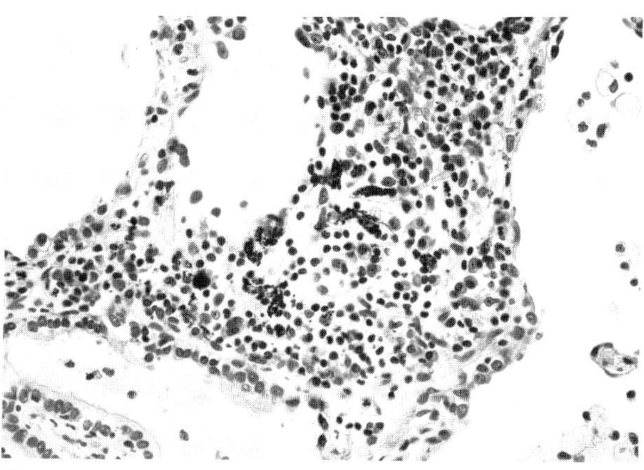

C

Figure 7–18   Extrinsic allergic alveolitis: *A*, lymphocytic and plasmacellular interstitial infiltrate; *B*, poorly formed granulomas with cholesterol clefts in giant cells; and *C*, mononuclear cell bronchiolitis.

fibrosing alveolitis, since the lymphocytic infiltrate diminishes and granulomas may not be apparent.

The clinical syndrome and lesions in avian allergic alveolitis are similar to those of farmer's lung. The allergens are bird proteins, and precipitating antibodies to extracts of feathers, droppings, serum, and egg white may be present in the blood (Moore et al, 1974). The condition has been found in pigeon breeders, pigeon racers, poultry farmers, and owners of parakeets. Extrinsic allergic alveolitis may also result from multiplication of thermophilic actinomycetes in humidifiers and air conditioners (Fink et al, 1971). This is an easily overlooked cause of extrinsic allergic alveolitis because no history of occupational exposure can be elicited.

It is probable that allergic alveolitis is similar in several other conditions, but the lesions and the serum findings are not fully described. These include pituitary snuff takers' lung (Mahon et al, 1967), furriers' lung, maple-bark strippers' lung (Emanuel et al, 1962), suberosis (cork workers' lung) (Pimental and Avila, 1973), sequoisis or redwood workers' lung (Cohen et al, 1967) and malt workers' lung (Grant et al, 1976). In maple-bark strippers' lung, granulomas containing spores of *Cryptostami (Coniosporum) corticale* are seen, although the condition is thought to result from hypersensitivity to the spores rather than from a direct effect. In sequoisis, foreign-body giant cells are described that contain doubly refractile material that dissolves during tissue processing. Lamellar bodies have been described resembling Schaumann bodies, which contain a central particle of redwood dust. Thesaurosis is sometimes thought of as a member of this group, although there is some question whether it exists, and it is not clear whether it is a form of allergic alveolitis. Thesaurosis is considered to be a result of inhalation of hair spray (Bergmann et al, 1962). The original description stressed the finding of alveolar macrophages containing PAS-positive material, together with interstitial granulomas resembling sarcoid. Epidemiologic studies showed no increased frequency of lung disease in hairdressers, who are most likely to have excess exposure to hair spray, and thus some do not believe that the condition exists (Gowdy and Wagstaff, 1972). However, one of us (WT) has seen two cases, in which the lung lesions appeared directly related to inhalation of hair spray and disappeared after cessation of exposure. The course of the disease and the lung lesions closely resembled sarcoid rather than allergic alveolitis.

Two relatively common conditions have features similar to extrinsic allergic alveolitis. Bagassosis is a lung disease caused by inhalation of sugar cane after the sugar has been extracted. The residue, bagasse, is compressed for various industrial uses, and the disease probably results from hypersensitivity to fungal spores that multiply during the storage of bagasse. Almost 50 percent of the workers exposed to high levels of bagasse develop symptoms resembling those of allergic alveolitis, and radiologic changes are more extensive in the upper zones of the lung (Spencer, 1977). Antibodies to thermophilic actinomycetes occur in about two thirds of the patients with bagassosis (Salvaggio et al, 1969). Lung lesions resemble those of extrinsic allergic alveolitis in the early stages, and giant cells containing spindle- and rod-shaped particles are found. Electron microscopically, bacteria and fungi in varying degrees of dissolution and undergoing phagocytosis are seen (Spencer, 1977). In the later stages of the disease, there is both extensive pulmonary fibrosis and emphysema.

Byssinosis results from inhalation of cotton dust, but the relationship to allergic alveolitis is far from established. The clinical features differ in that bronchoconstriction is a prominent feature and is found at the beginning of the work week and diminishes over the succeeding days. There is no serologic evidence for sensitivity to cotton dust, and extracts of the cotton bract of pods contain a substance that causes histamine release (Hitchcock et al, 1973). The lesions of the lung are not well described but the infiltrates appear different from those of allergic alveolitis. There is extensive lung pigmentation and peribronchial fibrosis with bronchial distortion, together with fibrous nodules throughout the lung. "Byssinosis bodies" have been described in the nodules. They are large, approximately 200 by 50 μm, with a central birefringent hematoxophil core that possibly represents a cotton fiber (Ruttner et al, 1968). The fiber is coated with brown, iron-containing pigment.

In cases in which occupational exposure is obvious, the diagnosis of EAA is ordinarily made without resorting to biopsy. Nevertheless, an occasional patient seemingly without relevant environmental exposure will have an open lung biopsy showing the typical findings of EAA. In the series of Coleman and Colby (1988), the causative antigen was identified in retrospect in only 37 percent of cases. Failure to identify the responsible agent did not appear to have adverse prognostic significance.

EOSINOPHILIC GRANULOMA

Eosinophilic granuloma (EG) of the lung has been considered to be one of the manifestations of "histiocytosis X," with the Hand-Schüller-Christian syndrome and Letterer-Siwe disease being the more severe variants. The feature common to them is proliferation of a particular type of histiocyte, at one time termed the "X cell" (Basset et al, 1976b). The "X cell" has been found to have immunologic and ultrastructural characteristics of Langerhans cells of the epidermis, and thus EG is more properly viewed as an infiltrative lung disease of Langerhans cells. Whether the nature of the disease is inflammatory or neoplastic is unresolved, and its precise relationship to the Hand-Schüller-Christian syndrome and Letterer-Siwe disease is uncertain.

EG is confined to the lung in about 80 percent of cases. Identical histologic lesions may be seen in the bones or elsewhere in the body, thus suggesting overlap with Hand-Schüller-Christian syndrome or Letterer-Siwe disease. Isolated involvement of the lung can occur at any age but is most common in young men (Lewis, 1964). Spontaneous pneumothorax is the presenting complaint in about 20 percent of cases; the patients usually have systemic complaints such as malaise, dyspnea and weight loss, and many have fever. The prognosis is not certain, and there is no series large enough to determine this precisely. It is regarded as favorable in perhaps three-fourths of patients with lesions limited to the lung by some (Colby and Lombard, 1983), but others have suggested that the prognosis is less favorable (Basset et al, 1978). Involvement of bones or systemic involvement carries with it a poorer prognosis.

Radiologically EG presents with nodules ranging from a few millimeters to over 1 cm in diameter, or a reticulonodular pattern with fine honeycombing (Friedman et al, 1981). The nodules have irregular margins and often a stellate appearance. The process is usually more severe in the upper and middle lung zones and is associated with normal or increased lung volumes (Friedman et al, 1981; Lacronique et al, 1982). On CT most patients have extensive honeycombing, the cystic airspaces usually measuring less than 10 mm in diameter, and many have nodules 1 to 5 mm in diameter (Moore et al, 1989) (Fig. 7–19). The nodules may have lucent centers.

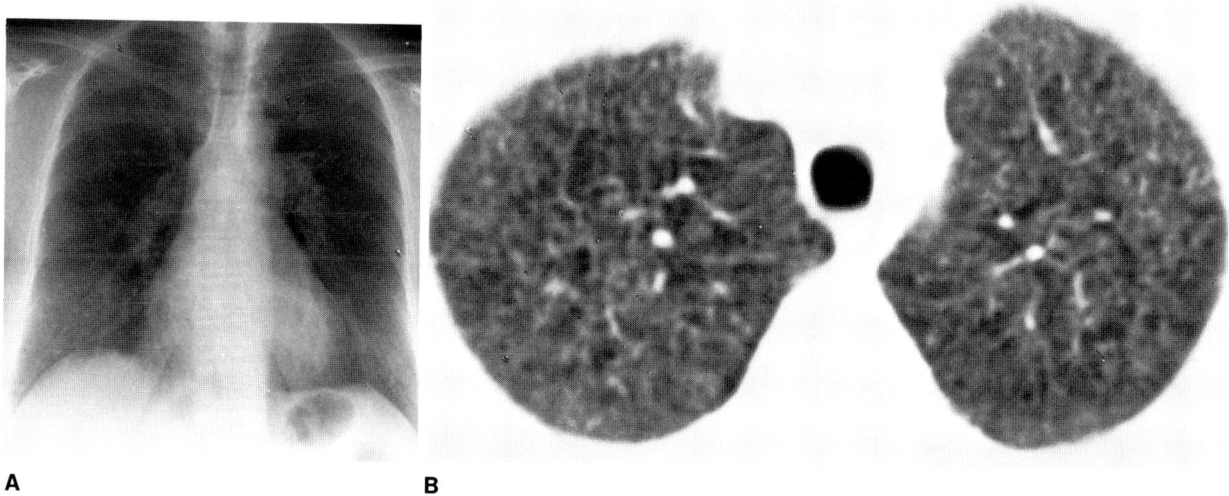

A   B

Figure 7–19   Severe, longstanding histiocytosis X in a 49-year-old woman. *A*, Chest radiograph shows evidence of pulmonary arterial hypertension. The parenchymal abnormalities appear to be mild on the radiograph and consist of irregular linear and a few nodular opacities, giving a reticulonodular appearance. *B*, 10-mm collimation CT scan immediately above the level of the aortic arch shows extensive bilateral changes. They involve the lungs diffusely at this level. On the conventional CT the findings appear to consist predominantly of ill-defined nodular densities. *C*, High resolution CT shows that the parenchymal changes consist of irregular linear densities and fine honeycombing. While the findings on the chest radiograph appear to be mild, it can be seen here that there is severe fibrosis and diffuse fine honeycombing. This patient illustrates the need to complement conventional radiography with CT and the need to complement conventional CT with several high-resolution images to assess the lung parenchyma adequately.

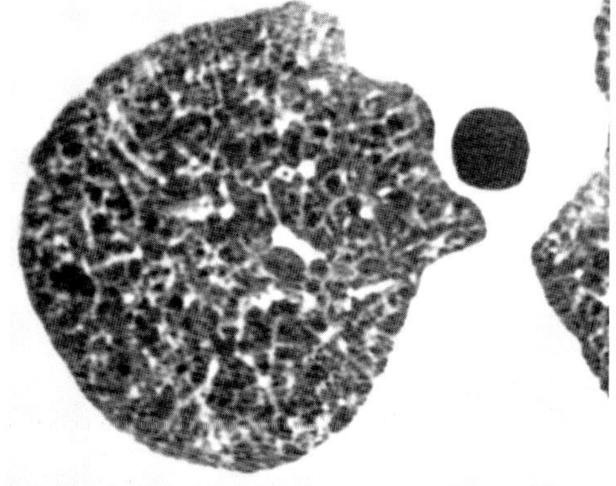

C

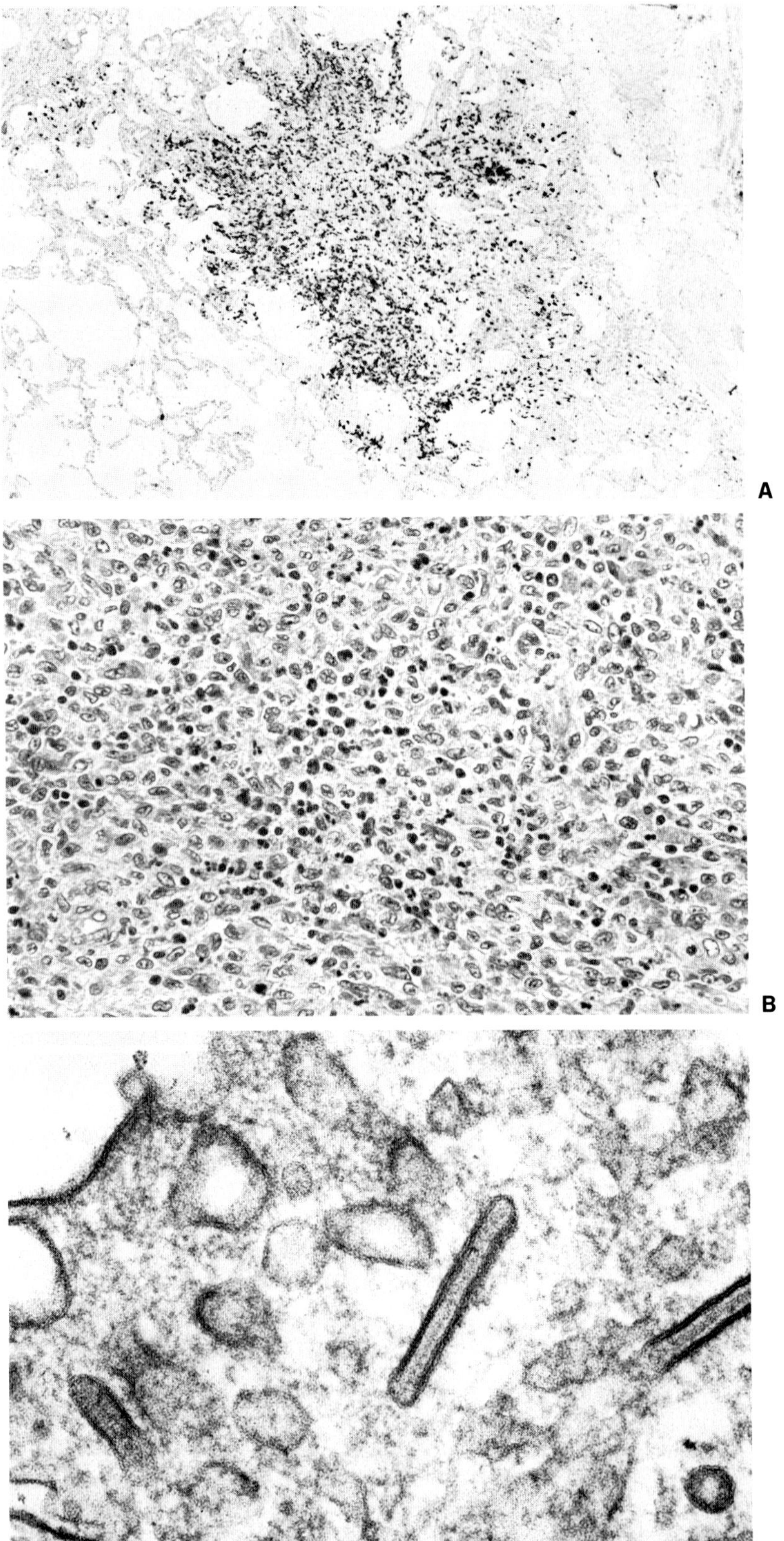

Figure 7–20 Eosinophilic granuloma. *A*, S100 stains highlight the stellate nature of an active lesion. *B*, cellular infiltrate consists of Langerhans histiocytes and eosinophils in early lesions. *C*, linear Birbeck granule in cytoplasm of Langerhans histiocyte.

In early cases, the nodules of EG are irregularly dispersed, affecting the proximal and distal parts of the acinus. Distal acinar subpleural involvement is the cause of spontaneous pneumothorax. Proximal acinar involvement may compress pulmonary arteries and bronchioles, leading to pulmonary hypertension and obstructive dysfunction.

The nodules of eosinophilic granuloma have irregular margins and a stellate shape (Fig. 7–20). In early stages, there is an admixture of eosinophils and Langerhans-type histiocytes. The latter cells have an indented nucleus with one or two nucleoli, and an abundant, finely vacuolated or faintly eosinophilic cytoplasm. These cells have characteristic ultrastructural cytoplasmic inclusions termed Birbeck granules, which consist of linear- or racket-shaped bodies continuous with the external cell membrane. The cells are strongly positive with immunoperoxidase stains for S100 protein. In addition to the eosinophils and Langerhans histiocytes, there is an admixture of lymphocytes, macrophages, and fibroblasts within the nodules of EG.

As the disease progresses, the eosinophils (eosinophils are absent in 20 to 30 percent of cases) and finally the Langerhans histiocytes disappear, and one is left with nonspecific fibrosis and cyst formation (Brody et al, 1974). At this point a definitive diagnosis may be impossible, although there are two clues to the diagnosis even in inactive cases. One clue is the stellate nature of the inactive scars (Fig. 7–21) and the other is the striking tendency to pan-upper-zonal honeycomb fibrosis with basal sparing.

The usual method of tissue diagnosis is open lung biopsy, since transbronchial biopsies are unlikely to be useful and may lead to an erroneous diagnosis of DIP due to the common phenomenon of a localized, severe, DIP-like reaction immediately adjacent to the nodules. It has been suggested (Hammar et al, 1978) that EG can be diagnosed by the finding of Langerhans histiocytes in sputum. This may not be so since these cells may be found in a variety of interstitial lung diseases (Kawanami et al, 1981) including UIP, DIP, collagen-vascular disease, extrinsic allergic alveolitis, and end-stage fibrosis. Webber et al (1985) also found that while in active EG there were more S100 positive cells present, the number of such cells were comparable between less active EG lesions and other forms of infiltrative lung disease. Langerhans cells also occur in the stroma of bronchoalveolar carcinoma (Hammar et al, 1986). Not

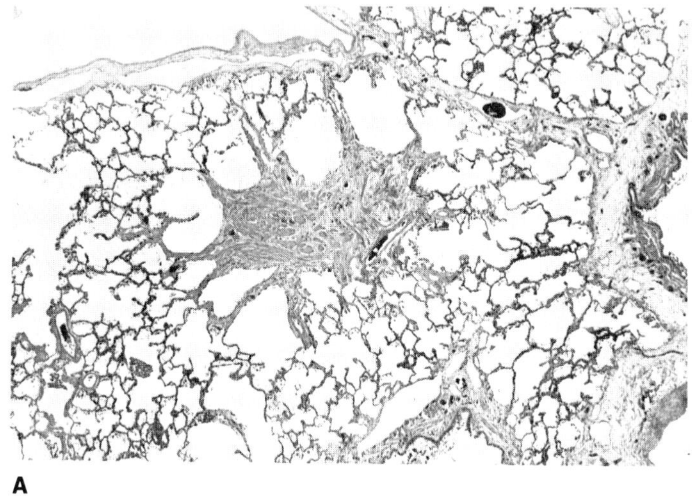

A

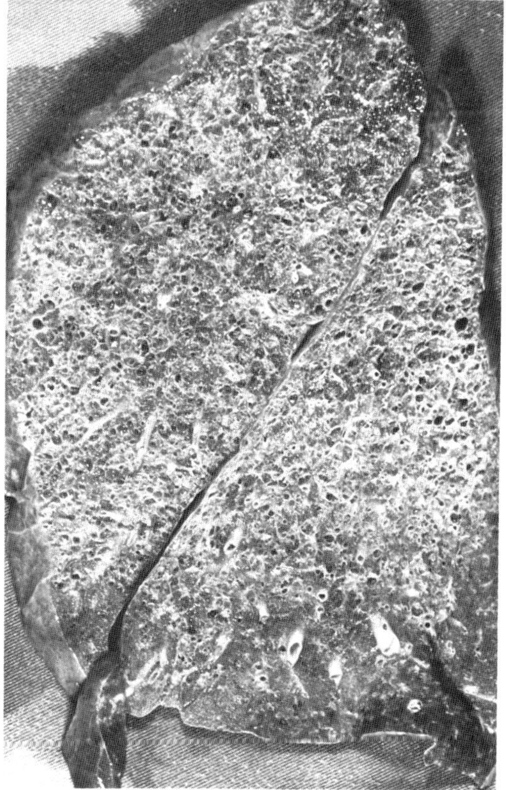

B

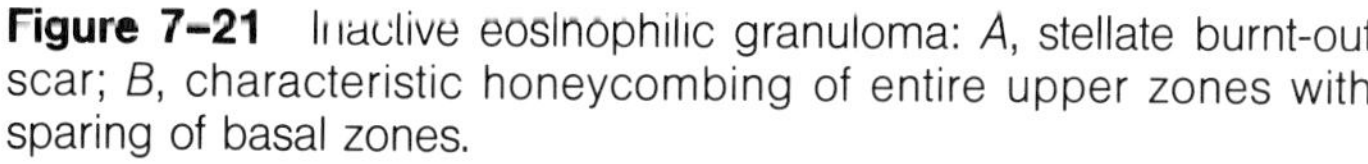

Figure 7–21 Inactive eosinophilic granuloma: *A*, stellate burnt-out scar; *B*, characteristic honeycombing of entire upper zones with sparing of basal zones.

only is the simple presence of Langerhans histiocytes in the lung not diagnostic of EG, but other cells within the lung stain positively for S100 protein, including myoepithelial cells of the tracheobronchial glands, cells of bronchial-associated lymphoid tissue, and cartilage. Thus, as is the case for most of the interstitial lung diseases, the pattern of lung involvement is as important as cytologic details in establishing the diagnosis of EG. An additional potential source of misdiagnosis in EG is eosinophilic infiltration of the pleura following an episode of spontaneous pneumothorax in young adults (Askin et al, 1977). In spontaneous pneumothorax, the eosinophilic infiltrate may extend into the underlying lung, which is usually fibrotic, but the absence of collections of Langerhans histiocytes and the presence of severe pleural reaction in spontaneous pneumothorax should be guides to the correct diagnosis. This is self limiting and should not be considered a *forme fruste* of EG.

TUBEROUS SCLEROSIS AND LYMPHANGIOLEIOMYOMATOSIS

Pulmonary lymphangioleiomyomatosis (LAM) is a rare syndrome characterized by a bizarre proliferation of smooth muscle in the interstitium at all levels of the acinus. Intrathoracic nodal involvement and thoracic duct involvement are also common. While dyspnea is the most common presenting symptom, pneumothorax, hemoptysis and chylous pleural effusions each occur in about half of patients during the course of their illness. Mechanical explanations for these complications have been postulated (Corrin et al, 1975; Basset et al, 1976a): bronchiolar obstruction has been claimed to be the cause of the dilated airspaces, venous lesions may lead to intra-alveolar hemorrhage and hemosiderosis, and involvement of the thoracic duct and major pulmonary lymphatics may cause chylous pleural effusions. Pulmonary function abnormalities may be either restrictive or obstructive or a mixture of the two. Most patients die within 10 years of diagnosis.

LAM is usually confined to women of childbearing age (although we have seen one case first presenting in a 58-year-old woman [Fig. 7–22]). Because of this peculiarity, the possibility of hormonal influence has been raised. More recently, emphasis has been placed on hormone receptors in the proliferating cells (Brentani et al, 1984; Graham et al, 1984) and on estrogen suppression as a possible treatment (Svendsen et al, 1984).

Initially, the radiologic appearance is that of fine linear densities, mainly at the bases, which progress to honeycomb changes throughout the lungs. In con-

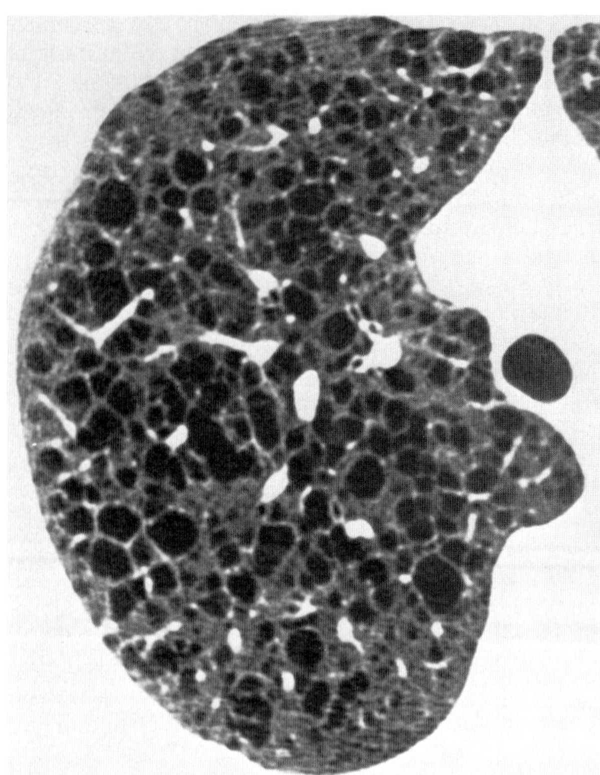

Figure 7–22   High-resolution CT in a 58-year-old woman with progressive shortness of breath. The diagnosis of lymphangioleiomyomatosis was first suggested by CT. The characteristic findings consist of cystic airspaces of various sizes with relatively normal intervening lung parenchyma. Even in retrospect the findings are difficult to appreciate on the chest radiograph.

trast to fibrosing alveolitis, lung volumes progressively increase radiologically. The pattern and extent of disease are easier to determine on CT (see Fig. 7–22). CT characteristically shows thin-walled cystic airspaces with normal intervening parenchyma (Templeton et al, 1989). The CT appearance is virtually pathognomonic, the only differential diagnostic consideration being eosinophilic granuloma.

The lung lesions are characterized by an "irrational" proliferation of smooth muscle involving all structures of the acinus, including bronchioles, vessels, lymphatics, and alveolar walls (Fig. 7–23). Widespread cystic change occurs throughout the lung with subpleural cysts grossly obvious in the event of open lung biopsy (see Fig. 7–23). Hemosiderosis is present in about half the cases. Lymphatic smooth muscle proliferation may lead to extrusion of lymph into alveoli, and dilated lymphatic channels may be apparent in the center of proliferations of smooth muscle. Ultrastructural examination of LAM has shown that

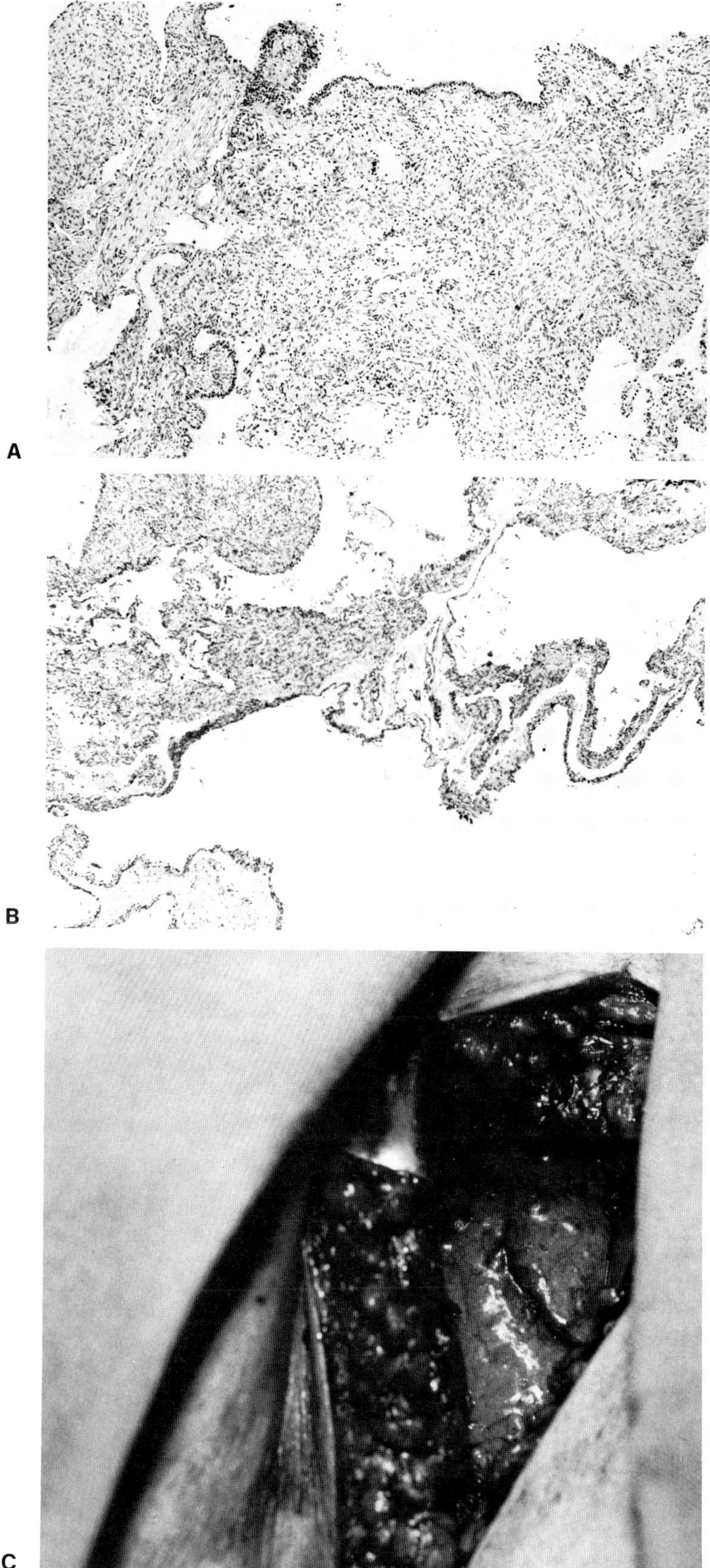

Figure 7–23 Lymphangioleiomyomatosis: bundles of smooth muscle proliferating in bronchiolar wall (*A*) and in cyst walls (*B*). *C*, Gross appearance at biopsy with multiple discrete cysts obvious on pleural surface.

the proliferating cells are primarily smooth muscle, with some admixed myofibroblasts and fibroblasts (Basset et al, 1976a).

The differential diagnosis includes UIP, in which extensive smooth muscle proliferation may occur in its later stages. However, this is accompanied by bronchiolectasis, type-II cell proliferation, fibrosis, and interstitial inflammation, none of which are features of LAM. The clinical course is different in that LAM is often associated with pleural effusion and pneumothorax. In "benign metastasizing leiomyomas" (see Chapter 9), the lesions are nodular and discrete, both pathologically and radiologically.

The relationship between tuberous sclerosis (TS) and LAM is not completely clear. The pulmonary lesions are identical although the syndrome of pulmonary LAM is quite different from TS (Corrin et al, 1975). The features of TS include dermal fibromas and angiofibromas, mental retardation, cerebral tumors, intracranial calcification, and seizures; none of these features are associated with pulmonary LAM. TS is familial in 25 percent of cases, whereas familial pulmonary LAM has not been described to date. Lung involvement occurs in only about 1 percent of patients with TS. TS has no sex predisposition. Nevertheless, there are obvious similarities between TS and LAM. Lung involvement in TS always occurs in female patients of childbearing age, and in these patients, the pathologic, clinical and radiologic changes are identical to those of LAM. Furthermore, renal angiomyolipomas are associated with both syndromes (Capron et al, 1983; Lack et al, 1986). The easiest concept is that TS and LAM represent variations of the same disease process, although it is not precise to regard lymphangiomyomatosis as a *forme fruste* of tuberous sclerosis.

EOSINOPHILIC PNEUMONIA

A number of different conditions have been described in which the airspaces of the lungs contain large numbers of eosinophils (Carrington et al, 1969; Liebow and Carrington, 1969b). It is better to think of them as variants of eosinophilic pneumonia than as separate disease entities. Löffler's syndrome is generally applied to the mildest form of the condition in which the patients are usually asymptomatic. The term "pulmonary infiltrates with eosinophilia" (PIE) has limitations because the same lung lesions and symptoms may occur with transient or even no blood eosinophilia. The presence of pulmonary infiltrates, often with eosinophilia, is well recognized in patients with asthma, and conversely 20 percent or more of patients with eosinophilic pneumonia have asthma. In the above-mentioned circumstances, the etiology of eosinophilic pneumonia is not known, but there are some well-recognized associations of eosinophilic pneumonia. The best examples include acute drug sensitivity to nitrofurantoin and other drugs. In some instances, these cases are referred to as hypersensitivity angiitis, and these should be regarded as a more specific cause of eosinophilic pneumonia (Table 7–5). Pulmonary infiltrates with peripheral eosinophilia are common in tropical countries and probably represent a reaction to migration of parasites through the lung. Eosinophilic pneumonia, usually with asthma, may be a manifestation of periarteritis nodosa (and this may or may not be the same as Churg-Strauss syndrome or allergic angiitis and granulomatosis; see Chapter 9). Finally, eosinophilic pneumonia, together with asthma, may be a manifestation of aspergillosis (allergic bronchopulmonary aspergillosis).

Patients with eosinophilic pneumonia often

TABLE 7–5

DRUGS CAUSING PULMONARY EOSINOPHILIA AND/OR POLYARTERITIS

	PULMONARY EOSINOPHILIA	POLYARTERITIS
Allopurinol		+
Aspirin	+	
Busulfan		+
Hydantoins		+
Hydralazine		+
Imipramine	+	
Iodides		+
Gold salts		+
Nitrofurantoin	+	+
Penicillins	+	+
Sulfonamides	+	+

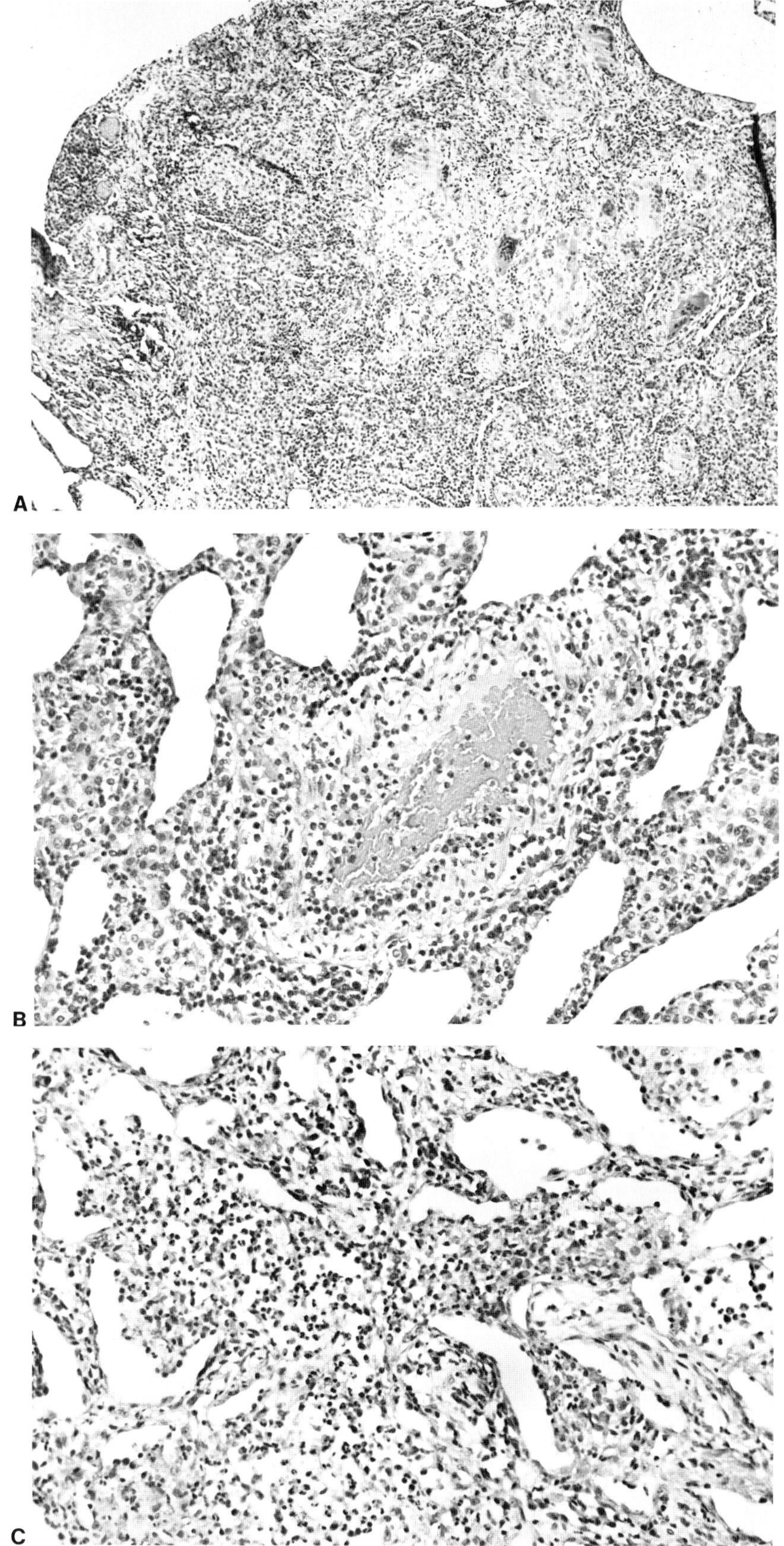

Figure 7–24 Eosinophilic pneumonia: *A*, sarcoid-like granulomas and adjacent alveolar filling with eosinophils and macrophages; *B*, mild eosinophilic angiitis; and *C*, alveolar wall thickening and early granulation tissue with intra-alveolar eosinophils.

show a typical clinical syndrome and radiographic appearance (Gaensler and Carrington, 1977). The condition is almost entirely confined to adults, being most common in middle age, with an average age of onset of 50 years. Eighty percent of the patients are women. Severe systemic effects of fever, sweats, and loss of weight are common, together with cough and dyspnea. Asthma occurs in about one-fourth of the cases and nasal symptoms in about one third. Eosinophilia of the blood is usually found, but it is important to recognize that this may be transient or absent. The chest radiograph usually shows subpleural parenchymal densities with poorly defined margins, involving mainly the upper lung zones. In the most extreme example, the infiltrates occur only in the peripheral portions of the lung and spare the central region, resulting in an appearance described as the "photographic negative of pulmonary edema" (Gaensler and Carrington, 1977). The infiltrates may disappear spontaneously and recur in the same position. About three-fourths of the cases have a distinctive radiograph. CT scans show the characteristic predominantly subpleural airspace consolidation even when this distribution is not apparent on the radiograph (Mayo et al, 1989). The response to steroids is dramatic and may even be used as a diagnostic test, since the symptoms may disappear within hours and the radiologic abnormalities within days. Lung biopsy can usually be avoided, but there are a sufficient number of atypical cases that biopsy is required from time to time to establish the diagnosis.

The histologic features are "flooding" of alveolar spaces with eosinophils and macrophages, and an associated mild interstitial pneumonia (Fig. 7–24). Sometimes, the interstitial pneumonia and diffuse alveolar damage may be severe, with type-II hyperplasia and large numbers of macrophages in the airspaces; this may lead to a mistaken diagnosis of desquamative interstitial pneumonia. Necrosis of the cellular exudate may occur, resulting in a granulomatous appearance. Sarcoid-like granulomas are found in approximately one fourth of cases (Carrington et al, 1969). Angiitis of small vessels was noted by Carrington et al (1969) in the majority of cases, and this may be the lesion responsible for hemoptysis, which occasionally is a serious complication. Bronchiolitis obliterans is present in a minority of cases and is usually mild and is particularly associated with the curious syndrome of rheumatoid arthritis and eosinophilic penumonia (Cooney, 1981). Occasionally, it may be severe, and it may be difficult to separate eosinophilic pneumonia from bronchiolitis obliterans. Eosinophilic infiltration of any degree of severity is not a feature of bronchiolitis obliterans. The histologic appearance of eosinophilic pneumonia is usually diagnostic, but it is important to recognize

that the features also include necrosis of the exudate, granulomas, diffuse alveolar damage, and bronchiolitis obliterans. These features may occasionally make the diagnosis very difficult to make.

ALVEOLAR PROTEINOSIS (LIPOPROTEINOSIS)

Pulmonary alveolar proteinosis is an infiltrative lung disease in which there is an intra-alveolar accumulation of lipoproteinaceous, surfactant-like material (Singh et al, 1983). The disease may be seen in one of four clinical settings: as an idiopathic disease, as an occupational disease (Miller et al, 1984), as a drug-induced disease, and as an infiltrate in the immunocompromised host (Bedrossian et al, 1980; Singh et al, 1983). In the idiopathic variety, there is a male predominance and the usual age of patients is 30 to 50 years. The presenting symptom is generally dyspnea; cough, while present, is often not as productive as one might predict from the histology (Davidson and MacLeod, 1969). Pulmonary alveolar proteinosis of occupational etiology is most commonly associated with silica, although other substances have also been implicated both experimentally and clinically (Miller et al, 1984). Lesions resembling proteinosis have been discussed previously in relation to amphophilic drugs. In the immunocompromised host the underlying diseases are usually either leukemia or lymphoma (Bedrossian et al, 1980; Green et al, 1980), and most of these patients have been treated with busulphan.

Radiologically, pulmonary alveolar proteinosis presents with bilateral perihilar, patchy, or diffuse airspace consolidation, which is generally worse in the lung bases (Prakash et al, 1987) (Fig. 7–25). Air bronchograms are rarely seen. Characteristically, the patients may have mild symptoms in spite of extensive radiologic abnormalities. The appearance on CT is nonspecific (see Fig. 7–25) except in a few patients in whom an unusual sharply demarcated border is present between the airspace consolidation and normal parenchyma, creating a geographic pattern (Godwin et al, 1988). CT may also demonstrate focal infiltrates that may not be visible on the radiograph (Godwin et al, 1988). Interestingly, pulmonary alveolar proteinosis can be readily differentiated from other diseases by magnetic resonance imaging (MRI) (Moore et al, 1986). Alveolar proteinosis is characterized on MRI by a lower T1 (400 to 500 msec) than other airspace consolidation (T1 > 600 msec).

The histologic appearance is similar in all of the clinical settings. The alveolar spaces are filled by granular, hypocellular, intensely eosinophilic material that is strongly PAS-positive, diastase-resistant

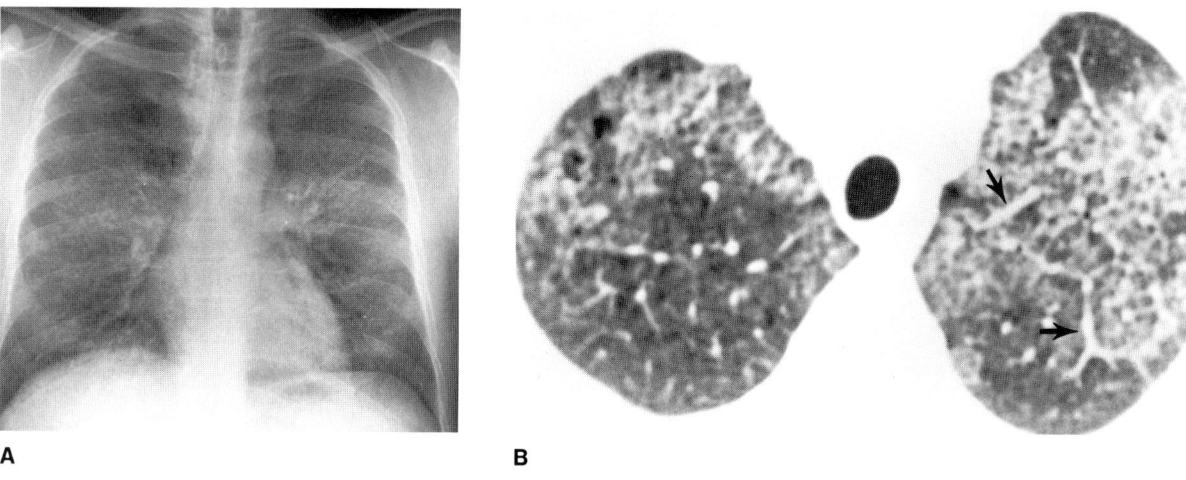

A   B

Figure 7–25   Pulmonary alveolar proteinosis in a 45-year-old man. *A*, Chest radiograph shows bilateral ground-glass increased density with relative sparing of the subpleural lung regions. *B*, High-resolution CT through the upper lobes in the same patient shows patchy distribution of the areas of ground-glass density. Also noted are extensive interstitial changes consisting of thickening of the interlobular septa in the left upper lobe (*arrow*). This thickening may be due to prominence of the lymphatics related to absorption of the surfactant-like material or it may represent fibrosis. *C*, CT scan in another patient with pulmonary alveolar proteinosis shows patchy distribution of the areas of airspace opacification.

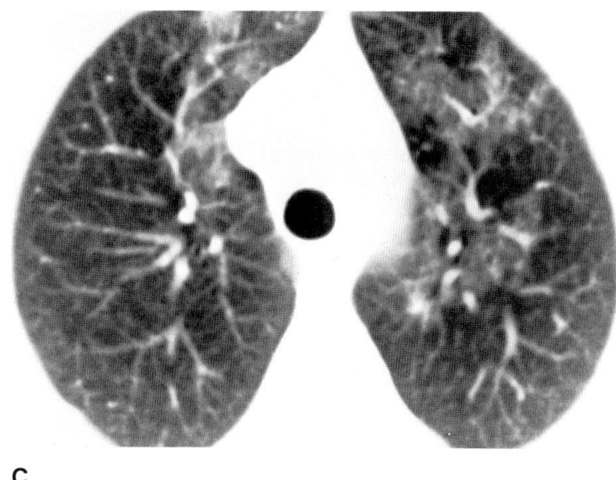

C

(Fig. 7–26). There may be some degree of type-II pneumonocyte proliferation, but interstitial and intra-alveolar inflammation is usually absent. Discrete eosinophilic bodies may be seen within airspaces by light microscopy. By electron microscopy, the granular material consists of myelin-like figures and laminated bodies, membrane bound vacuoles, and electron-dense debris. Immunohistochemistry shows the intra-alveolar material to contain surfactant apoprotein, although this reaction is said to be more strongly and diffusely positive in the idiopathic and occupational varieties than in the immunocompromised host (Singh et al, 1983; Miller et al, 1984). It is of importance to investigate all patients, and immunocompromised patients in particular, with pulmonary alveolar proteinosis for superinfection. The lipoproteinaceous material serves as a good culture medium and a variety of associated fungal, viral, mycobacterial, nocardial, and protozoal superinfec-

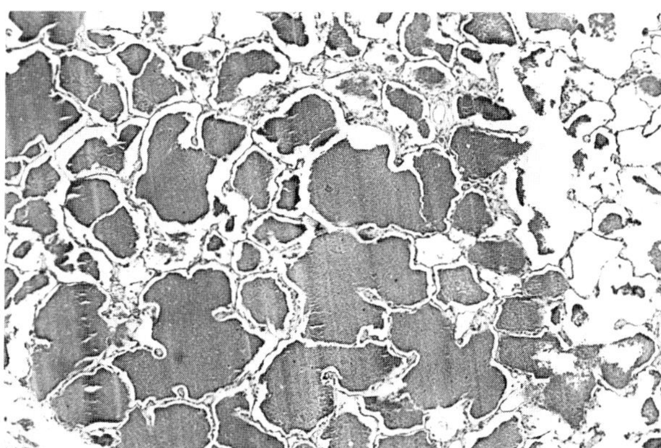

Figure 7–26   Alveolar proteinosis showing accumulation of intra-alveolar eosinophilic material with almost no inflammatory reaction.

tions have been observed (Bedrossian et al, 1980; Green et al, 1980).

The pathogenesis of the disease is uncertain. There is no real evidence of excessive surfactant production. The defect appears to be a failure of surfactant clearance, which is normally a function of alveolar macrophages (Miller et al, 1984). The surfactant-like material itself has been found to be directly toxic to macrophages. Abnormalities of macrophage number, morphology, and phagocytic function have been shown in patients with alveolar proteinosis. Function of normal macrophages exposed in vitro to lavage fluid from patients with alveolar proteinosis has been shown to be abnormal (Gonzales-Roth and Harris, 1986). The current belief is that nonspecific factors lead to a transient localized surfactant clearance failure, and before this failure is corrected, the material accumulates sufficiently to directly suppress clearance mechanisms.

The usual means of diagnosis is open lung biopsy. Transbronchial lung biopsy and examination of bronchoalveolar lavage fluid (Martin et al, 1980) may be diagnostic but do not provide information about superimposed infection. Treatment with lavage usually induces remission with excellent long-term survival, particularly in nonimmunocompromised patients.

PULMONARY ALVEOLAR MICROLITHIASIS

Alveolar microlithiasis is rare. Approximately 150 cases have been reported (Mascie-Taylor et al, 1985), and about half are familial (Ravines, 1969). The Mayo Clinic recorded only eight cases in 46 years (Prakash et al, 1983). Although it has often been described in siblings, there is only one recorded instance of its occurrence in both a parent and a child. Most cases are diagnosed in adult life, but microlithiasis may occur in stillborns (Caffrey and Altman, 1965); a number of cases in children have been reported. It is probable that the condition is a congenital metabolic disorder usually with a slowly progressive course. In some instances, however, there is a rapid course; alternatively, it may not present until old age (Sears et al, 1971). The chest radiograph may also be unchanged for many years. The patients may be asymptomatic but usually have varying degrees of dyspnea and finally die of respiratory failure at a mean age in the early 40s (Mascie-Taylor et al, 1985). In the past, treatment has been supportive only, although more recently repeated lavage and transplantation have been suggested as treatment options (Mascie-Taylor et al, 1985).

The respiratory defect is characteristically mild compared with the appearance of the chest radiograph, especially in young patients (Fuleihan et al, 1969). The chest radiograph is usually immediately diagnostic with an appearance of sand-like micronodular opacities involving both lungs, the lower zones being more opaque than the upper. The lungs may appear almost completely opaque on routine radiographs, but discrete opacities can be seen on overexposed films. There are no reports yet of CT or MRI, but it is likely that both will be diagnostic.

Grossly, the lung tissue is firm and gritty and maintains its shape and may have to be cut with a band-saw. Histologically, the airspaces contain large numbers of concentrically laminated calcified bodies, which show radial striations. They are referred to as calcispherites and contain calcium and phosphorus, in the same concentration as found in bone, together with small amounts of magnesium and iron. They are fairly uniform in size and are about 0.25 mm in diameter, but some may be as large as 1 mm or more. Ossification may occur. The calcispherites are nearly all in airspaces, but a few occur in the interstitium. In the stillborn infants referred to (Caffrey and Altman, 1965), the calcispherites appeared to form in the alveolar epithelium and were extruded into the airspaces. The intervening alveolar wall is relatively normal (Sosman et al, 1957), but there is interstitial fibrosis with a mild chronic inflammatory cell infiltrate, particularly when there are large aggregates of calcispherites. Calcispherites have to be distinguished from the corpora amylacea that are found in the airspaces of the lung, especially in patients with chronic heart failure. Corpora amylacea are laminated but are smaller, not calcified, and usually contain a central black core.

PULMONARY CALCIFICATION

Pulmonary calcification occurs in a number of clinical settings in which disturbances of calcium phosphate or parathyroid hormone metabolism are found. These include primary or secondary hyperparathyroidism, ectopic parathyroid hormone production by a malignancy, various infectious and neoplastic osteodestructive processes, sarcoidosis, and milk-alkali syndrome (Gilman et al, 1980). Of these, by far the most common setting is chronic renal failure with secondary hyperparathyroidism. Pulmonary calcification may develop in these patients whether they are untreated, treated with transplantation, or treated with dialysis. Conger et al (1975) found pulmonary calcification in 60 percent of patients dying of chronic renal failure treated by long-term dialysis. The measurable abnormalities of calcium, phosphates, and parathyroid hormone are often remarkably mild or absent in the face of progressive calcification (Conger et al, 1975; Gilman et al, 1980; Faubert et al, 1980), and the process can be unresponsive to parathyroid resection. The reason for the discrepancy between the degree of serum abnormalities and the degree of tissue abnormalities is unknown. The course of pulmonary calcification is usually benign, and only with a considerable amount of calcification are pulmonary function test abnormalities the rule (Conger et al, 1975). Accelerated life-threatening progression may occur with acute failure of a transplanted kidney (Breitz et al, 1987).

The radiologic appearance is variable. Patients with mild interstitial calcification usually have a normal radiograph. Moderate calcification tends to cause a reticular pattern, whereas more severe calcification often is seen as mottled areas of increased density simulating airspace disease (Sanders et al, 1987) (Fig. 7–27). The calcific nature of the infiltrates is rarely detected on the radiograph but can be readily seen on CT, digital chest radiography (Sanders et al, 1987), or nuclear medicine scans using bone imaging agents such as ^{99m}Tc diphosphonate (Faubert et al, 1980). Metastatic pulmonary calcification characteristically involves predominantly the upper lung zones (Jost and Sagel, 1979). This is presumably because the lung apex has a higher ventilation/perfusion ratio than the lower lung zones, leading to a lower PCO_2 and a relative alkalinity which favors calcium deposition.

Histologically, the calcification involves otherwise normal interstitial tissue. For this reason, the terminology "metastatic calcification" is often used, to distinguish the process from "dystrophic calcification," which is calcification of previously abnormal areas of fibrosis, scarring, granulomatous inflammation, etc. In milder cases, the calcium is distributed as fine thin deposits along alveolar walls without inflammation or fibrosis (Fig. 7–28). Greater amounts of calcification result in broader alveolar wall deposits, bronchiolar and vascular deposits, and relatively mild but definite fibrosis. Inflammatory reaction is not found in uncomplicated metastatic calcification.

AMYLOIDOSIS

Amyloidosis of the lower respiratory tract has a variety of different pathologic patterns (Celli et al, 1978; Thompson and Citron 1983; Cordier et al, 1986; Colby and Carrington, 1988). In the proximal airways, amyloid may be found as a single nodule in the major bronchi; such nodules are almost always small asymptomatic lesions incidentally found at bronchoscopy. They require no specific therapy and have a good prognosis. Proximal airway amyloidosis may also take the form of multiple submucosal infiltrative plaques; this form may result in functional obstruction (Fig. 7–29). Endoscopic resection of these plaques is sometimes successful, but lung resection may be necessary. This form also has a good prognosis. There is some question about the relationship of this form of amyloid and tracheobronchiopathica osteoplastica. In the more peripheral lung zones,

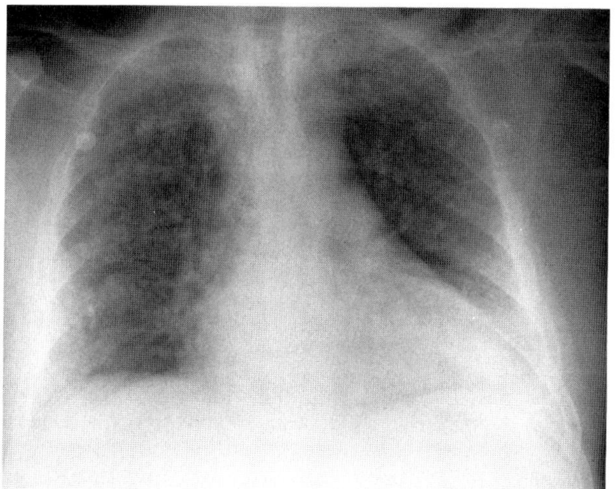

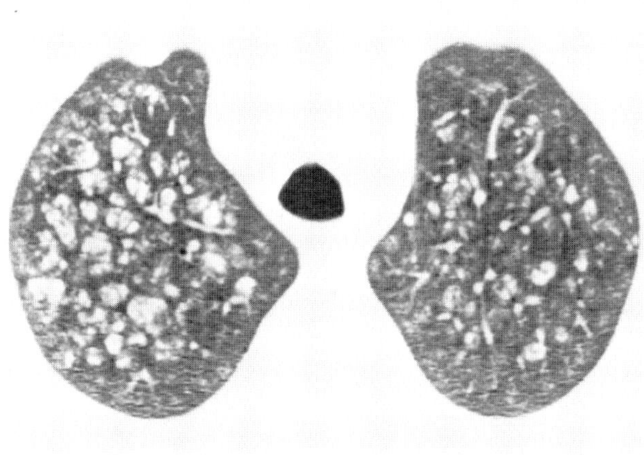

A   **B**

Figure 7–27   Metastatic calcification due to renal failure in a 42-year-old woman. *A*, Radiograph shows mottled areas of increased density in the upper lung zones. *B*, These are better delineated on high resolution CT. Calcification was seen on the mediastinal window.

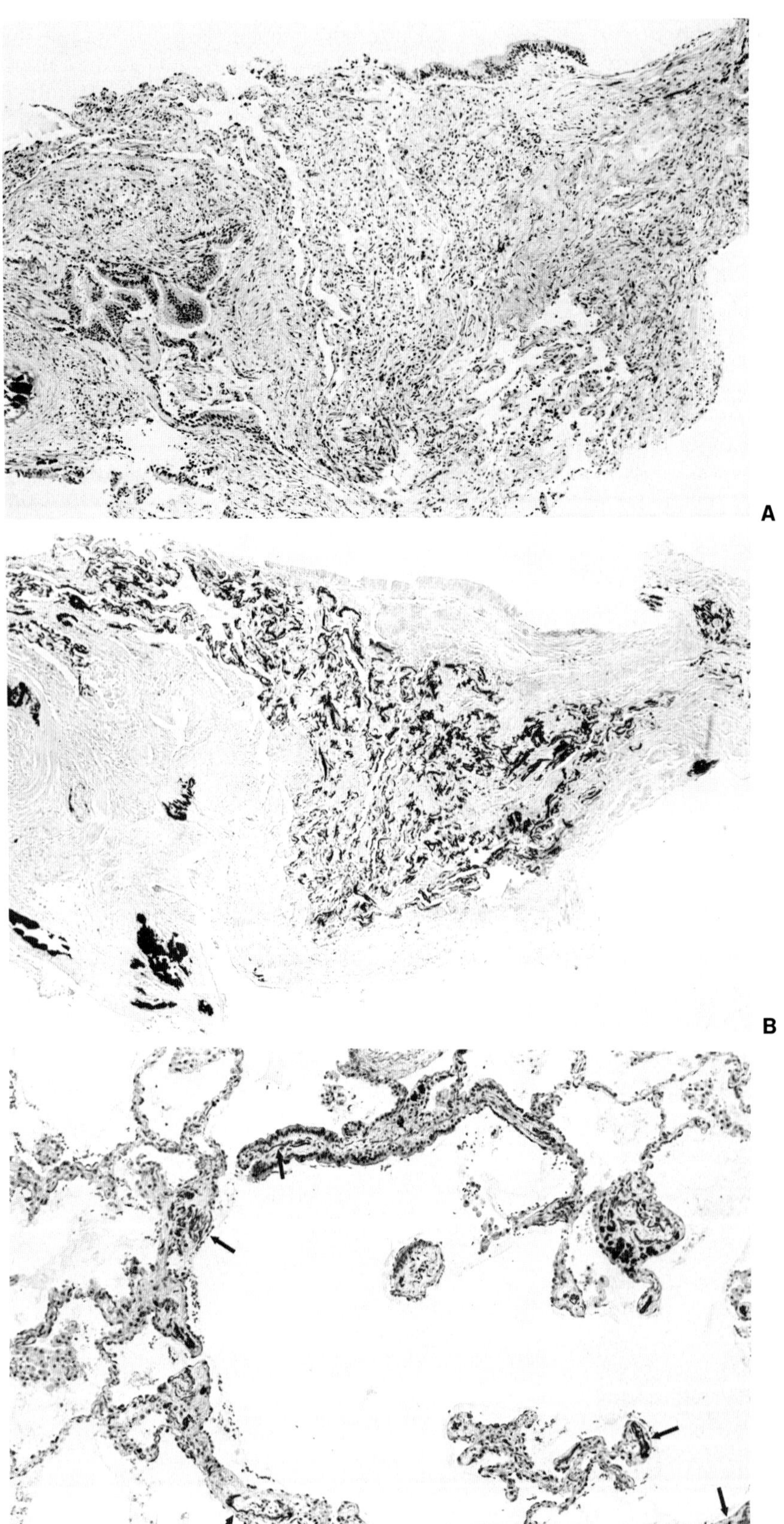

Figure 7–28 Metastatic calcification. *A*, H&E stain of transbronchial biopsy showing the usual degree of collapse, with very subtle linear calcification and no cellular reaction. *B*, Von Kossa stain for calcium highlights the mineral deposits. *C*, Another renal transplant patient with thicker calcifications and bronchiolar calcifications (*arrows*).

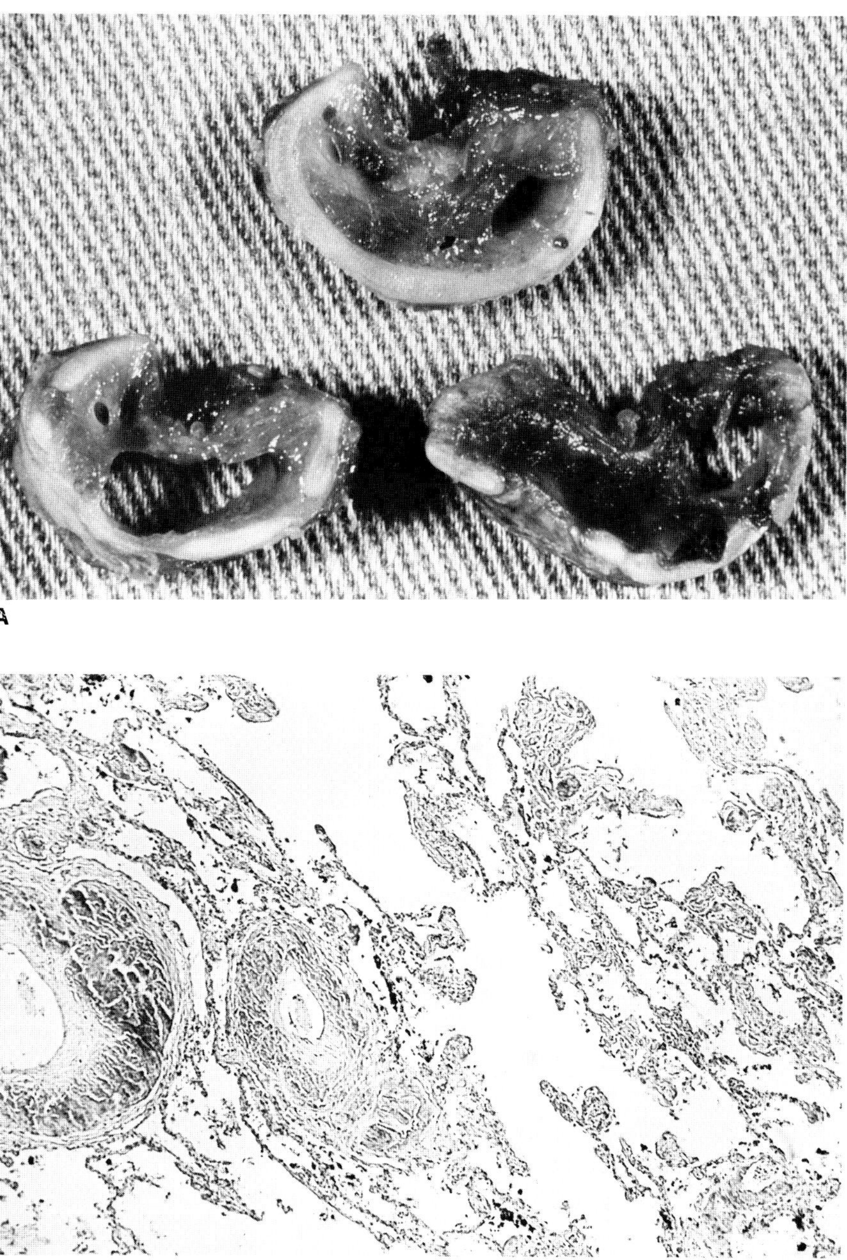

Figure 7–29 *A*, Bronchial plaque form of amyloidosis totally obstructs the bronchus in this patient, ultimately necessitating resection. *B*, Vascular amyloid in a patient with primary amyloidosis.

amyloid may take the form of one or more nodules, simulating neoplasms. These nodules can reach several centimeters in diameter and can also cavitate. Specific treatment is probably not necessary, although some patients come to resection because of an uncertain diagnosis preoperatively. The prognosis of this form of amyloidosis is also good. The most common pathologic pattern of lower respiratory tract amyloidosis is that of diffuse parenchymal infiltrates in alveolar walls, vessel walls, and bronchiolar walls

(see Fig. 7–29). There is no effective therapy for this condition and the prognosis is poor.

The clinical settings correlate to some extent with the pathologic patterns of disease. While patients with generalized primary amyloidosis usually have lower respiratory tract involvement of the diffuse parenchymal type, their respiratory symptoms tend to be greatly overshadowed by their cardiac disease. Patients with generalized amyloidosis secondary to chronic inflammatory disease very seldom have symptoms referable to respiratory tract amyloid and tend to have scant lung deposits pathologically (Celli et al, 1978). Patients with amyloidosis secondary to plasma cell dyscrasias often have diffuse parenchymal respiratory tract amyloid. In contrast, localized pulmonary amyloid confined to the lung usually takes one of the more indolent pathologic patterns as described above—namely, localized tracheobronchial, plaque-like tracheobronchial or parenchymal pseudotumor(s)—but occasionally localized pulmonary amyloidosis takes the diffuse parenchymal form and this has a poor prognosis.

"Amyloid" as a substance may be divided into amyloid of light-chain proteins (AL) and amyloid of serum acute-phase proteins (AA). AA amyloidosis is found in amyloidosis secondary to chronic inflammatory disorders, and AL amyloid comprises the deposits in primary generalized and plasma cell dyscrasia–associated amyloidosis. For all practical purposes, the type of amyloid found in amyloid localized to the respiratory tract, as well as clinically significant respiratory tract amyloid associated with other diseases, is AL amyloid (Costa and Corrin, 1985; Gertz and Greipp, 1986).

REFERENCES

Abdi EA, Nguyen GK, Ludwig RN, Dickout WJ. Pulmonary sarcoidosis following interferon therapy for advanced renal cell carcinoma. Cancer 1987; 59:896-900.

Anderson LG, Talal N. The spectrum of benign and malignant lymphoproliferation in Sjögren's syndrome. Clin Exp Immunol 1972; 9:199-205.

Askin FB, McCann BG, Kuhn C. Reactive eosinophilic pleuritis: a lesion to be distinguished from pulmonary eosinophilic granuloma. Arch Pathol Lab Med 1977; 101:187-191.

Barrowcliff DF, Arblaster PG. Farmer's lung: a study of an early acute fatal case. Thorax 1968; 23:490-500.

Basset F, Corrin B, Spencer H, et al. Pulmonary histiocytosis "X". Am Rev Respir Dis 1978; 188:811-820.

Basset F, Soler P, Marsac J, Corrin B. Pulmonary lymphangiomyomatosis—three new cases studied with electron microscopy. Cancer 1976a; 38:2357-2366.

Basset F, Soler P, Wyllie L, et al. Langerhans' cells and lung interstitium. Ann NY Acad Sci 1976b; 278:499-508.

Bedrossian CWM, Luna MA, Conklin RH, Hiller WC. Alveolar proteinosis as a consequence of immunosuppression: a hypothesis based on clinical pathologic observations. Hum Pathol 1980; 11:527-535.

Bergmann M, Flance IJ, et al. Thesaurosis due to inhalation of hair spray: report of twelve new cases, including three autopsies. N Engl J Med 1962; 266:750-755.

Bitterman PB, Rennard SI, Keogh BA, et al. Familial idiopathic pulmonary fibrosis. N Engl J Med 1986; 314:1343-1347.

Bone RC, Wolfe J, Sobonya RE, et al. Disquamative interstitial pneumonia following long-term nitrofurantoin therapy. Am J Med 1976; 60:697-701.

Breitz HB, Sirotta PS, Nelp WB, et al. Progressive pulmonary calcification complicating successful renal transplantation. Am Rev Respir Dis 1987; 136:1480-1482.

Brentani MM, Carvalho RR, Saldiva PH, et al. Steroid receptors in pulmonary lymphangiomyomatosis. Chest 1984; 85:96-99.

Brody AR, Kanich RE, Graham WG, et al. Cyst wall formation in pulmonary eosinophilic granuloma. Chest 1974; 66:576-578.

Caffrey PR, Altman RS. Pulmonary alveolar microlithiasis occurring in premature twins. J Pediatr 1965; 66:758-761.

Camp M, Mehta JB, Whitson M. Bronchiolitis obliterans and *Nocardia asteroides* infection of the lung. Chest 1987; 92:1107-1108.

Camus P, Lombard J-N, Perrichon M, et al. Bronchiolitis obliterans–organizing pneumonia in patients taking acebutolol or amiodarone. Thorax 1989; 44:711-715.

Capron F, Ameille J, Leclerc P, et al. Pulmonary lymphangioleiomyomatosis and Bourneville's tuberous sclerosis with pulmonary involvement: the same disease? Cancer 1983; 52:851-855.

Carrington CB, Addington WW, Goff AM, et al. Chronic eosinophilic pneumonia. N Engl J Med 1969; 289:787-798.

Carrington C, Gaensler EA, Coutu RE, et al. Natural history and treated course of usual and desquamative interstitial pneumonia. N Engl J Med 1978; 298:801-810.

Carrington CB, Gaensler EA. Clinical-pathologic approach to diffuse infiltrative lung disease. In Thurlbeck WM, Abell MR, eds. The lung: structure, function and disease. Baltimore: Williams & Wilkins, 1978:58-87.

Carrington CB, Liebow AA. Lymphocytic interstitial pneumonia [Abstract]. Am J Pathol 1966; 48:36.

Celli BR, Rubinow A, Cohen AS, Brody JS. Pattern of pulmonary involvement in systemic amyloidosis. Chest 1978; 74:543-547.

Chamberlain DW, Hyland RM, Ross DJ. Diphenylhydantoin-induced lymphocytic interstitial pneumonia. Chest 1986; 90:458-460.

Churg AM. Pulmonary angiitis and granulomatosis revisited. Hum Pathol 1983; 14:868-883.

Coates EO, Watson JHL. Diffuse interstitial lung disease in tungsten carbide workers. Ann Intern Med 1971; 75:709-716.

Cohen HL, Merigan TC, Kosek JC, Eldridge F. A granulomatous pneumonitis associated with redwood sawdust inhalation. Am J Med 1967; 43:785-794.

Colby TV, Carrington CB. Infiltrative lung disease. In Thurlbeck WM, ed. Pathology of the lung. New York: Thieme, 1988:425-517.

Colby TV, Carrington CB. Lymphoreticular tumors and

infiltrates of the lung. In Sommers S, ed. Pathology annual 1983, part I. Norwalk CT: Appleton-Century-Crofts, 1983.

Colby TV, Lombard C. Histiocytosis X presenting in the lung. Hum Pathol 1983; 14:847–856.

Coleman A, Colby TV. Histologic diagnosis of extrinsic allergic alveolitis. Am J Surg Pathol 1988; 12:514–518.

Conger JD, Hammond WS, Alfrey AC, et al. Pulmonary calcification in chronic dialysis patients. Ann Intern Med 1975; 83:330-336.

Cook PG, Wells IP, McGavin CR. The distribution of pulmonary shadowing in farmer's lung. Clin Radiol 1988; 39:21–27.

Cooney TP. Inter-relationship of chronic eosinophilic pneumonia, bronchiolitis obliterans and rheumatoid disease: a hypothesis. J Clin Pathol 1981; 34:129–137.

Cordier JF, Loire R, Brune J. Amyloidosis of the lower respiratory tract. Chest 1986; 90:827–831.

Corrin B, Liebow AA, Friedman PJ. Pulmonary lymphangiomyomatosis. Am J Pathol 1975; 79:348–382.

Corrin B, Price AB. Electron microscopic studies in desquamative interstitial pneumonia associated with asbestos. Thorax 1977; 27:324–331.

Costa PD, Corrin B. Amyloidosis localized to the lower respiratory tract: probably immunoamyloid nature of the tracheobronchial and nodular pulmonary forms. Histopathology 1985; 9:703–710.

Crystal R, Bitterman PB, Rennard SI, et al. Interstitial lung diseases of unknown cause: disorders characterized by chronic inflammation of the lower respiratory tract. N Engl J Med 1984; 310:154–166.

Crystal R, Fulmer JD, Roberts WC, et al. Idiopathic pulmonary fibrosis: clinical histologic, radiographic, physiologic, scintigraphic, cytologic and biochemical aspects. Ann Intern Med 1976; 85:769–788.

Daniele RP, Rossman MD, Kern JA, Elias JA. Pathogencsis of sarcoidosis. Chest 1986; 89:174S-177S.

Davidson JM, MacLeod WM. Pulmonary alveolar proteinosis. B J Dis Chest 1969; 63:13–28.

Davison AG, Heard BE, McAllister WC, Turner-Warwick MEH. Cryptogenic organizing pneumonitis. Q J Med 1983; 52 (new series), No. 207:382–393.

Donohue WL, Laski B, Uchida I, Munn JD. Familial fibrocystic pulmonary dysplasia and its relation to the Hamman-Rich syndrome. Pediatrics 1959; 24:786–813.

Dreisin RB, Schwarz MI, Theophilopoulos AN, et al. Circulating immune complexes in the idiopathic interstitial pneumonia. N Engl J Med 1978; 298:353–357.

Emanuel DA, Lawton BR, Wenzel FJ. Maple-bark disease: pneumonitis due to *Coniosporium corticale*. N Engl J Med 1962; 266:333–337.

Epler GR, Colby TV, McLoud TC, et al. Bronchiolitis obliterans–organizing pneumonia. N Engl J Med 1985; 312:152–158.

Farr GH, Harley RA, Hennigar GR. Desquamative interstitial pneumonia: an electron microscopic study. Am J Pathol 1970; 60:347–358.

Faubert PF, Shapiro WB, Porush JG, et al. Pulmonary calcification in hemodialyzed patients detected by technetium-99m diphosphonate scanning. Kidney Int 1980; 18:95–102.

Fink JN, Banaszak EF, Thiede WH, Barboriak JJ. Interstitial pneumonitis due to hypersensitivity to an organism contaminating a heating system. Ann Intern Med 1971; 74:80-83.

Fink JN. Clinical features of hypersensitivity pneumonitis. Chest 1986; 89:193S-195S.

Fort GJ, Scovern H, Abruzzo JL. Intravenous cyclophosphamide and methylprednisolone for the treatment of bronchiolitis obliterans and interstitial fibrosis associated with crysotherapy. J Rheumatol 1988; 15:850–864.

Friedman PJ, Liebow AA, Sokoloff J. Eosinophilic granuloma of lung: clinical aspects of primary pulmonary histiocytosis in the adult. Medicine 1981; 60:385–396.

Fuleihan FJD, Abboud RT, Balikian JP, et al. Pulmonary alveolar microlithiasis: lung function in five cases. Thorax 1969; 24:84-90.

Fulmer JD, Crystal RG. The biochemical basis of pulmonary function. In Crystal RG, ed. The biochemical basis of pulmonary function. New York: Marcel Dekker, 1976:419.

Gadek JE, Kelman JA, Fells G, et al. Collagenase in the lower respiratory tract of patients with idiopathic pulmonary fibrosis. N Engl J Med 1979; 301:737–742.

Gaensler EA, Carrington CB. Peripheral opacities in chronic eosinophilic pneumonia: the photographic negative of pulmonary edema. Am J Roentgenol Radium Ther Nucl Med 1977; 128:1-13.

Gardiner IT, Uff JS. "Blue bodies" in a case of cryptogenic fibrosing alveolitis (desquamative type)—an ultrastructural study. Thorax 1978; 33:806–813.

Genereux GP: The end-stage lung: pathogenesis, pathology, and radiology. Radiology 1975; 116:279–289.

Gertz MA, Greipp PR. Clinical aspects of pulmonary amyloidosis (editorial). Chest 1986; 90:790-791.

Gibbs AR, Seal RME. Primary lymphoproliferative conditions of the lung. Thorax 1978; 33:140-152.

Gilman M, Nissim J, Terry P, Whelton A. Metastatic pulmonary calcification in the renal transplant recipient. Am Rev Respir Dis 1980; 121:415–419.

Godwin JD, Müller NL, Takasugi JE. Pulmonary alveolar proteinosis: CT findings. Radiology 1988; 169:609–613.

Gonzales-Roth RJ, Harris JO. Pulmonary alveolar proteinosis: further evaluation of abnormal alveolar macrophages. Chest 1986; 90:656–661.

Gosink BB, Friedman PJ, Liebow AA. Bronchiolitis obliterans: roentgenologic-pathologic correlation. Am J Roentgenol Radium Ther Nucl Med 1973; 117:816–832.

Gowdy JM, Wagstaff MJ. Pulmonary infiltration due to aerosol thesaurosis: a survey of hairdressers. Arch Environ Health 1972; 25:101-108.

Graham ML, Spelsberg TC, Dines DE, et al. Pulmonary lymphangiomyomatosis, with particular reference to steroid-receptor assay studies and pathologic correlation. Mayo Clin Proc 1984; 59:3–11.

Grant IW, Blackadder ES, Greenberg M, Blyth W. Extrinsic allergic alveolitis in Scottish maltworkers. Br Med J 1976; 1:490-493.

Green D, Dighe P, Ali NO, Katele GV. Pulmonary alveolar proteinosis complicating chronic myelogenous leukemia. Cancer 1980; 46:1763-1766.

Grieco MH, Chinoy-Acharya P. Lymphoid interstitial pneumonia associated with the acquired immune deficiency syndrome. Am Rev Respir Dis 1985; 131:952-955.

Guerry-Force ML, Müller NL, Wright JL, et al. A comparison of bronchiolitis obliterans with organizing pneumonia, usual interstitial pneumonia and small airways disease. Am Rev Respir Dis 1987; 135:705-712.

Hamman L, Rich AR. Acute diffuse intestitial fibrosis of the lungs. Bull Johns Hopkins Hosp 1944; 74:177-212.

Hammar S, Bockus D, Remington F. Metastatic tumor of unknown origin. Ultra Pathol 1986; 10:281-288.

Hammar SP, Winterbauer R, Bockus D. Diagnosis of pulmonary eosinophilic granuloma by ultrastructural examination of sputum [letter]. Arch Pathol Lab Med 1978; 102:606.

Hitchcock M, Piscetelli DM, Bouhuys A. Histamine release from human lung by a component of cotton bracts. Arch Environ Health 1973; 26:177-182.

Hunninghake GW. Staging of pulmonary sarcoidosis. Chest 1986; 89:178S-181S.

Israel HL, Pachefsky AS, Saldana MJ. Wegener's granulomatosis, lymphomatoid granulomatosis and benign lymphocytic angiitis and granulomatosis. Ann Intern Med 1977; 87:691-699.

Joshi VV, Oleske JM. Pulmonary lesions in children with the acquired immunodeficiency syndrome: a reappraisal based on data in additional cases and follow-up study of previously reported cases. Hum Pathol 1986; 17:641-642.

Joshi VV, Oleske JM, Minnefor AB, et al. Pathologic pulmonary findings in children with the acquired immunodeficiency syndrome. Hum Pathol 1985; 16:241-246.

Jost RG, Sagel SS. Metastatic calcification in the lung apex. AJR 1979; 133:1188-1190.

Kapanci Y, Costabella PM, Gabbiani G. Location and function of contractile interstitial cells of the lungs. In Bouhuys A, ed. Lung cells in disease. Amsterdam: North-Holland, 1976: 69.

Katzenstein A-LA, Myers JL, Mazur MT. Acute interstitial pneumonia: a clinicopathologic, ultrastructural and cell kinetic study. Am J Surg Pathol 1986a; 10:256-267.

Katzenstein A-LA, Myers JL, Prophet WD, et al. Bronchiolitis obliterans and usual interstitial pneumonia: a comparative clinicopathologic study. Am J Surg Pathol 1986b; 10:373-381.

Kawanami O, Basset F, Barrios R, et al. Hypersensitivity pneumonitis in man: light and electron microscopic studies of 18 lung biopsies. Am J Pathol 1983; 110:275-289.

Kawanami O, Basset F, Ferrans VJ, et al. Pulmonary Langerhans' cells in patients with fibrotic lung disorders. Lab Invest 1981; 44:227-233.

Koss MN, Hochholzer L, Feigin DS, et al. Necrotizing sarcoid-like granulomatosis: clinical, pathologic and immunopathologic findings. Hum Pathol 1980; 11(S):510-519.

Kravis TC, Ahmed A, Brown TE, et al. Pathogenic mechanisms in pulmonary fibrosis: collagen-induced migration inhibition factor production and cytotoxicity mediated by lymphocytes. J Clin Invest 1976; 58:1223-1232.

Lack EE, Dolan MF, Finisio J, et al. Pulmonary and extrapulmonary lymphangioleiomyomatosis. Am J Surg Pathol 1986; 10:650-657.

Lacronique J, Roth C, Battesti J-P, et al. Chest radiological features of pulmonary histiocytosis X: a report based on 50 adult cases. Thorax 1982; 37:104-109.

Leavitt RY, Fauci AS. Pulmonary vasculitis. Am Rev Respir Dis 1986; 134:149-166.

Lewis JG: Eosinophilic granuloma and its variants with special reference to lung involvement: a report of twelve patients. Q J Med 1964; 33:337-359.

Liebow AA. Pulmonary angiitis and granulomatosis. Am Rev Respir Dis 1973; 108:1-20.

Liebow AA, Carrington CB. The interstitial pneumonias. In Simon M, Potchen EJ, LeMay M, eds. Frontiers of pulmonary radiology: pathophysiologic, roentgenographic and radioisotopic considerations. New York: Grune & Stratton, 1969a: 102-141.

Liebow AA, Carrington CH. The eosinophilic pneumonias. Medicine 1969b; 48:251-272.

Liebow AA, Carrington CB. Diffuse pulmonary lymphoreticular infiltrations associated with dysproteinaemia. Med Clin North Am 1973; 57:809-843.

Liebow AA, Steer A, Billingsley JG. Desquamative interstitial pneumonia. Am J Med 1965; 39:369-404.

Mahon WE, Scott DJ, Ansell G, et al. Hypersensitivity to pituitary snuff with miliary shadowing in the lungs. Thorax 1967; 22:13-20.

Martin RJ, Coalson JJ, Rogers RM, et al. Pulmonary alveolar proteinosis: the diagnosis by segmental lavage. Am Rev Respir Dis 1980; 121:819-825.

Mascie-Taylor BH, Wardman AG, Madden CA, Page RL. A case of alveolar microlithiasis: observation over 22 years and recovery of material by lavage. Thorax 1985; 40:952-953.

Mason AMS, McIllmurray MB, Golding PL, Hughes DTD. Fibrosing alveolitis associated with renal tubular acidosis. Br Med J 1970; 4:596-599.

Massaro D, Katz S. Fibrosing alveolitis: its occurrence, roentgenographic pathologic features in von Recklinghausen's neurofibromatosis. Am Rev Respir Dis 1966; 93:934-942.

Mathieson JM, Mayo JR, Staples CA, Müller NL. Chronic diffuse infiltrative lung disease: diagnostic accuracy of computed tomography versus chest radiography. Radiology 1989; 171:111-116.

Mayo JR, Müller NL, Road J, et al. Chronic eosinophilic pneumonia: CT findings in six cases. AJR 1989; 153:727-730.

McCann BG, Brewer DB. A case of desquamative interstitial pneumonia progressing to "honeycomb lung." J Pathol 1974; 112:199–202.

Miller RR, Churg AM, Hutcheon M, Lam S. Pulmonary alveolar proteinosis and aluminum dust exposure. Am Rev Respir Dis 1984; 130:312–315.

Moore ADA, Godwin DJ, Müller NL, et al. Pulmonary histiocytosis X: comparison of radiographic and CT findings. Radiology 1989; 172:249–254.

Moore EH, Webb WR, Müller NL, Sollitto R. MRI of pulmonary airspace disease: experimental model and preliminary clinical results. AJR 1986; 146:1123–1128.

Moore VL, Fink JN, Barboriak JJ, et al. Immunologic events in pigeon breeders' disease. J Allergy Clin Immunol 1974; 53:319–328.

Morris JC, Rosen MJ, Marchevsky A, Teirstein AS. Lymphocytic interstitial pneumonia in patients at risk for the acquired immune deficiency syndrome. Chest 1987; 91:63–67.

Müller NL, Guerry-Force ML, Staples CA, et al. Differential diagnosis of bronchiolitis obliterans with organizing pneumonia: clinical, functional and radiologic findings. Radiology 1987b; 162:151–156.

Müller, NL, Kullnig P, Miller RR. The CT findings of pulmonary sarcoidosis: analysis of 25 patients. AJR 1989; 152:1179–1182.

Müller NL, Miller RR, Webb WR, et al. Fibrosing alveolitis: CT-pathologic correlation. Radiol 1986; 160:585–588.

Müller NL, Staples CA, Miller RR, et al. Disease activity in idiopathic pulmonary fibrosis: CT and pathologic correlation. Radiology 1987a; 165:731–734.

Murray JC, Laurent GJ. Editorial: what is pulmonary fibrosis? Thorax 1988;43:9–11.

Ohori NP, Sciurba FC, Owens GR, et al. Giant cell interstitial pneumonia and hard-metal pneumoconiosis: a clinicopathologic study of four cases and review of the literature. Am J Surg Pathol 1989; 13:581–587.

Ostrow D, Cherniack RM. Resistance to airflow in patients with diffuse interstitial lung disease. Am Rev Respir Dis 1973; 108:205–211.

Patchefsky AS, Israel HL, Hoch G, et al. Desquamative interstitial pneumonia: relationship to interstitial fibrosis. Thorax 1973; 28:680-685.

Patel RC, Dutta D, Schonfeld SA. Free-base cocaine associated with bronchiolitis obliterans–organizing pneumonia. Ann Intern Med 1987; 107:186–187.

Perreault C, Cousineau S, D'Angelo G, et al. Lymphoid interstitial pneumonia after allogeneic bone marrow transplantation. Cancer 1985; 55:1–9.

Pimentel JC, Avila R. Respiratory disease in cork workers ("suberosis"). Thorax 1973; 28:409–423.

Prakash UBS, Barham SS, Carpenter HA, et al. Pulmonary alveolar phospholipoproteinosis: experience with 34 cases and a review. Mayo Clin Proc 1987; 62:499–518.

Prakash UBS, Barham SS, Rosenow EC, et al. Pulmonary alveolar microlithiasis. Mayo Clin Proc 1983; 58:290–300.

Pratt D, Schwartz M, May J, Dreisen R. Rapidly fatal pulmonary fibrosis: the accelerated variant of interstitial pneumonitis. Thorax 1979; 34:587–593.

Ravines HT. Pulmonary alveolar microlithiasis: report of nine cases with a familial incidence in seven of the nine cases among three families. Am J Clin Pathol 1969; 52:767–775.

Reid L Mc A. Reduction in bronchial subdivisions in bronchiectasis. Thorax 1950; 5:233–247.

Reyes CN, Wenzel FJ, Lawton BR, Emanuel DA. Pulmonary pathology in farmers' lung. Chest 1982; 81:142–146.

Reynolds HY, Di Sant'Agnese PA, Zierdt CH. Analysis of cellular and protein content of broncho-alveolar lavage fluid from patients with idiopathic pulmonary fibrosis and chronic hypersensitivity pneumonitis. J Clin Invest 1977; 59:165–175.

Roethe RA, Fuller PB, Byrd RB, Hafermann DR. Transbronchial biopsy in sarcoidosis: optimal number and sites for diagnosis. Chest 1980; 77:400-402.

Ruttner JR, Spycher MA, Engeler M-L. Pulmonary fibrosis induced by cotton fibre inhalation. Pathol Microbiol 1968; 32:1–15.

Saltzstein SL. Pulmonary malignant lymphomas and pseudolymphomas: classification, therapy, and prognosis. Cancer 1963; 16:928–955.

Salvaggio J, Arquembourg GP, Seabury J, Buechner H. Bagassosis: IV—precipitins against extracts of thermophilic actinomycetes in patients with bagassosis. JAMA 1969; 46:538–544.

Salvaggio JE, Karr RM: Hypersensitivity pneumonitis: state of the art. Chest 1979; 75 [suppl 2]:270–274.

Salvaggio JE, de Shazo RD. Pathogenesis of hypersensitivity pneumonitis. Chest 1986; 89:190S–193S.

Sanders C, Frank MS, Rostand SG, et al. Metastatic calcification of the heart and lungs in end-stage renal disease: detection and quantification by dual-energy digital chest radiography. AJR 1987; 149:881–887.

Scadding JG, Mitchell DN, eds. Sarcoidosis. London: Chapman and Hall Medical, 1985:101–180.

Sears MR, Change AR, Taylor AJ. Pulmonary alveolar microlithiasis. Thorax 1971; 26:704–711.

Silver SF, Müller NL, Miller RR, Lefcoe MS. Computed tomography in hypersensitivity pneumonitis. Radiology 1989; 173:441–445.

Singh G, Katyal SL, Bedrossian CWM, Rogers RM. Pulmonary alveolar proteinosis; staining for surfactant apoprotein in alveolar proteinosis and in conditions simulating it. Chest 1983; 83:82–86.

Singh N, Cole S, Krause PJ, et al. Necrotizing sarcoid granulomatosis with extrapulmonary involvement. Am Rev Respir Dis 1981; 124:189–192.

Smith MJL, Benson MK, Strickland ID. Coeliac disease and diffuse interstitial lung disease. Lancet 1971; 1:473–475.

Sokolowski JW, Cordray DR, Cantow EF, et al. Giant cell interstitial pneumonia: a report of a case. Am Rev Resp Dis 1972; 105:417–420.

Solal-Celigny P, Coudere LJ, Herman D, et al. Lymphoid interstitial pneumonitis in acquired immunodeficiency syndrome–related complex. Am Rev Respir Dis 1985; 131:956–960.

Solliday NH, Williams JA, Gaensler EA, et al. Familial chronic interstitial pneumonia. Am Rev Resp Dis 1973; 108:193-204.

Sosman MC, Dodd GD, Jones WD, et al. The familial occurrence of pulmonary alveolar microlithiasis. AJR 1957; 77:947-1012.

Spencer H. Pathology of the lung (excluding pulmonary tuberculosis). 3rd ed. Vols. 1 and 2. Philadelphia: WB Saunders, 1977.

Stack BHR, Choo-Kang YFJ, Heard BE. The prognosis of cryptogenic fibrosing alveolitis. Thorax 1972; 27:535-542.

Staples CA, Müller NL, Vedal S, et al. Usual interstitial pneumonia: correlation of CT with clinical findings and radiologic findings. Radiology 1987; 162:377-381.

Strimlan CV, Rosenow EC III, Weiland LH, et al. Lymphocytic interstitial pneumonitis: review of 13 cases. Ann Intern Med 1978; 88:616-622.

Svendsen TL, Viskym K, Hansborg N, et al. Pulmonary lymphangiomyomatosis: a case of progesterone receptor-positive lymphangiomyomatosis treated with medroxprogesterone, oophorectomy and tamoxifen. Br J Dis Chest 1984; 78:264-271.

Swinburn CR, Jackson GJ, Gobden I, et al. Bronchiolitis obliterans-organizing pneumonia in a patient with ulcerative colitis. Thorax 1988; 43:735-736.

Templeton PA, McLoud TC, Müller NL, et al. Pulmonary lymphangioleiomyomatosis: CT and pathologic findings. J Comput Assist Tomogr 1989; 13:54-57.

Thomas PD, Hunninghake GW. Current concepts of the pathogenesis of sarcoidosis. Am Rev Respir Dis 1987; 135:747-760.

Thompson PJ, Citron KM. Amyloid and the lower respiratory tract. Thorax 1983; 38:84-87.

Tubbs RR, Benjamin SP, Osborne DG, Barenburg S. Surface and transmission ultrastructural characteristics of desquamative interstitial pneumonia. Hum Pathol 1978; 9:693-702.

Turner-Warwick M. Interstitial lung disease. Semin Resp Med 1984; 6:1-102.

Turner-Warwick M, Haslam P, Weeks J. Antibodies in some chronic fibrosing lung diseases: II—immunofluorescent studies. Clin Allergy 1971; 1:209-219.

Vedal S, Welsh EV, Miller RR, Müller NL. Desquamative interstitial pneumonia: computed tomographic findings before and after treatment with corticosteroids. Chest 1988; 93:215-217.

Watters LC, King TE, Schwarz MI, et al. A clinical, radiographic and physiologic scoring system for the longitudinal assessment of patients with idiopathic pulmonary fibrosis. Am Rev Respir Dis 1986; 133:97-103.

Watters LC, Schwarz MI, Cherniack RM, et al. Idiopathic pulmonary fibrosis: pretreatment bronchoalveolar lavage cellular constituents and their relationship with lung histopathology and clinical response to therapy. Am Rev Respir Dis 1987; 135:696-704.

Webb WR, Goodman PC. Fibrosing alveolitis in patients with neurofibromatosis. Radiology 1977; 122:289-293.

Webber D, Tron V, Askin F, Churg A. S-100 staining in the diagnosis of eosinophilic granuloma of the lung. Am J Clin Pathol 1985; 84:447-453.

Weisbrodt IM. Lymphomatoid granulomatosis of the lung, associated with a long history of benign lymphoepithelial lesions of the salivary glands and lymphoid interstitial pneumonitis: report of a case. Am J Clin Pathol 1976; 66:792-801.

Wilen SB, Rabinowitz JG, Ulreich S, Lyons HA. Pleural involvement in sarcoidosis. Am J Med 1974; 57:200-209.

Williams T, Eidus L, Thomas P. Fibrosing alveolitis, bronchiolitis obliterans and sulfasalazine therapy. Chest 1982; 81:766-768.

Zalin AM, Weeple J, Gumpel M. Fibrosing alveolitis and renal tubular acidosis. Br Med J 1970; 4:804-806.

CHAPTER 8

COLLAGEN VASCULAR DISEASE

All collagen vascular diseases may involve the respiratory system, but each may affect the respiratory system in several different ways. With a few exceptions (e.g., rheumatoid nodules), the morphologic abnormalities are not specific for collagen vascular disease in general, or for any one collagen vascular disease in particular. Ultrastructurally tubular inclusions within endothelial cells have been described (Hammar et al, 1983) in a variety of collagen vascular diseases, but these are not diagnostic. Immune complexes are not reliably present in lung tissue by either ultrastructural or immunohistochemical techniques.

RHEUMATOID ARTHRITIS

At least half of patients with rheumatoid arthritis (RA) have one or more forms of rheumatoid lung disease (Hunninghake and Fauci, 1979). In general, patients with severe joint involvement are more likely to develop pleuropulmonary manifestations, which usually, but not always, follow the development of clinical arthropathy. At least seven forms of pleuropulmonary disease have been established in association with RA: pleural effusions/pleuritis, rheumatoid lung nodules, Caplan's syndrome, fibrosing alveolitis, lymphoid hyperplasia with germinal centers, pulmonary hypertension, and obliterative bronchiolitis (see Chapter 12).

Pleural Effusions/Pleuritis

Pleural effusions/pleuritis are the most common complications of RA and may be found in up to 50 percent of patients at autopsy. Clinically, most patients have no symptoms; radiologically detected pleural effusions occurred in 7.9 percent of men and 1.6 percent of women in one large series (Walker and Wright, 1968). The majority of effusions are unilateral (Carr and Mayne, 1962). In most cases, pleural effusion is the only radiologically detectable abnormality in the chest. The effusion may precede other clinical findings of RA or be present in patients with only mild symptoms, but it is more common in patients with exacerbation of arthritis and with subcutaneous nodules (Campbell and Ferrington, 1968; Carr and Mayne, 1962).

Rheumatoid Lung Nodules

Rheumatoid lung nodules are the most distinctive histologic lesions in the biopsied lungs of patients with RA (Yousem et al, 1985). In most series, rheumatoid (necrobiotic) lung nodules are a rare manifestation of rheumatoid disease and are usually associated with subcutaneous nodules and advanced RA (Fraser et al, 1989). Radiologically, multiple well-defined nodules, ranging from a few millimeters to several centimeters in diameter, are seen throughout the lung; occasionally the nodules are solitary. Cavitation is not uncommon. Rheumatoid nodules in the lung occur almost exclusively in patients with subcutaneous nodules, and the lung nodules may wax and wane with the skin nodules (Portner and Gracie, 1966). Radiologically, the differential diagnosis is bronchogenic carcinoma or metastatic disease. Jolles and colleagues (1989) described seven patients with seropositive RA and subcutaneous nodules who developed new pulmonary nodules on chest radiographs. Four had solitary nodules, and three had multiple nodules. In all seven patients the nodules were due to primary or metastatic carcinoma, indicating that histologic proof of presumed rheumatoid lung nodules is required. Rheumatoid nodules may also be seen as reticular or airspace infiltrates and, when microscopic, are not radiographically apparent (Yousem et al, 1985).

The histologic appearance is similar to that of rheumatoid nodules elsewhere, and the major histologic differential diagnosis is with infectious granulomas. In view of the potential for steroid therapy, accuracy of diagnosis is obviously of the utmost importance. The histologic distinction may not be easy, but the characteristic palisading, the presence of few giant cells, and the absence of organisms are important criteria for favoring a diagnosis of rheumatoid nodules.

Caplan's Syndrome

Caplan's syndrome is the occurrence of necrobiotic nodules in the lung of industrially exposed workers. First described in coal miners, the syndrome is characterized by the rapid development of single or multiple nodules that are 1 to 5 cm in diameter. Similar nodules have been described in subjects exposed to silica, aluminum, asbestos, and roof tiles, as well as in boiler scalers (Hunninghake and Fauci, 1979). Radiologically, the nodules are similar to the ones seen in RA without pneumoconiosis. Histologically, the lesion consists of a central necrotic area together with dust and collagenization. The necrotic area is surrounded by palisaded fibroblasts, and very characteristically there is an accumulation of polymorphonuclear leukocytes at the junction of the two zones, often in the region of a cleft-like space. Endarteritis is common and is usually seen in and adjacent to the nodules.

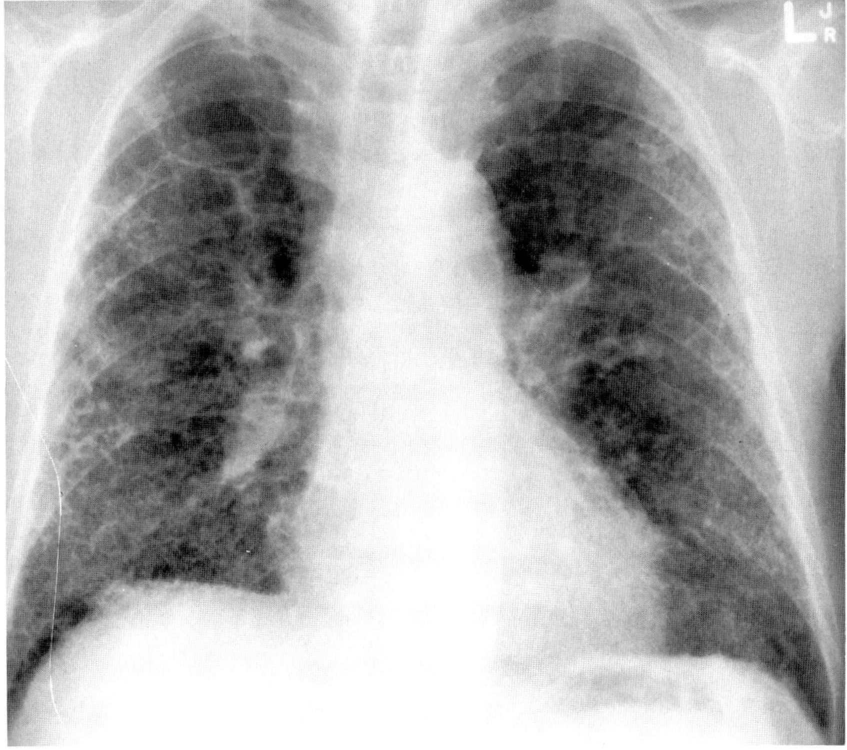

Figure 8–1 Longstanding rheumatoid arthritis and end-stage fibrosing alveolitis in a 60-year-old man. *A*, Chest radiograph shows reticular densities and honeycomb cysts throughout both lungs. *B*, High-resolution CT through the lung bases demonstrates almost complete replacement of lung parenchyma by cystic airspaces. *C*, High-resolution CT at the level of the tracheal carina shows honeycombing predominantly in the subpleural lung regions.

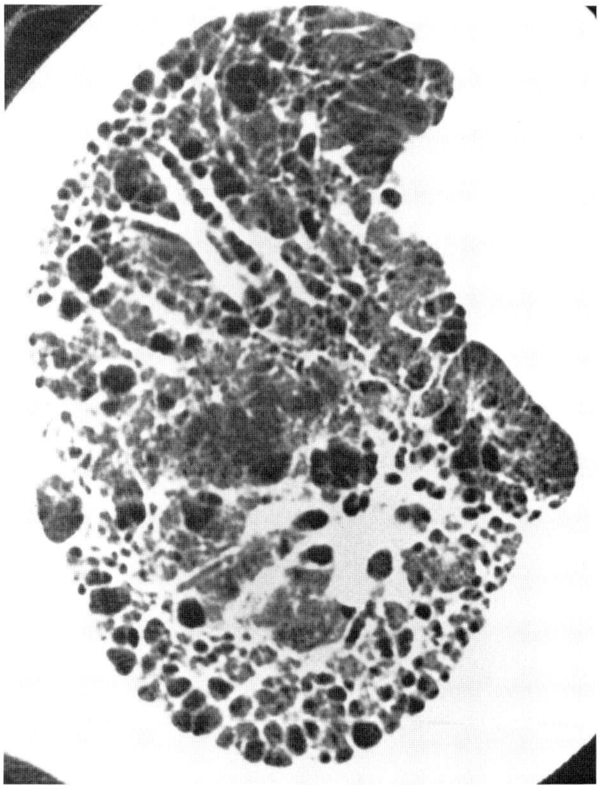

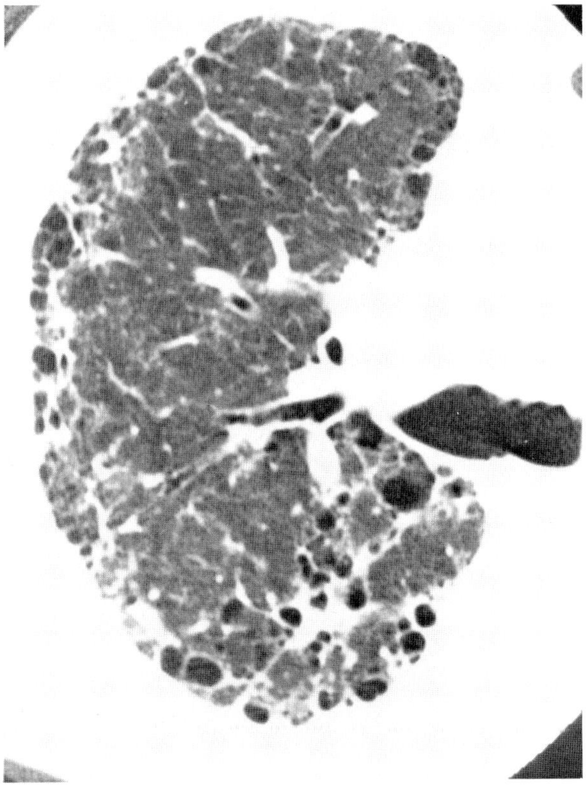

A

B

C

Fibrosing Alveolitis

The prevalence of fibrosing alveolitis in patients with rheumatoid arthritis is uncertain, the frequency of lung involvement in various studies being markedly dissimilar. Walker and Wright (1967) found that 1.6 percent of patients had radiologic evidence of fibrosing alveolitis, whereas radiologic evidence of parenchymal disease was present in 9 percent of patients in the series by Frank and colleagues (1973), and 80 percent of patients in the series by Cervantes-Perez and coworkers (1980). Probably the most representative data are those of Jurik and colleagues (1982), who compared the chest radiographs of 309 patients with RA with sex- and age-matched controls. A reticulondular pattern of fibrosis was seen in 4.5 percent of patients with RA as compared with 0.3 percent of the controls. Abnormalities in pulmonary function that suggested fibrosing alveolitis were found in 30 to 40 percent of patients with RA (Frank et al, 1973; Laitinen et al, 1975). In about half of these patients, the chest radiograph was normal, and the majority showed interstitial fibrosis if biopsies were performed (Frank et al, 1973). The observed difference in frequency may depend on the nature of the patients studied—e.g., the more severe the RA, the more frequently will fibrosing alveolitis be found. Radiologically and histologically, the lesions are usually indistinguishable from those of usual interstitial pneumonia (UIP) (Fig. 8–1). However, nodules may be seen in the lung parenchyma and occasionally in the walls of airways. In some instances, the infiltrate may be quite cellular with little fibrosis ("cellular interstitial pneumonia"), and occasionally a desquamative interstitial pneumonia pattern may be seen (Yousem et al, 1985). Foci of lymphocytes with germinal centers are often seen in biopsies of patients with RA, but are by no means specific for RA.

Lymphoid Hyperplasia with Germinal Centers

Lymphoid hyperplasia with germinal centers may be found distributed along bronchovascular bundles and interlobular septa (Yousem et al, 1985). (See the section on follicular bronchitis/bronchiolitis in Chapter 12.) If accompanied by a cellular or fibrotic interstitial infiltrate, the appearance merges with cellular interstitial pneumonia or with UIP as described above. Radiologically, lymphoid hyperplasia presents as a reticulonodular or nodular pattern (Yousem et al, 1985) (Fig. 8–2).

Pulmonary Hypertension

Pulmonary hypertension is the rarest (Hunninghake and Fauci, 1979) of the pulmonary disorders seen in association with RA. The clinical presentation is that of primary pulmonary hypertension, and the lesions are indistinguishable histologically.

SYSTEMIC LUPUS ERYTHEMATOSUS

Systemic lupus erythematosus (SLE) commonly involves the lungs and pleura (Hunninghake and Fauci, 1979). The radiologic findings in SLE are nonspecific. Acute lupus pneumonitis and pulmonary hemorrhage may present as patchy areas of consolidation, usually most prominent in the lung bases. Diaphragmatic dysfunction may lead to elevation of the diaphragm, low lung volumes, and areas of plate-like atelectasis (Fig. 8–3). Plate-like atelectasis is a common finding in lupus, particularly in patients with pleuritis, pleural effusion, or diaphragmatic dysfunction (Hunninghake and Fauci, 1979). Pleural effusions are common and usually bilateral.

Although a variety of different morphologic lesions are described in autopsied patients with SLE, many of these lesions are probably coincidental (Haupt et al, 1981). Even the lesions apparently due to SLE are not morphologically specific (Miller et al, 1985).

Painful pleuritis with or without effusion is the most common abnormality, occurring in approximately 50 to 75 percent of patients (Haupt et al, 1981). The histologic abnormalities in pleural biopsies are nonspecific and include fibrinous exudate, chronic inflammation, and fibrosis.

Fibrosing alveolitis is relatively uncommon. Eisenberg and coworkers (1973) estimated that diffuse interstitial disease due to SLE occurred in less than 5 percent of their outpatients with SLE. Haupt and colleagues (1981) found interstitial pneumonitis due to SLE in 9 percent of patients in one autopsy series, with progression to fibrosis in only 4 percent.

Acute lupus pneumonitis is a potentially disastrous complication, characterized usually by diffuse alveolar damage with or without capillaritis, vascular thrombosis, and bronchiolitis (Matthay et al, 1974). Mortality is cited as 50 percent in the acute episode of this complication; progression to chronic interstitial pneumonitis or fibrosis is common in the survivors.

Diffuse pulmonary hemorrhage is another potentially life-threatening complication of SLE that presents acutely (see chapter 6). In addition to recent hemorrhage and hemosiderosis, the characteristic (but not pathognomonic) finding is acute capillaritis with karyorrhexis of neutrophils, alveolar wall necrosis, and neutrophilic arteriolitis (Myers and Katzenstein, 1986).

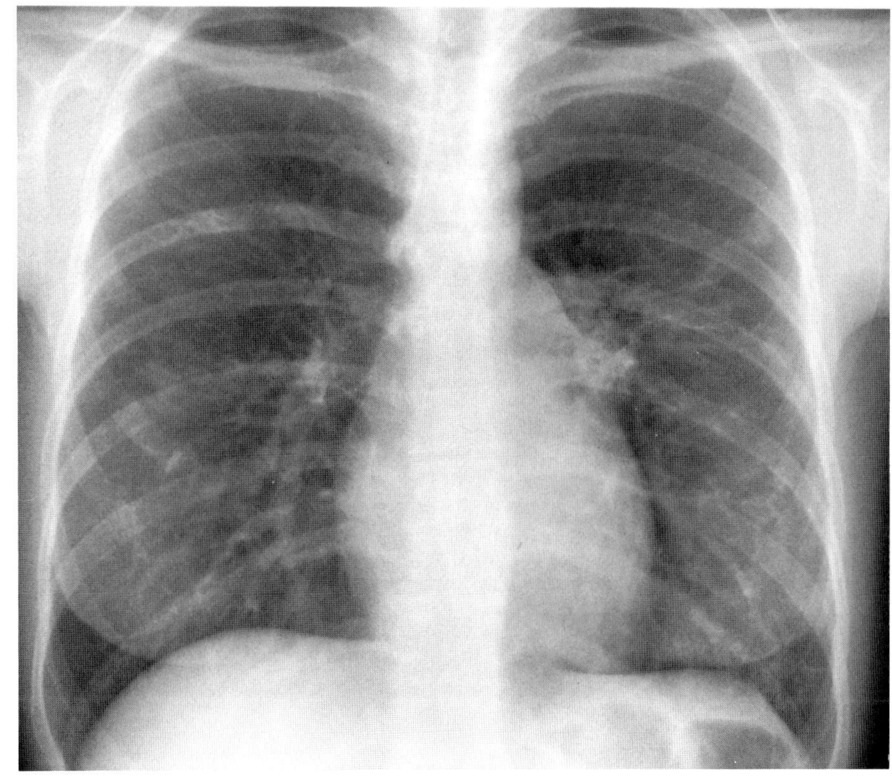

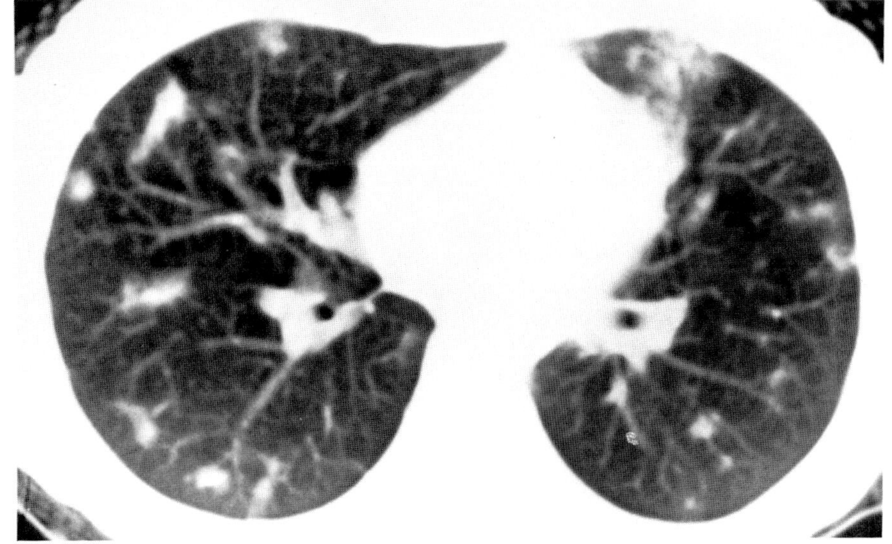

Figure 8–2 Rheumatoid arthritis and biopsy-proven pulmonary lymphoid hyperplasia in a 24-year-old woman. *A*, Chest radiograph demonstrates bilateral, ill-defined, small nodular opacities. *B*, A 10-mm collimation CT scan demonstrates the nodular densities and their irregular margins. A small area of consolidation is seen in the lingula.

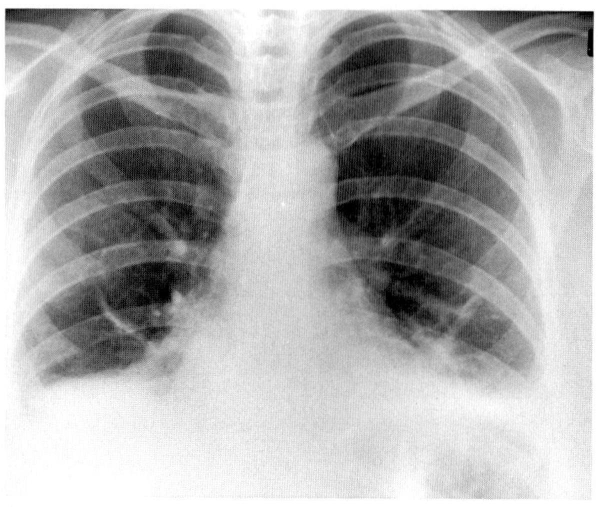

A

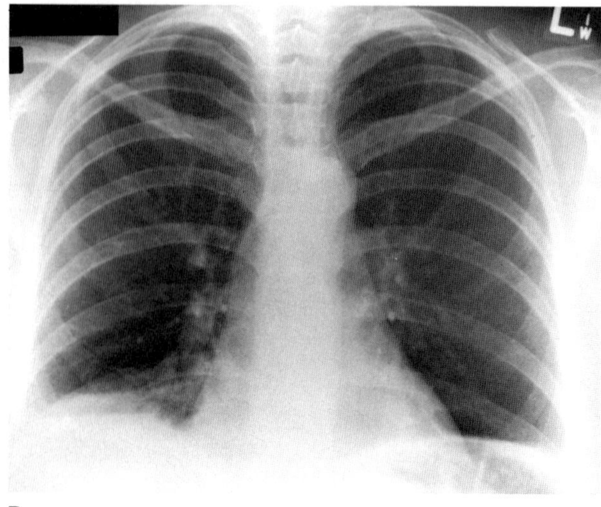

B

Figure 8–3 Systemic lupus erythematosus in a 29-year-old woman who presented with a 3-week history of intermittent pleuritic chest pain and progressive shortness of breath. *A,* Initial chest radiograph shows bilateral pleural effusions, areas of plate-like atelectasis, and decreased lung volumes. *B,* Chest radiograph following one week of treatment with corticosteroids shows clearing of the plate-like atelectasis and almost complete resolution of the pleural effusions. However, the low lung volumes persist.

PROGRESSIVE SYSTEMIC SCLEROSIS

Progressive systemic sclerosis (PSS) involves the lung in the majority of cases (Owens and Follansbee, 1987) of both the classic diffuse form of the disease and the generally more indolent "CREST" variant (calcinosis, Raynaud's phenomenon, esophageal dysfunction, sclerodactyly without truncal dermal abnormalities, and telangiectasias.). Dyspnea develops in over 60 percent of patients during the course of their disease. Over 70 percent of patients experience functional abnormalities, the most common being reduced diffusing capacity. Autopsy shows morphologic abnormalities of the lungs in 70 percent. The most common pathologic processes are vasculopathy, fibrosing alveolitis, small airways disease, and carcinoma (Yousem, 1990).

Vasculopathy

In Yousem's series (1990), almost all patients had some degree of vasculopathy, characterized by myxomatous fibrosis of the intima of arterioles. Scattered inflammatory cells were sometimes seen in the intima, but transmural vasculitis was not observed. These vascular abnormalities eventually led to pulmonary hypertension in the majority of cases.

Fibrosing Alveolitis

PSS-associated fibrosing alveolitis is morphologically indistinguishable from UIP. Typically, the inflammatory component is relatively mild compared with the fibrosing component, although some degree of disease activity is usually demonstrable by biopsy, gallium scans, or bronchoalveolar lavage (Rossi et al, 1985). Concurrent vasculopathy is almost always found in patients with PSS-associated fibrosing alveolitis. The incidence of radiographically recognizable interstitial disease is probably around 20 percent, although various studies quote an incidence ranging from 10 to 80 percent (Taormina et al, 1981). The radiographic findings of interstitial fibrosis in PSS are identical to those of UIP. The clinical response to steroids is poor.

Small Airways Disease

The small airways disease of PSS is characterized by submucosal fibrosis and bronchiolectasis with a variable degree of chronic inflammation. Most patients with PSS-related small airways disease are cigarette smokers (Yousem, 1990). Patients with long-standing PSS-related fibrosis, especially those who are smokers, are at high risk for the development of bronchogenic carcinoma, which may be of any of

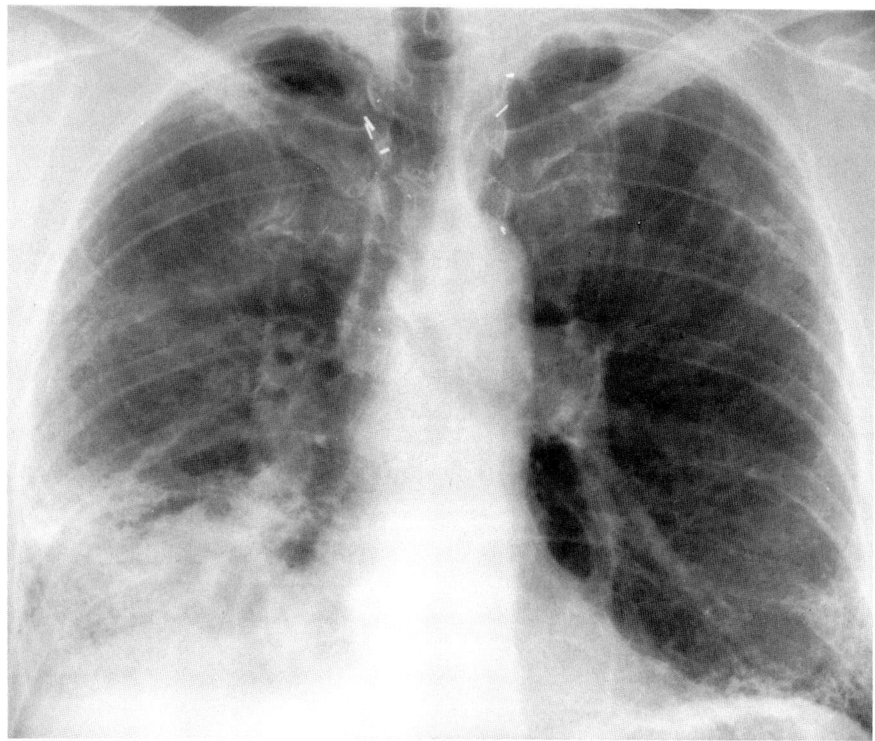

Figure 8–4   Progressive systemic sclerosis in a 63-year-old man. Chest radiograph shows bilateral reticular densities involving predominantly the lower lung zones. A large cell bronchogenic carcinoma (5 cm in diameter) is present in the right lower lobe. The surgical clips are related to a previous sympathectomy.

the usual cell types (Fig. 8–4). Pleural disease is considerably less common in PSS than in RA or SLE.

ANKYLOSING SPONDYLITIS

Ankylosing spondylitis is associated with extensive upper zonal pulmonary fibrosis and bullae, which usually develop 10 years or more after the onset of the disease. The precise frequency of pulmonary involvement is not known, but a range of up to 30 percent has been reported. The largest single series indicates a frequency of about 1 percent (Rosenow et al, 1977). Most patients with this complication are male. Radiologically, the process begins as apical pleural involvement, followed by an apical infiltrate, and progressing to cyst formation. Generally, the disease begins unilaterally and becomes bilateral, although involvement of the lower lobes is rare. The chest radiograph may closely mimic that of tuberculosis. While the decreased thoracic wall complicance resulting from the joint disease may cause restrictive dysfunction and dyspnea, uncomplicated fibrobullous disease itself is usually asymptomatic. Symptoms such as fever, cough, and hemoptysis may develop in the event of secondary infection of the bullae, which is relatively common. *Aspergillus* and atypical species of mycobacteria are the most frequent offenders. The histologic findings in uncomplicated fibrobullous disease are nonspecific inflammation and fibrosis.

MIXED CONNECTIVE TISSUE DISEASE

Mixed connective tissue disease (MCTD) is often associated with radiologic and/or functional evidence of interstitial pulmonary disease (Hunninghake and Fauci, 1979; Prakash et al, 1985). The abnormalities usually respond quite well to corticosteroid therapy, but in a few instances severe and progressive pulmonary disease (either fibrosing alveolitis or pulmonary hypertension) occurs (Wiener-Kronish et al, 1981). We have seen one patient with MCTD associated with recurrent diffuse pulmonary hemorrhage (Fig. 8–5).

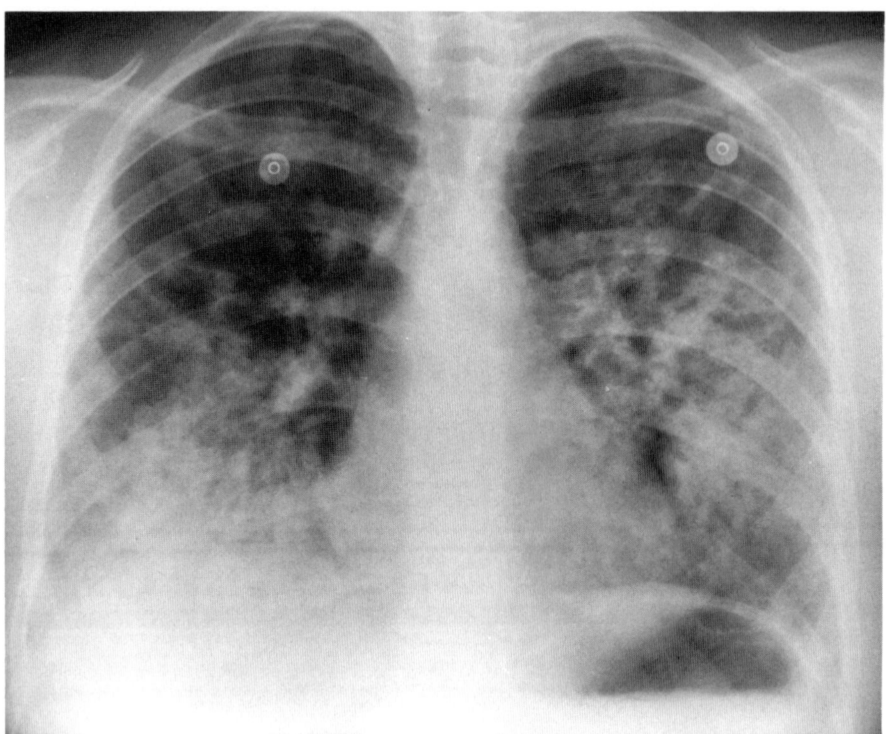

Figure 8–5 Mixed collagen vascular disease and recurrent pulmonary hemorrhage in a 17-year-old woman. Chest radiograph shows bilateral airspace consolidation.

SJÖGREN'S SYNDROME

The common pulmonary lesions of Sjögren's syndrome are analogous to the lesions of the salivary gland, namely a marked lymphoreticular infiltrate in the submucosal glands of the tracheobronchial tree (Hunninghake and Fauci, 1979). A lymphoproliferative disorder involving the pulmonary interstitium, ranging from relatively low-grade lymphoid interstitial pneumonia to a high-grade malignant lymphoma, may develop (see Chapter 7). Fibrosing alveolitis and pleural disease are seen in patients with other concurrent autoimmune features such RA or SLE.

BEHÇET'S DISEASE

Behçet's disease is an uncommon disease that involves the lung in approximately 5 percent of cases (Raz et al, 1989; Yazici et al, 1990; O'Duffy, 1990). Although the major components of the syndrome are oral and genital ulcers and iridocyclitis, multiorgan involvement on the basis of an immune complex vasculopathy is well recognized. The characteristic lung abnormalities include a necrotizing mononuclear, nongranulomatous vasculitis involving all sizes of the arterial and venous network. A poly-

morphonuclear leukocyte infiltrate is believed to follow, rather than precede, the mononuclear cell component. Elastin and muscle destruction occurs and leads to the development of aneurysms, arterial and venous thromboses, and pulmonary infarcts. Characteristically, disease activity is episodic so that a wide range of active and healed lesions are identified in tissue. Fibrosing alveolitis and pleural disease are not features of this disorder. Aphthous ulcers are occasionally found in the proximal tracheobronchial tree.

Erosion of aneurysms into adjacent bronchi leads to hemoptysis, which is a common presentation of pulmonary involvement by Behçet's disease. This complication, usually seen in young adult men, is often massive and life-threatening (Raz et al, 1989). Treatment is surgical if the process is localized, and steroid therapy is usually helpful if it is not. Anticoagulation to prevent thrombosis of the aneurysm has been associated with marked deterioration in several patients.

The radiologic findings are nonspecific. Transient areas of airspace consolidation, presumably representing hemorrhage or infarction, occur. Lobar or segmental artery aneurysms may be seen as small or large central nodular opacities. The diagnosis of pulmonary artery aneurysm is usually made by angiography, although occasionally the diagnosis can be made by computed tomography (Winer-Muram and Gavant, 1989).

POLYMYOSITIS/DERMATOMYOSITIS

Polymyositis/dermatomyositis (PM/DM) is uncommonly associated with pulmonary involvement, the reported incidence of significant radiologic abnormalities being only approximately 5 percent (Frazier and Miller, 1974). There is no relationship between the extent, severity, or duration of muscle disease and the development of lung disease. Some patients present with simultaneous dermal/muscle and lung disease; others present with dermal/muscle disease preceding any radiologic evidence of lung disease; in a few patients, the appearance of lung disease precedes detectable dermal/muscle abnormalities (Frazier and Miller, 1974; Tazelaar et al, 1990).

Tazelaar and colleagues (1990) described the histologic patterns of reaction seen in specimens from lung biopsy of 14 patients and autopsy of one patient with symptomatic PM/DM-related interstitial disease. Six patients had a cellular bronchiolitis obliterans–organizing pneumonia (BOOP) reaction pattern with little fibrosis, and these patients tended to do well with steroid therapy. Five patients had a variably cellular UIP reaction, and three of these died. Three patients with a diffuse alveolar damage died. One patient had diffuse "cellular interstitial pneumonia" and did well with steroid therapy. We have also seen a case with a diffuse cellular interstitial reaction simulating lymphoid interstitial pneumonitis (LIP) in a patient with dermatomyositis. Tazelaar and colleagues (1990) make the point that in PM/DM-associated interstitial lung disease, the degree of cellularity or disease activity is probably less useful as a prognostic indicator than is reaction pattern. Nevertheless, steroids and immunosuppressive agents are prescribed, regardless of the pattern. In addition, if another major disease process such as aspiration pneumonia, malignancy, or infection is suspected, open biopsy is recommended.

REFERENCES

Campbell GD, Ferrington E. Rheumatoid pleuritis with effusion. Chest 1968; 53:521–527.

Carr DT, Mayne JG. Pleurisy with effusion in rheumatoid arthritis, with reference to the low concentration of glucose in pleural fluid. Am Rev Respir Dis 1962; 85:345–350.

Cervantes-Perez P, Toro-Perez AH, Rodriguez-Jurado P. Pulmonary involvement in rheumatoid arthritis. JAMA 1980; 243:1715–1719.

Eisenberg H, Dubois EL, Sherwin RP, Balchum OJ. Diffuse interstitial lung disease in systemic lupus erythematosus. Ann Intern Med 1973; 79:37–45.

Frank ST, Weg JG, Harkleroad LE, Fitch RF. Pulmonary dysfunction in rheumatoid disease. Chest 1973; 63: 27–34.

Fraser RG, Paré JAP, Paré PD, et al. Diagnosis of diseases of the chest. 3rd ed. Philadelphia: WB Saunders, 1989:1189–1239.

Frazier AR, Miller RD. Interstitial pneumonitis in association with polymyositis and dermatomyositis. Chest 1974; 65:403–407.

Hammar SP, Winterbauer RH, Bockus D, et al. Endothelial cell damage and tubuloreticular structures in interstitial lung disease associated with collagen vascular disease and viral pneumonia. Am Rev Respir Dis 1983; 127:77–84.

Haupt HM, Moore GW, Hutchins GM. The lung in systemic lupus erythematosus. Am J Med 1981; 71:791–798.

Hunninghake GW, Fauci AS. Pulmonary involvement in the collagen vascular diseases. Am Rev Respir Dis 1979; 119:471–503.

Jolles H, Moseley PL, Peterson MW. Nodular pulmonary opacities in patients with rheumatoid arthritis—a diagnostic dilemma. Chest 1989; 96:1022–1025.

Jurik AG, Davidsen D, Graudal H. Prevalence of pulmonary involvement in rheumatoid arthritis and its relationship to some characteristics of the patients—a radiological and clinical study. Scand J Rheumatol 1982; 11:217–224.

Laitinen O, Nissila M, Salorinne Y, et al. Pulmonary involvement in patients with rheumatoid arthritis. Scand J Respir Dis 1975; 56:297–304.

Matthay RA, Schwarz MI, Petty TL, et al. Pulmonary manifestations of systemic lupus erythematosus: review of twelve cases of acute lupus pneumonitis. Medicine 1974; 54:397–409.

Miller LR, Greenberg SD, McLarty JW. Lupus lung. Chest 1985; 88:265–269.

Myers JL, Katzenstein ALA. Microangitis in lupus-induced pulmonary hemorrhage. Am J Clin Pathol 1986; 85:552–556.

O'Duffy JD. Behçet's syndrome. N Engl J Med 1990; 323:326–327.

Owens GR, Follansbee WP. Cardiopulmonary manifestations of systemic sclerosis. Chest 1987; 91:118–127.

Portner MM, Gracie WA. Rheumatoid lung disease with cavitary nodules, pneumothorax, and eosinophilia. N Engl J Med 1966; 275:697–700.

Prakash UBS, Luthra HS, Divertie MB. Intrathoracic manifestations in mixed connective tissue disease. Mayo Clin Proc 1985; 60:813–821.

Raz I, Okon E, Chajek-Shaul T. Pulmonary manifestations in Behçet's syndrome. Chest 1989; 95:585–589.

Rosenow EC, Strimlan CV, Muhm JR, Ferguson RH. Pleuropulmonary manifestations of ankylosing spondylitis. Mayo Clinic Proc 1977; 52:641–649.

Rossi GA, Bitterman PB, Rennard SI, et al. Evidence for chronic inflammation as a component of the interstitial lung disease associated with progressive systemic sclerosis. Am Rev Respir Dis 1985; 131:612–617.

Slavin RE, de Groot WJ. Pathology of the lung in Behçet's disease. Am J Surg Pathol 1981; 5:779–788.

Taormina VJ, Miller WT, Gefter WB, Epstein DM. Progressive systemic sclerosis subgroups: variable pulmonary features. AJR 1981; 137:227–285.

Tazelaar HD, Viggiano RW, Pickersgill J, Colby TV. Interstitial lung disease in polymyositis and dermatomyositis. Am Rev Respir Dis 1990; 141:727–733.

Walker WC, Wright V. Rheumatoid pleuritis. Ann Rheum Dis 1967; 26:467.

Walker WC, Wright V. Pulmonary lesions and rheumatoid arthritis. Medicine 1968; 47:501–520.

Wiener-Kronish JP, Solinger AM, Warnock ML, et al. Severe pulmonary involvement in mixed connective tissue disease. Am Rev Respir Dis 1981; 124:499–503.

Winer-Muram HT, Gavant ML. Pulmonary CT findings in Behçet disease. J Comput Assist Tomogr 1989; 13:346–347.

Yazici H, Pazarli H, Barnes CG, et al. A controlled trial of azathiaprine in Behçet's syndrome. N Engl J Med 1990; 322:281–285.

Yousem SA. Pulmonary pathologic manifestations of the CREST syndrome. Hum Pathol 1990; 21:467–474.

Yousem SA, Colby TV, Carrington CB. Lung biopsy in rheumatoid arthritis. Am Rev Respir Dis 1985; 131:770–777.

CHAPTER 9

TUMORS

Most types of primary and metastatic carcinomas and sarcomas result in one or more masses in the lung. The types of tumors that may be expected to give rise to a clinical and radiologic pattern of bilateral infiltrative lung disease include lymphangitic carcinomatosis, multicentric bronchioloalveolar carcinoma, lymphoma and leukemia, Kaposi's sarcoma, and "benign metastasizing leiomyoma."

PULMONARY LYMPHANGITIC CARCINOMATOSIS

Pulmonary lymphangitic carcinomatosis (PLC) is characterized by metastatic tumor growth primarily in lymphatic channels. Adenocarcinomas are usual, although neuroendocrine carcinoma and squamous cell carcinoma have been described. The most common primary sites are lung, breast, gastrointestinal tract, and pancreas (Munk et al, 1988). The prognosis is poor, and long-term survival is exceptional.

Because the pulmonary lymphatics are located in the bronchovascular bundles, interlobar septa, and pleura, the macroscopic appearance of PLC is one of thickening of these structures (Fig. 9-1). Microscopically, the diagnostic feature is the presence of tumor cells within the lumen of lymphatic vessels (Fig. 9-2). Variable amounts of edema, fibrosis, inflammation, and intra-alveolar tumor may also be seen. The presence of tumor cells in peribronchial lymphatics explains the high yield of transbronchial lung biopsy (TLB) in the diagnosis of PLC (Fig. 9-3), 80 percent in one series (Wall et al, 1981).

At autopsy, the distribution of disease is typically bilateral and diffuse. However, early in the course of disease, the distribution of PLC may be localized to one lobe. In the series by Munk and colleagues (1988), 10 of 21 patients had localized PLC at the time of diagnosis. It seems possible that the yield of TBB could be enhanced by the use of computed tomography (CT) to guide the bronchoscopist to the most severely affected area (Fig. 9-4).

The pathogenesis of PLC is thought to be related to the seeding of lymphatics from blood vessel tumor emboli, which are almost always obvious in these cases (Janower and Blennerhassett, 1971). However, the propensity for tumor growth within lymphatic vessels is unexplained. Retrograde growth of tumor due to blocked mediastinal nodes seems unlikely since, in at least half the cases, the nodes are not massively involved (Janower and Blennerhassett, 1971).

The radiologic manifestations of PLC include a reticular, reticulonodular or nodular pattern; septal (Kerley) lines; and thickening of the interlobar fissures (Trapnell, 1964; Munk et al, 1988) (Fig. 9-5). Unilateral or bilateral hilar adenopathy is present in 30 to 40 percent of patients (Janower and Blennerhassett, 1971; Munk et al, 1988). Approximately 30 percent of patients have unilateral or bilateral pleural effusions. The radiologic findings, however, are nonspecific; even symptomatic patients may have a normal chest radiograph (Janower and Blennerhassett, 1971; Munk et al, 1988). Recently, CT has been shown to be helpful in the diagnosis of PLC (Munk et al, 1988; Mathieson et al, 1989). The findings on CT

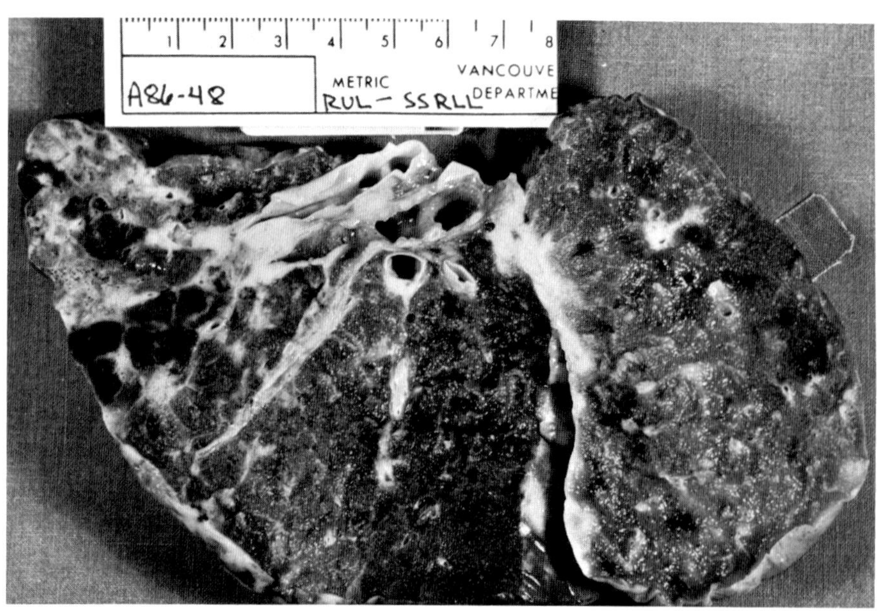

Figure 9-1 Gross appearance of lymphangitic carcinomatosis with thickening of bronchovascular bundles and nodular expansion of interlobular septa and pleura.

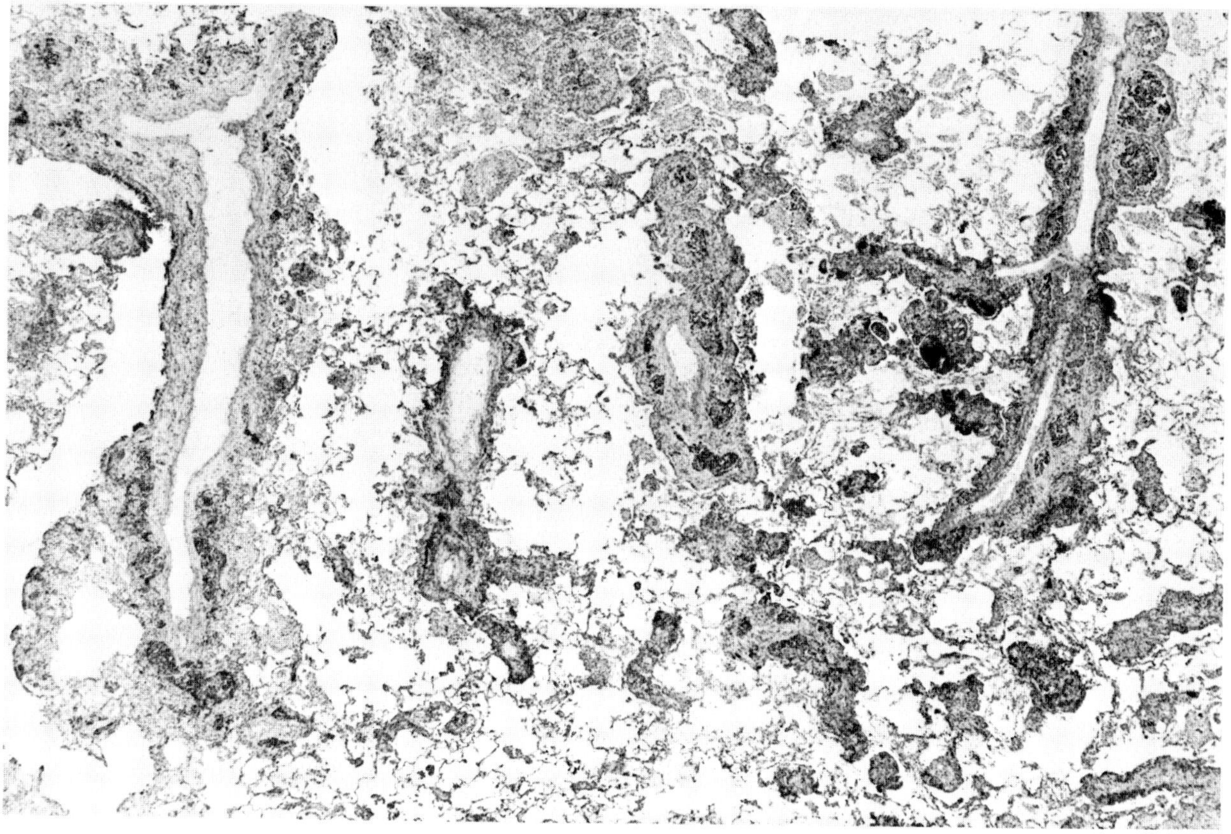

Figure 9–2   Microscopically, the interstitial thickening in pulmonary lymphangitic carcinomatosis is due primarily to plugs of tumor cells in lymphatic channels.

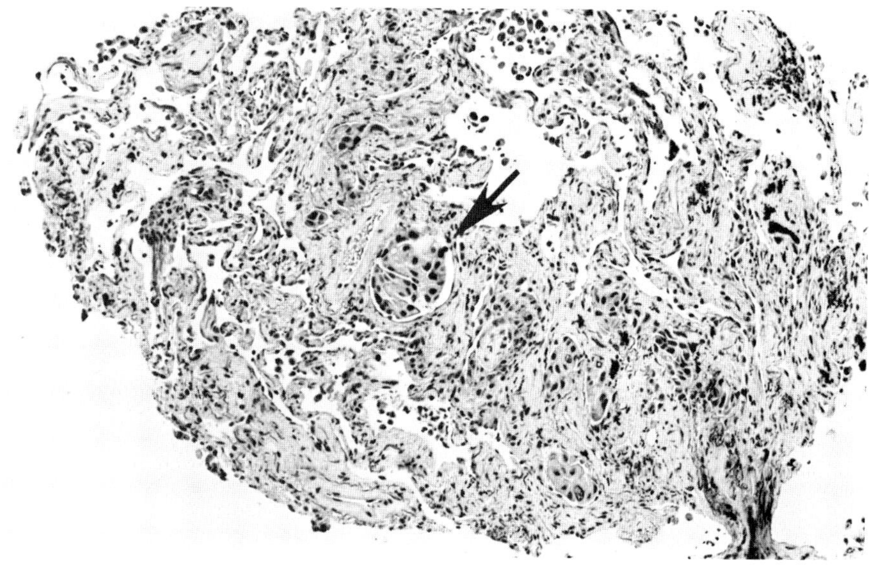

Figure 9–3   Transbronchial lung biopsy diagnostic of pulmonary lymphangitic carcinomatosis.

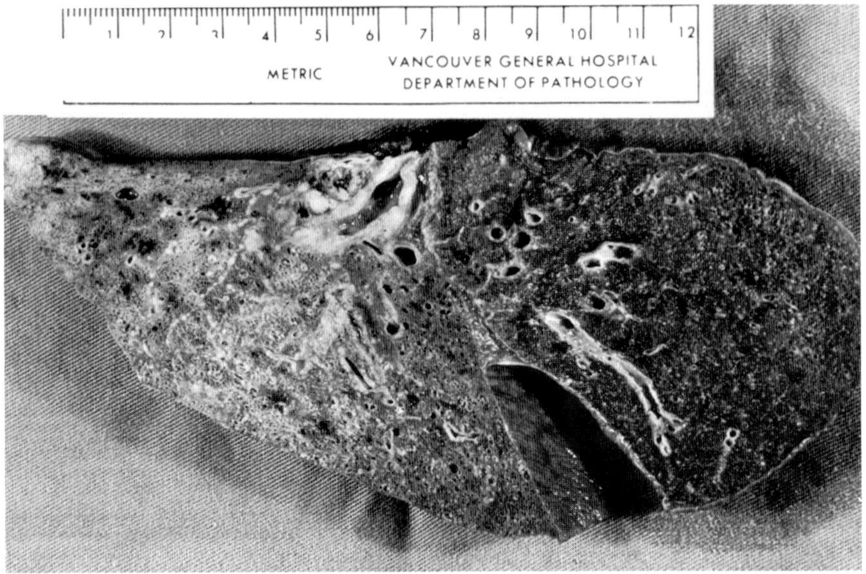

Figure 9–4 This patient died with pulmonary lymphangitic carcinomatosis localized to the right upper lobe. CT can be useful in directing the biopsy site in such cases.

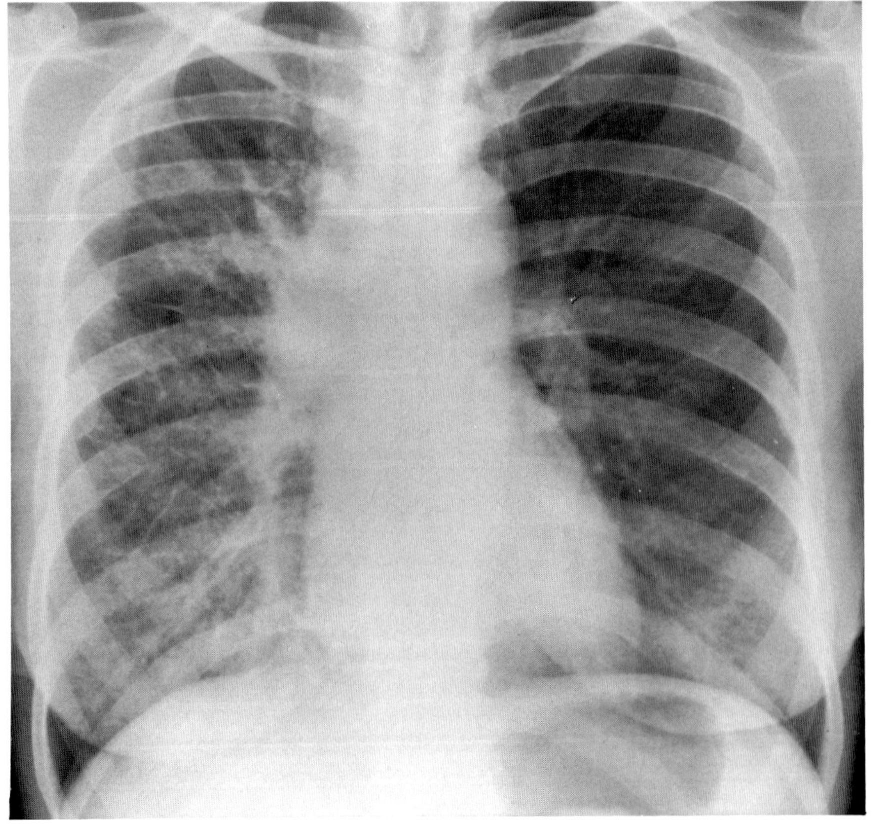

Figure 9–5 Unilateral lymphatic spread of bronchogenic carcinoma in a 47-year-old woman. Chest radiograph shows right hilar and paratracheal adenopathy and linear densities representing thickened interlobular septa.

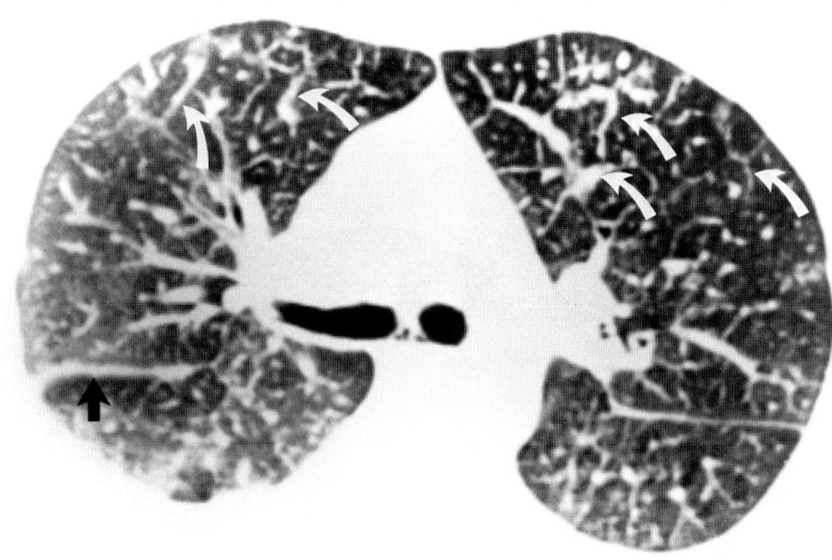

Figure 9–6 Pulmonary lymphatic spread from gastric carcinoma in a 55-year-old woman. A 1.5-mm collimation CT scan shows uneven beaded thickening of interlobular septa (*curved arrows*), centrilobular core structures, and right major fissure (*black arrow*).

consist of uneven, nodular thickening of the bronchovascular bundles and uneven thickening of the interlobular septa, giving the appearance of polygonal lines (Fig. 9–6). These findings often allow a confident radiologic diagnosis with CT even when the chest radiograph is normal or shows nonspecific findings (Munk et al, 1988; Stein et al, 1987).

Dyspnea, nonproductive cough, and usually anorexia with weight loss are the primary symptoms associated with PLC. All three of these may precede the roentgenographic changes, and the dyspnea may be out of proportion to what is seen on the chest roentgenogram. Fever, chills, and sweats are uncommon with this diffuse disease as is chest pain unless there is associated chest wall invasion. The cough may not respond to the usual antitussive medications, including strong narcotics. Pulmonary function studies show a restrictive pattern with impaired diffusion, again with the diffusion impairment possibly greater than what would be expected from the chest roentgenogram. Hemoptysis is rare unless there is an associated separate endobronchial lesion.

BRONCHIOALVEOLAR CARCINOMA

Bronchioalveolar carcinoma (BAC) is a subtype of adenocarcinoma of the lung characterized by growth of tumor cells along pre-existent alveolar septa. Liebow coined the term "lepidic" for this growth pattern to connote tumor cells alighting on alveolar walls as butterflies alighting on shrubbery. Most cases of BAC are characterized grossly by one

or more nodules; uninodular BAC occurs two to three times more frequently than multinodular BAC. A few cases result in a macroscopic pattern of bilateral pneumonia-like infiltrates. These less common, bilateral, multinodular and pneumonic forms enter into the differential diagnosis of diffuse lung disease.

Grossly, diffuse pneumonic BAC has ill-defined borders and occupies much of the lobe(s), thus mimicking pneumonia. The cut surface is gray-white and fleshy to overtly mucoid (Fig. 9–7). Microscopically, the classic appearance is one of well-differentiated, highly mucinous cells, reminiscent of colloid carcinoma of the colon, growing on pre-existent alveolar walls (Fig. 9–8). In multinodular cases, the proportion of nonmucinous tumors is high (Tao et al, 1978; Manning et al, 1984; Clayton, 1986). Our cases of multinodular BAC were not particularly mucinous (Miller et al, 1988) (Fig. 9–9). We concur with the opinion that multinodular BAC is usually nonmucinous and that diffuse pneumonic BAC is mucinous in the majority of instances (Edgerton et al, 1981).

The pathogenesis of diffuse BAC is not entirely clear. The diffuse pneumonic pattern of mucinous BAC is generally interpreted as aerogenous spread or aspiration-implantation (Clayton, 1986; Manning et al, 1984). Multinodular nonmucinous BAC sometimes spreads in the same way, although actual multicentric origin seems more likely in many cases (Miller et al, 1988).

Radiologically BAC may present as a single nodule; as multiple nodules; or as localized, patchy, or diffuse airspace consolidation (Hill, 1984) (Figs. 9–10, 9–11). BAC that presents initially as a single nodule, if left untreated, may progress either to a mass, to

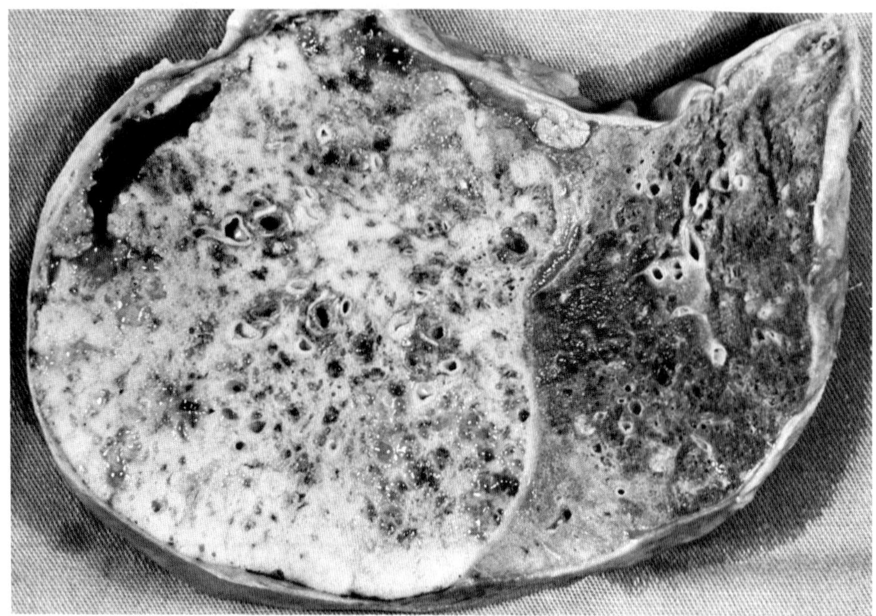

Figure 9–7   Pneumonic bronchioalveolar carcinoma occupying nearly all of the lower lobe with remarkable sparing of the middle lobe (specimen cut transversely in orientation of CT scan).

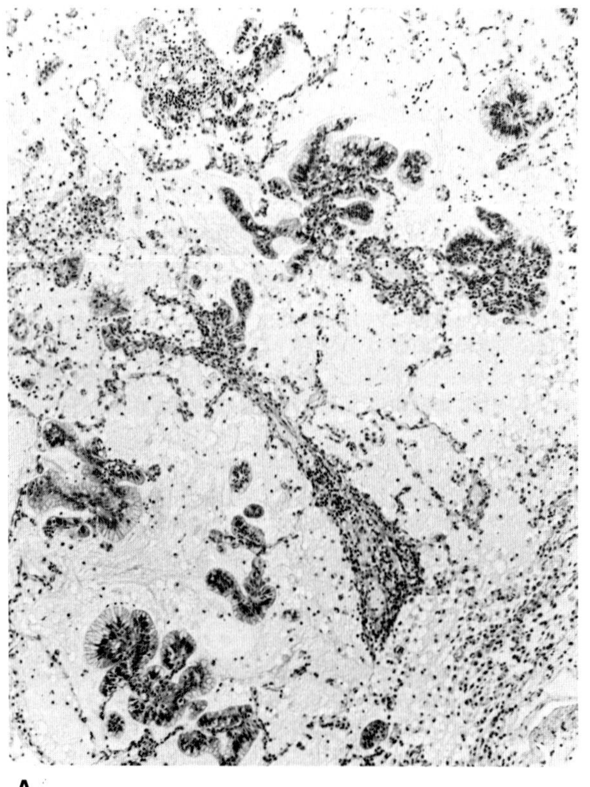

A

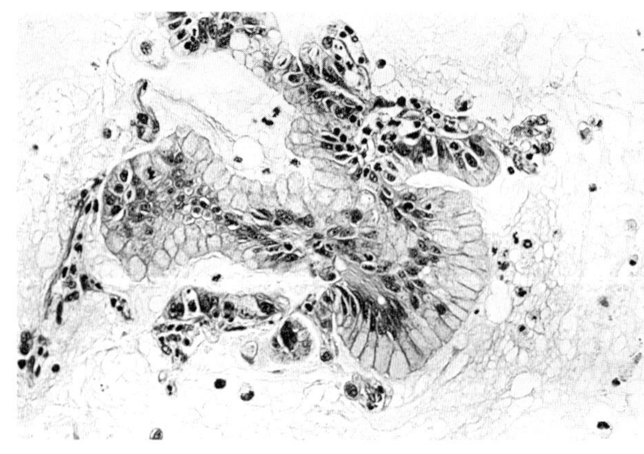

B

Figure 9–8   *A*, Mucinous bronchioalveolar carcinoma characterized by tumor cells on alveolar walls, and abundant intra-alveolar mucin and muciphages. *B*, Tumor cells resemble those of colloid carcinoma with mucinous cytoplasm and basal nuclei.

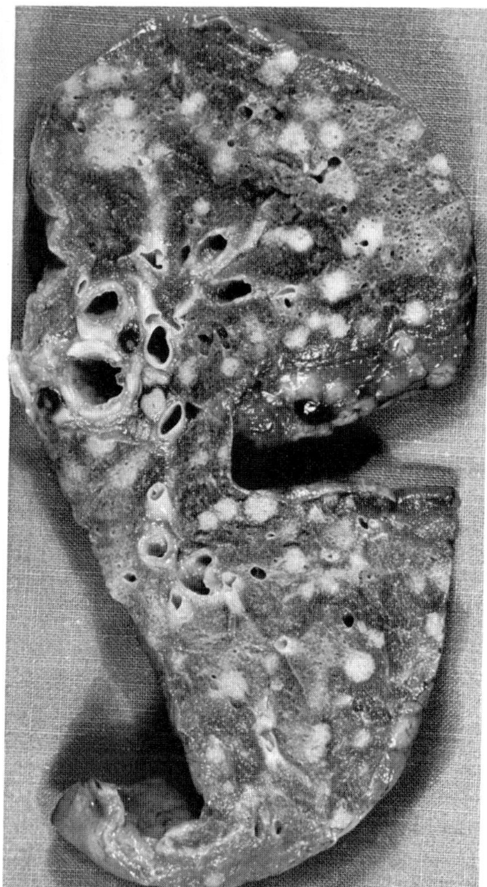

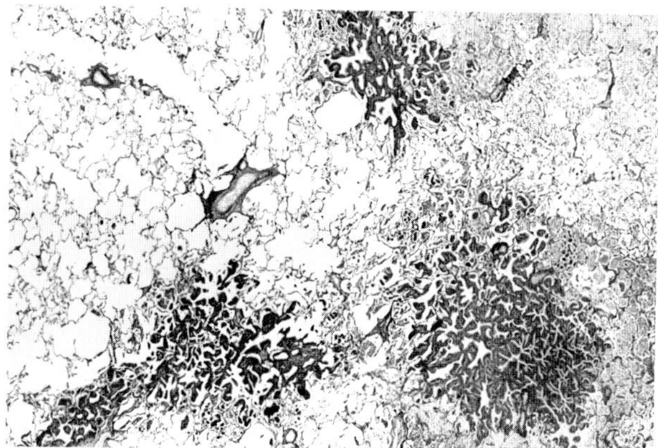

Figure 9–9 *A*, Autopsy appearance of advanced multinodular bronchioalveolar carcinoma, nonmucinous type. *B*, Relatively scant apical mucin production in this not overtly mucinous multicentric bronchioalveolar carcinoma (PAS and diastase). *C*, Three nodules of bronchioalveolar carcinoma, not particularly mucinous.

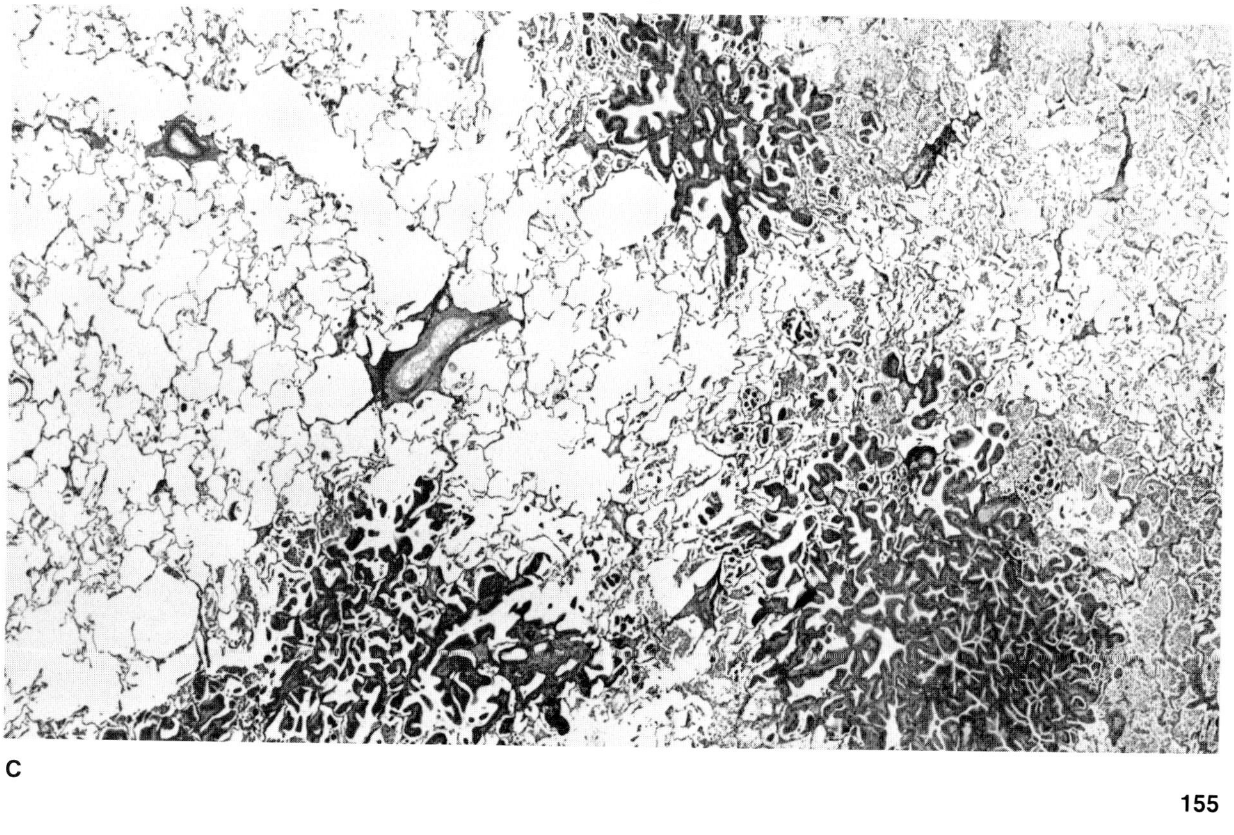

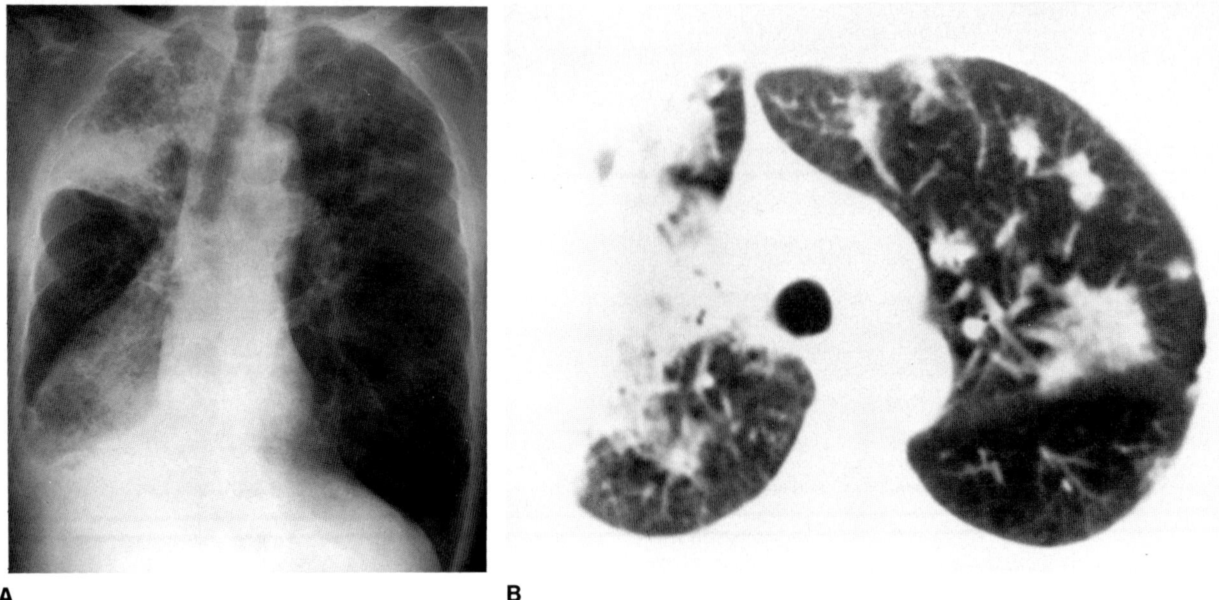

A   **B**

Figure 9–10   *A*, Bronchioalveolar carcinoma in an 86-year-old man. Chest radiograph shows extensive airspace consolidation in the right upper and right lower lobes with associated loss of volume. The process is sharply marginated by the minor and major fissures. Patchy airspace consolidation is present in the left upper lobe. *B*, CT scan better delineates the nodular densities with ill-defined irregular margins in the left upper lobe.

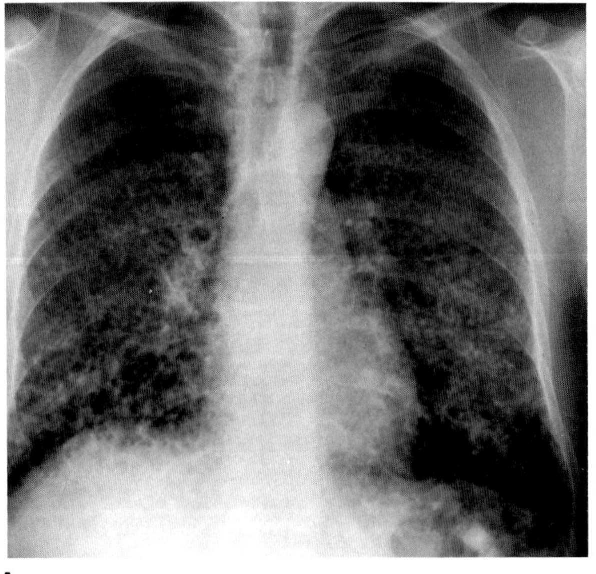

A

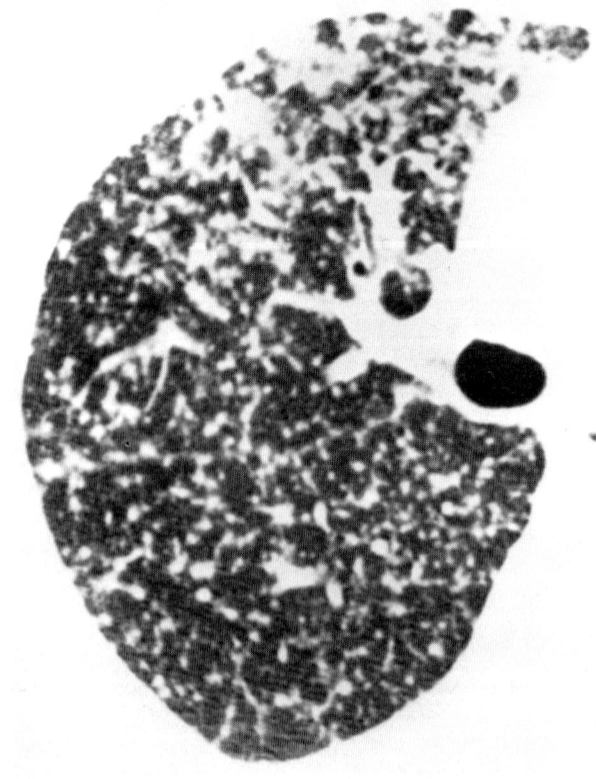

Figure 9–11   Bronchioalveolar carcinoma in a 38-year-old man. *A*, Chest radiograph shows sharply marginated small nodules bilaterally. There is relative sparing of the lung apices. *B*, High-resolution CT through the right mid-lung zone better delineates the small nodules. Confluence of the nodules is present anteriorly.

B

localized or diffuse consolidation, or to diffuse nodular involvement of the lungs (Hill, 1984). Cavitation of the nodules or areas of consolidation, associated hilar lymphadenopathy, pleural effusion, or atelectasis are uncommon but may occur (Hill, 1984). When BAC presents as diffuse nodules these may coalesce or may remain sharply marginated to simulate metastatic disease. Because BAC tends to grow around bronchi rather than to obstruct them, air bronchograms are often seen within the nodules, or as mass-like lesions, and areas of airspace consolidation.

Dyspnea is the most common presenting symptom of diffuse BAC. Unless there is excessive production of mucus, cough is not a common presentation. Contrary to lymphangitic carcinoma, where the symptoms can precede the radiologic changes, almost always the chest roentgenogram is abnormal at the time of earliest symptoms. Hemoptysis is rare. The course of BAC can vary from only a few weeks to 2 to 4 years from the time of initial roentgenographic change. As the dyspnea progresses, anorexia and weight loss eventually occur.

LYMPHOMA

Lymphomatous involvement of the lung may occur either as pulmonary involvement in a patient with established extrapulmonary lymphoma or less frequently as primary pulmonary lymphoma (Koss et al, 1983). Pulmonary involvement by systemic lymphoma is common, particularly in non-Hodgkin's lymphoma (Palosaari and Colby, 1986).

The distinction between primary and secondary pulmonary lymphoma cannot be made on pathologic examination of lung tissue only (Kennedy et al, 1985), as a variety of gross patterns of disease (solitary or multiple nodules, solitary infiltrate, or multiple infiltrates with or without hilar or mediastinal adenopathy) may be seen in either setting. Four reports (Turner et al, 1984; Koss et al, 1983; Kennedy et al, 1985; Weiss et al, 1985) described 291 patients with pulmonary lymphoma and indicated that approximately 40 percent of patients have a solitary nodule and the remaining 60 percent (approximately 20 percent each) have either a solitary infiltrate, multiple nodules, or multiple infiltrates. The 60 percent of patients in the latter three groups are most likely to present with the overall features of infiltrative lung disease.

Lymphoma involving the lung has a striking propensity for lymphangitic distribution, along bronchovascular bundles, interlobular septa, and pleura. For this reason, lymphoma can grossly mimic lymphangitic carcinomatosis. This pattern of distribution has been repeatedly emphasized (Colby and Carrington 1983a, 1983b, Turner et al, 1984; Palosaari and Colby, 1986) and described as lymphangitic "tracking." In cases of solitary or multiple nodules, the lymphangitic distribution cannot be discerned in the center of the nodules but can almost always be found at the edge of the nodule(s) (Fig. 9–12) (Turner et al, 1984). In cases of solitary or multiple infiltrates, the infiltrates are most prominent along lymphatics (Fig. 9–13). Because of the lymphangitic involvement of the pleura, pleural effusions commonly occur in patients with pulmonary lymphoma, particularly non-Hodgkin's lymphoma (Sahn, 1988). For the same

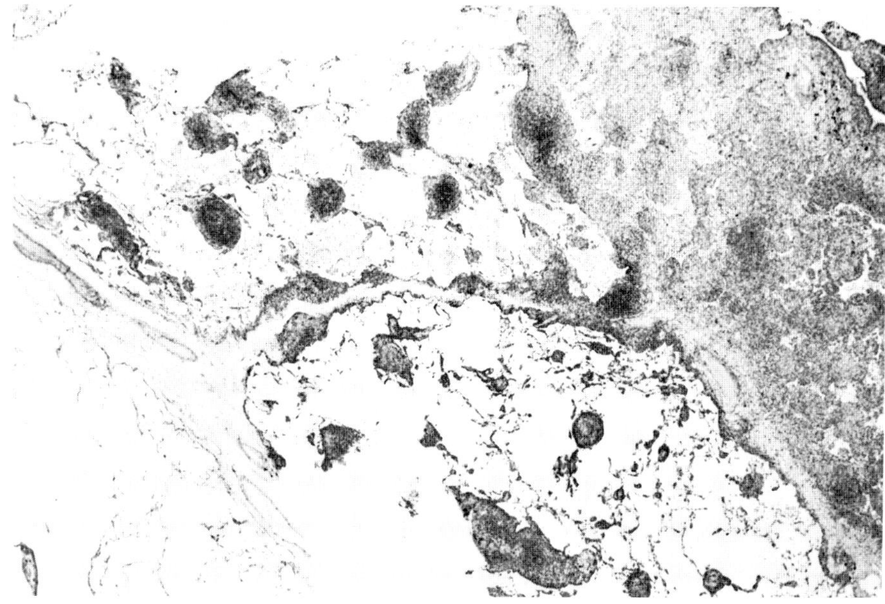

Figure 9–12 Small cell lymphoma of lung with "tracking" at the edge of a solid nodule.

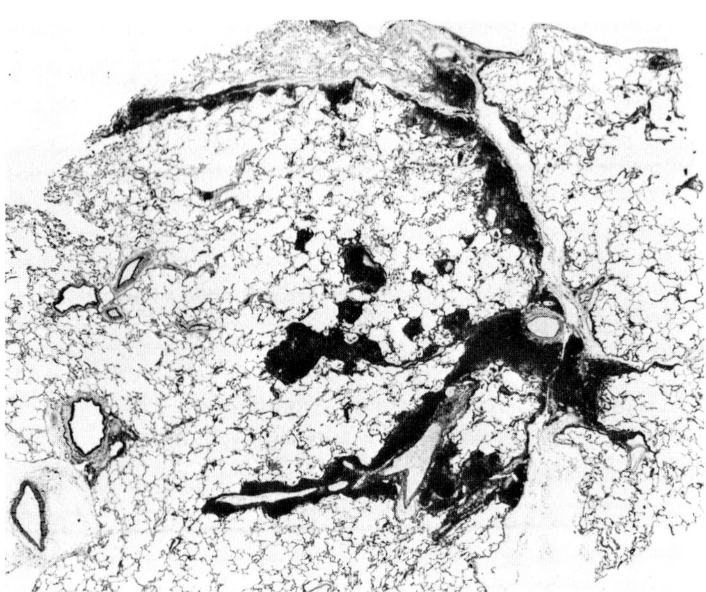

Figure 9–13   Lymphangitic infiltrates of low-grade lymphoma.

reason, bronchial and bronchiolar involvement is also common. It has been postulated (Rose et al, 1986; Isaacson and Wright, 1984) that there is an affinity of lymphomatous cells for bronchial-associated lymphoid tissue (BALT). Occasionally, lymphomatous growth in the walls of conducting airways may be very dramatic with multiple submucosal plaques, endobronchial masses (Rose et al, 1986), or diffuse small airway infiltrates leading to obstructive symptoms (Palosaari and Colby, 1986).

As is the case for other extranodal lymphomas (Evans, 1982), the criteria for diagnosis of pulmonary lymphoma is not so well established as the criteria for nodal malignancy. For many years, the criteria for malignancy were those of Saltstein and included absent germinal centers, definite cytologic atypia, and nodal or pleural invasion (Saltstein, 1963). These criteria have been revised in recent years to incorporate the hematopathologic tenets of clonality, immunologic markers, and natural history of various specific types of lymphomas. Although architectural effacement cannot be assessed in the usual sense, it has been suggested that "tracking" is a reliable substitute (Colby and Carrington, 1983a, 1983b). Visceral pleural invasion and bronchial cartilaginous erosion are now regarded as nonspecific architectural abnormalities seen in approximately 70 percent of lymphomas (Koss et al, 1983) but these are also

seen in a significant proportion of benign lymphoproliferative lesions. Parietal pleural invasion (Fig. 9–14) is said to be diagnostic of lymphoma (Koss et al, 1983). Contiguous nodal involvement is a specific indicator of malignancy but is seen in only one-fourth to one-third of patients (Koss et al, 1983).

The relative incidence of bland-looking small lymphocytic and small cleaved-cell lymphomas compared with intermediate- and high-grade lymphomas varies among series from a minority (Weiss et al, 1985) to the vast majority (Koss et al, 1983; Turner et al, 1984). The distinction between benign lymphocytic infiltration and well-differentiated lymphoma may be difficult or even impossible. Current recommendations are that monomorphous infiltrates and especially monoclonal infiltrates are indicative of lymphoma. The cytologic criteria are also complicated by the fact that residual BALT or reactive infiltrates may be present in and around a lymphoma, giving it a deceptively polymorphous appearance (Colby and Carrington, 1983a, 1983b). Nevertheless, monomorphous or monoclonal infiltrates that are present take precedence in terms of diagnostic significance.

Along with these changes in diagnostic criteria, there have been changes in the approach to treatment and expected prognosis. Specifically, the vast majority of cytologically bland lesions are indolent,

Figure 9–14   *A,* Visceral pleural involvement by low-grade lymphoma (open lung biopsy). *B,* Parietal pleural involvement by low-grade lymphoma (pleural biopsy).

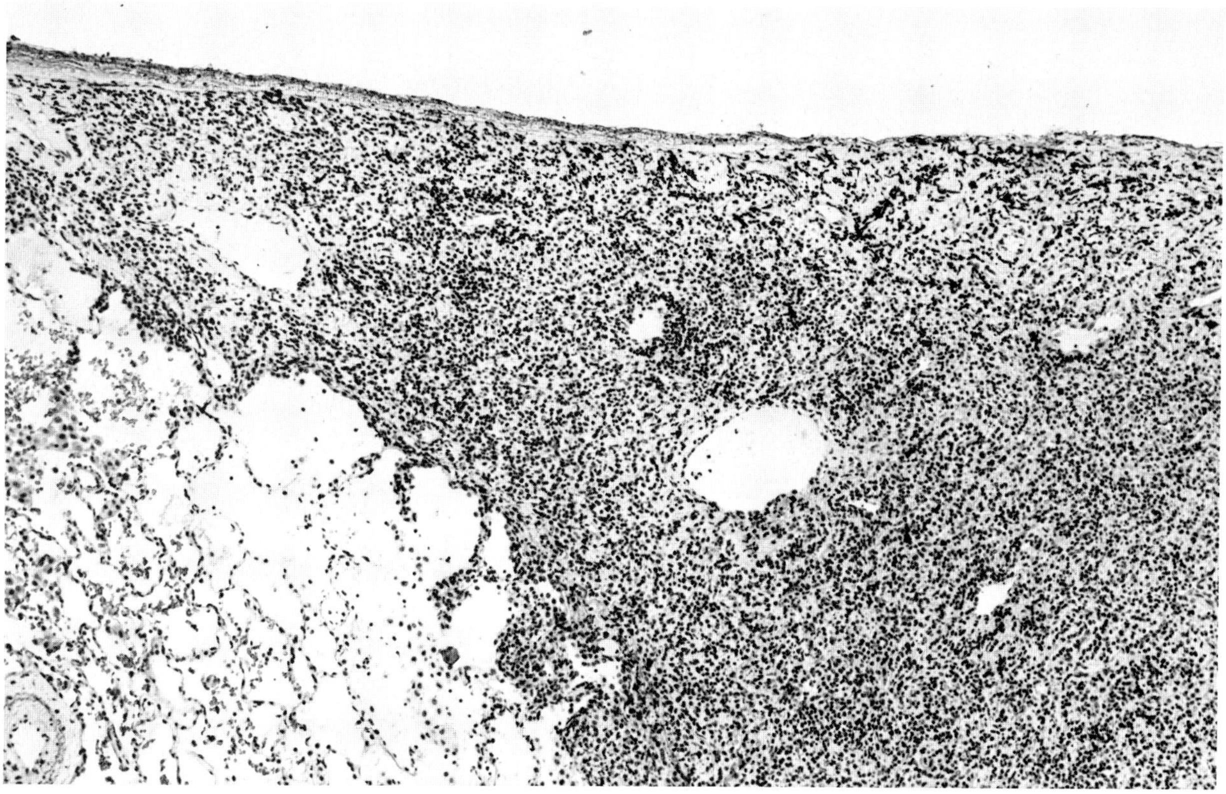

A

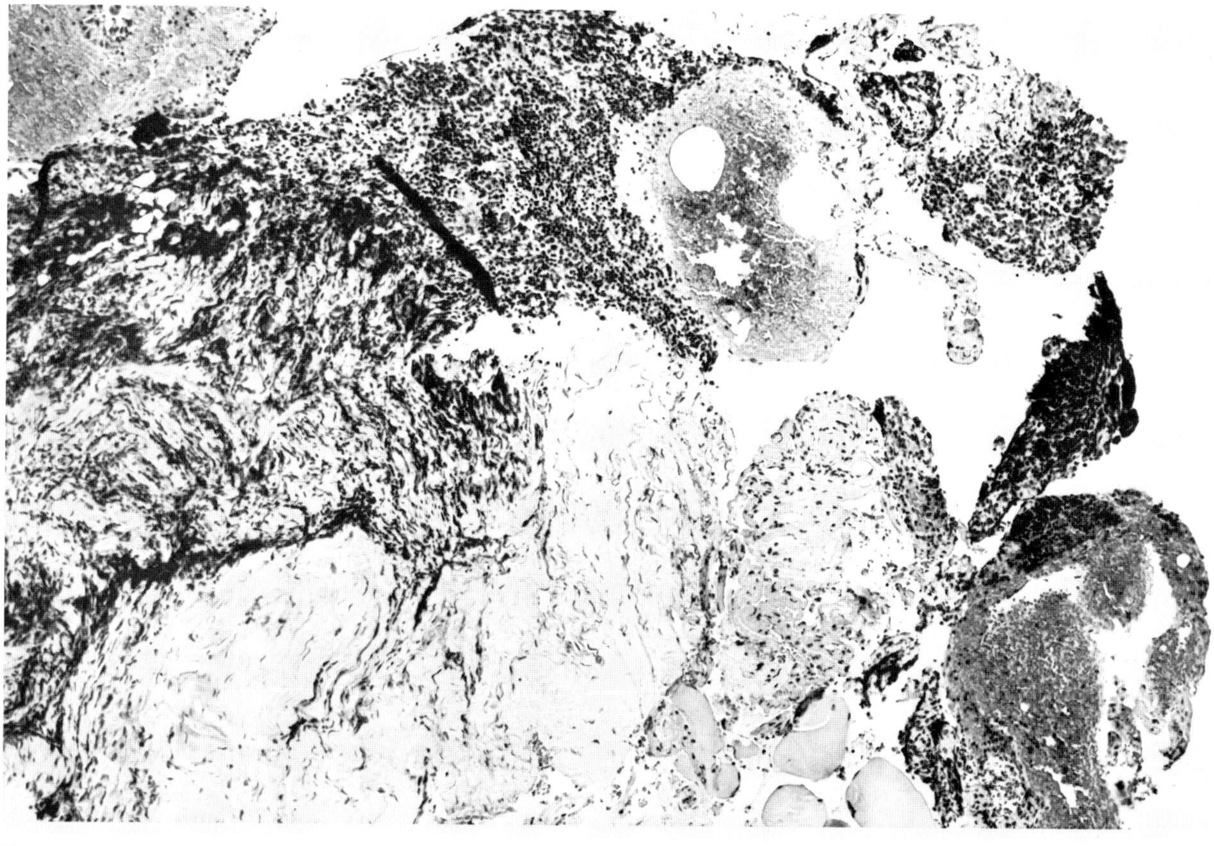

B

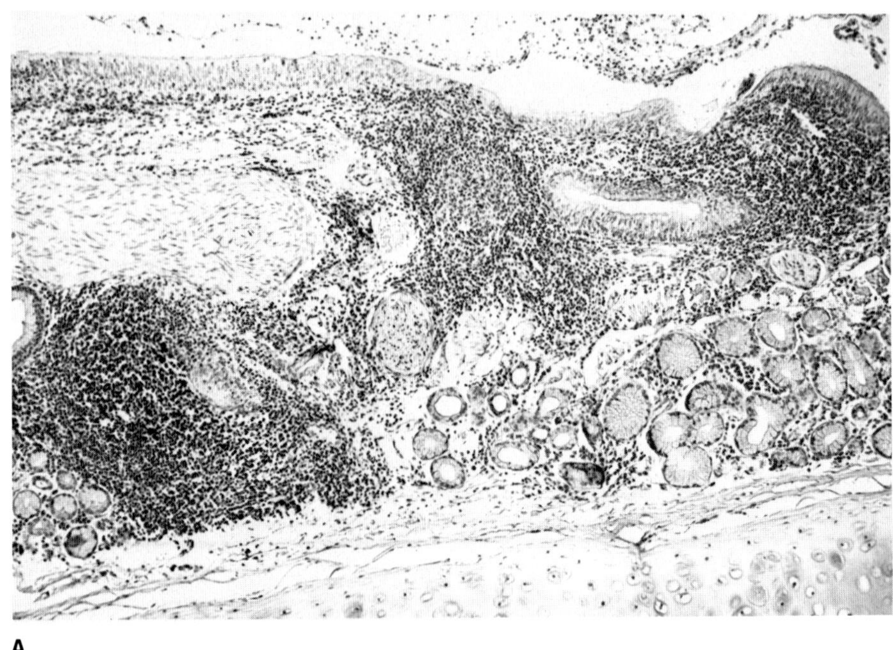

A

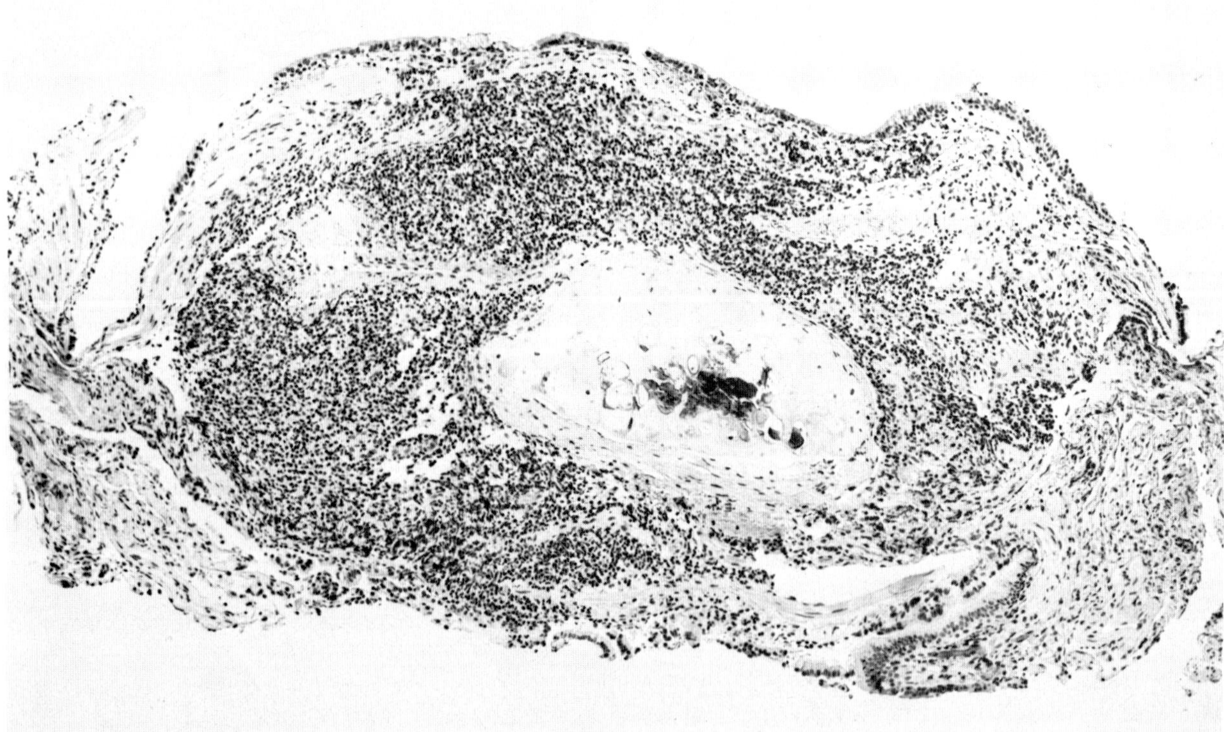

B

Figure 9–15 *A*, Marked bronchial inflammation in patient with broncholith shows germinal center formation and intact bronchial glands and perichondrium. *B*, Bronchial lymphoma (bronchial biopsy).

with occasional exceptions that cannot be predicted on histologic grounds. Localized lesions are best treated with surgical resection (Peterson et al, 1985), and multiple or bilateral infiltrates are best treated with chemotherapy.

One might expect that like lymphangitic carcinomatosis, the diagnosis of pulmonary lymphoma may be readily established by TBB, but this is not the case (Churg, 1988): TBBs cannot demonstrate tracking, and the cytologic monotony is especially likely to be obscured by secondary inflammation or BALT. Furthermore, TBB yields insufficient material for typing of lymphocytes and clonal studies. Nevertheless, we believe that the diagnosis of lymphoma may be strongly suspected in bronchial and transbronchial lung biopsy material because of the characteristics of the infiltrate (Fig. 9–15).

Radiologically, the lungs are involved at initial presentation in 12 percent of patients with Hodgkin's lymphoma and 4 percent of patients with non-Hodgkin's lymphoma (Blank and Castellino, 1980). Pulmonary lymphoma may present on the chest radiograph and on CT with findings similar to lymphangitic carcinomatosis: a reticular, reticulonodular, or nodular pattern with thickening of the bronchovascular bundles, septal lines, with or without associated lymphadenopathy or pleural effusion (Müller et al, 1987; Bergin and Müller, 1987) (Fig.

9–16). These findings reflect the propensity of lymphoma, like lymphangitic carcinomatosis, to extend along the lymphatics. Other manifestations include single or multiple nodules or masses that may cavitate, and localized or multiple areas of airspace consolidation, sometimes with air bronchograms (Blank and Castellino, 1980). In Hodgkin's disease, lung involvement is virtually always accompanied by radiographically demonstrable hilar and mediastinal lymphadenopathy (Castellino, 1986). Non-Hodgkin's lymphoma may involve the mediastinal nodes and lungs or may be limited to the lung. Primary lymphoma of the lung may have radiologic manifestations similar to those of Hodgkin's or non-Hodgkin's lymphoma (Fig. 9–17). However, by definition, lymphadenopathy is not present. Most commonly, primary lymphoma of the lung presents as a large confluent area of airspace consolidation. The course of the disease is indolent, with the pulmonary infiltrates remaining unchanged over several years.

The differential diagnosis of pulmonary lymphoma should include lymphoid interstitial pneumonia, pseudolymphoma, lymphomatoid granulomatosis, and follicular bronchiolitis (Turner et al, 1984; Weiss et al, 1985). Lymphoid interstitial pneumonia (LIP) (see Chapter 7) is a rare form of chronic infiltrative lung disease characterized by a diffuse interstitial infiltrate of polymorphous and polyclonal

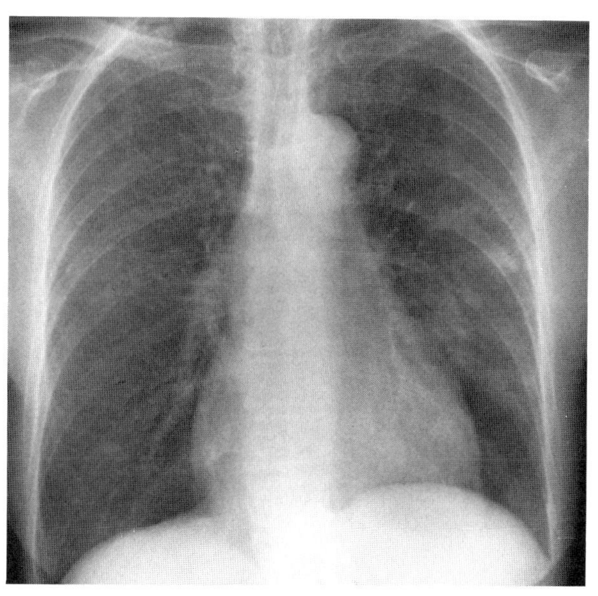

A

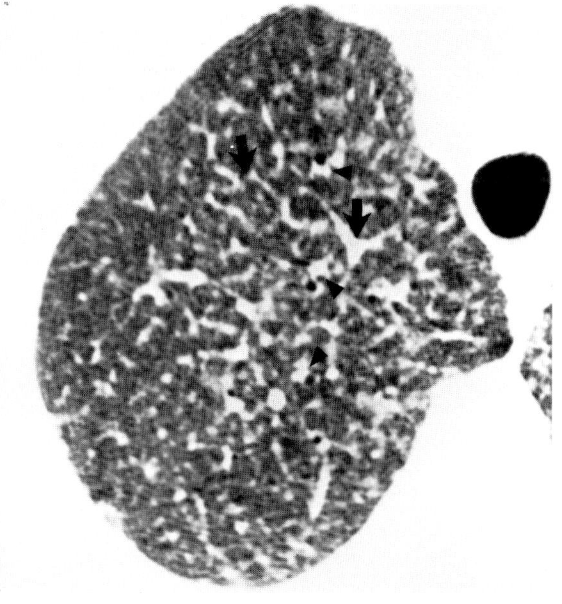

B

Figure 9–16   Small cleaved B-cell lymphoma in a 76-year-old woman. *A,* Chest radiograph shows bilateral reticulonodular pattern. *B,* High-resolution CT through the right upper lobe shows nodular thickening of interlobular septa (*arrows*) and bronchovascular bundles (*arrowheads*).

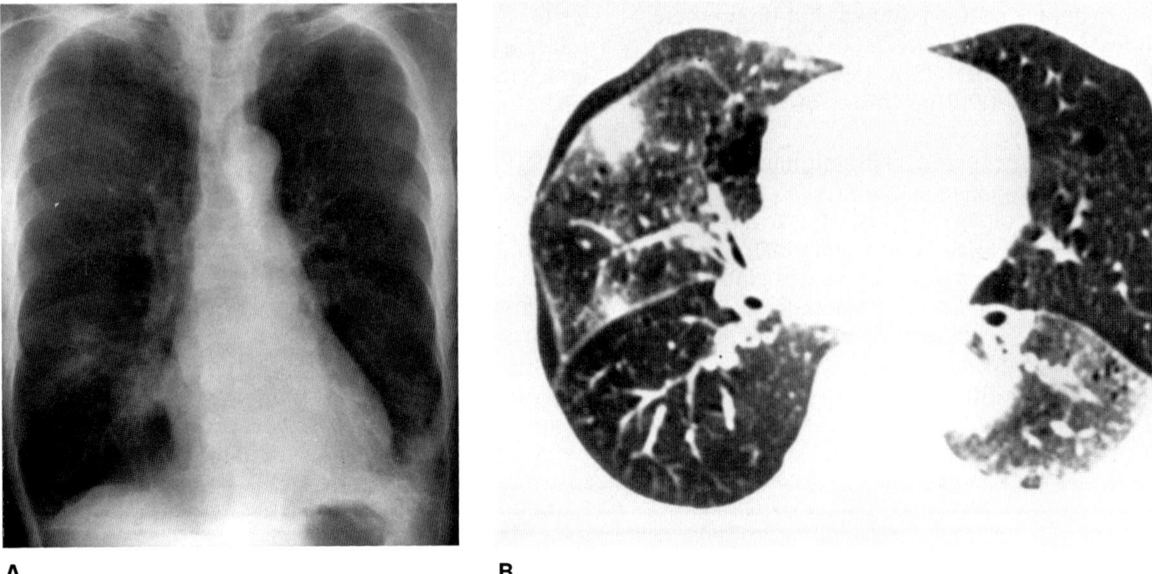

Figure 9–17   Primary lymphocytic lymphoma of the lung in a 79-year-old man. *A,* Chest radiograph shows ill-defined bilateral infiltrates. *B,* A 1.5-mm collimation CT scan through the lower lung zones shows areas of airspace consolidation and nodular densities in the right middle and left lower lobes.

lymphoreticular cells. Patients with LIP often have immunologic abnormalities such as AIDS, Sjögren's syndrome, or apparently benign gammopathies, but by definition should not have evidence of systemic lymphoma. Histologically, the differential diagnosis between LIP and lymphoma is both architectural (absence of tracking and of transpleural and nodal involvement in LIP) and cytologic (polymorphous in LIP, monomorphous in lymphoma).

Pseudolymphoma refers to a localized mass lesion composed of a lymphoreticular infiltrate which, like LIP, is polymorphous. Experts in this field (Turner et al, 1984, Colby and Carrington, 1983a, 1983b; Marchevsky et al, 1983) believe that most cases of pseudolymphoma of the lung are indistinguishable from well differentiated monoclonal lymphoma with indolent behavior.

Lymphomatoid granulomatosis (LYG) is characterized by multiple pulmonary nodules of polymorphous atypical lymphoreticular cells with angiodestruction and consequent necrosis. As described elsewhere, LYG is probably best considered to be a lymphoma from the outset (see Chapter 10).

Follicular bronchiolitis (FB) is characterized by an intense polymorphous inflammatory infiltrate with germinal centers, primarily involving the airways and giving rise to bilateral infiltrates (Yousem et al, 1985). The bronchiolar distribution of this lesion results in a low-power appearance of tracking along broncho-

vascular bundles. Furthermore, FB has been associated with immune-deficiency states, including acquired immunodeficieny syndrome (AIDS), in which there is an increased risk of development of lymphoma. FB is distinguished from lymphoma by the presence of many germinal centers and obvious polymorphism of the infiltrate (see Chapter 12).

LEUKEMIA

Leukemic infiltration of the lungs is seen microscopically at autopsy in 10 to 50 percent of patients with leukemia (Blank and Castellino, 1980; Klatte et al, 1963; Maile et al, 1983). However, leukemic infiltration is rarely symptomatic or grossly apparent and rarely causes any radiologic manifestations except for hilar and mediastinal adenopathy (Blank and Castellino, 1980; Maile et al, 1983). In the few cases in which leukemic infiltrates were the sole or the main manifestation, the radiographic findings consisted of peribronchial infiltration or ill-defined patchy opacities (Blank and Castellino, 1980; Klatte et al, 1963; Maile et al, 1983). Dugdale and colleagues (1987) described one case of endobronchial chloroma in a patient with acute myelogenous leukemia causing symptomatic airway obstruction. Kovalski and coworkers (1990) described three patients with symptomatic and radiologically apparent leukemic infiltrates, in whom the diagnosis was established by TBB and the infiltrates resolved with appropriate chemotherapy. These cases notwithstanding, by far the most common causes of pulmonary infiltrates in leukemia are infection and pulmonary hemorrhage (Blank and Castellino, 1980).

KAPOSI'S SARCOMA

Kaposi's sarcoma (KS) involving the lung is most commonly seen in patients with AIDS and rarely occurs sporadically (Purdy et al, 1986). The cited incidence of pulmonary KS in patients with AIDS varies from 3 percent (Murray et al, 1984) to 90 percent (Purdy et al, 1986) depending both on whether the series is based on autopsy or biopsy specimens and on the diagnostic criteria used. The vast majority of patients with AIDS-related pulmonary KS have evidence of previously established or concurrent KS of skin or lymph nodes (Garay et al, 1987; Purdy et al, 1986; Hamm et al, 1987; Zibrak et al, 1986), although a patient with pulmonary KS may have no other sites of involvement (Nash and Fligiel, 1984; Talavera et al, 1988). Approximately 80 percent of patients with AIDS-related pulmonary KS have previous or concurrent pulmonary infection (Garay et al, 1987). The distinction of pulmonary KS from pulmonary infection is important, as the latter can be treated, at least temporarily, with antibiotics. There is no effective chemotherapy for pulmonary KS at the present time.

Like lymphangitic carcinomatosis and lymphoma, pulmonary KS has a tendency to grow along lymphatic routes in the bronchovascular bundles, interlobular septa, and pleura (Purdy et al, 1986) (Fig. 9–18). The histologic lesion of pulmonary KS is similar to the appearance of KS of any site (Fig. 9–19). Ill-defined nodules of tumor are composed primarily of spindled mesenchymal cells with nuclear atypia and mitotic activity. Vascular clefts, extravasated red blood cells, and hemosiderin are usually obvious. Variable numbers of lymphocytes, plasma cells, and histiocytes are present, but in a classic lesion these cells do not obscure the spindle cell component.

Because of its lymphangitic growth pattern, patients with pulmonary KS may occasionally present with hemoptysis (Nash and Figiel, 1984) or hemorrhagic pleural effusions (Garay et al, 1987; Talavera et al, 1988; Hamm et al, 1987). In instances of involvement of proximal bronchi, erythematous plaques may be found on bronchoscopy. While some investigators believe that this bronchoscopic appearance alone is sufficiently diagnostic and that biopsy, with its attendant risk of hemorrhage, is not necessary (Zibrak et al, 1986), others believe that bronchial biopsy of these plaques is a low-risk, high-yield procedure (Hamm et al, 1987). In the absence of hemorrhagic plaques, TBB may be diagnostic,

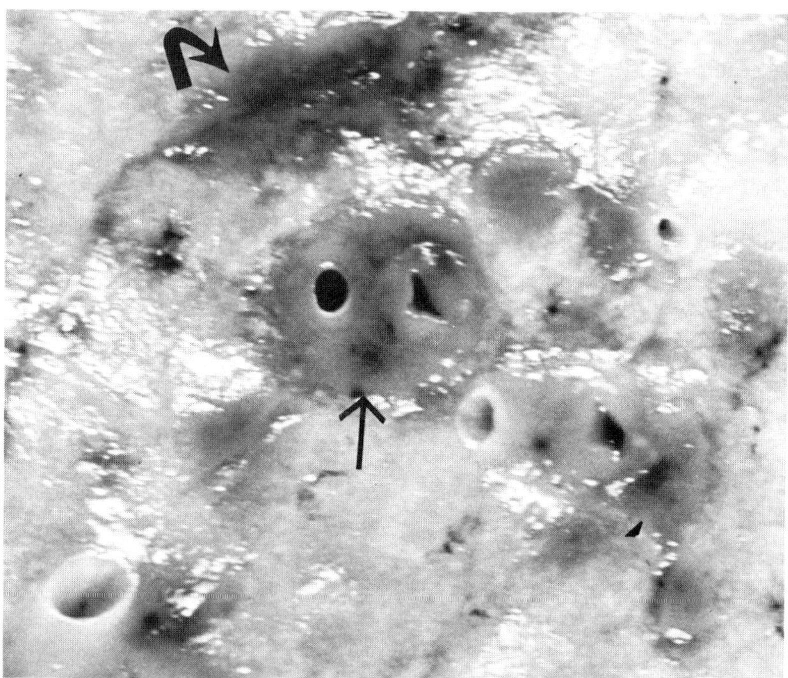

Figure 9–18   Gross appearance of Kaposi's sarcoma showing hemorrhagic tumor around bronchovascular bundle (*straight arrow*) and interlobular septa (*curved arrow*).

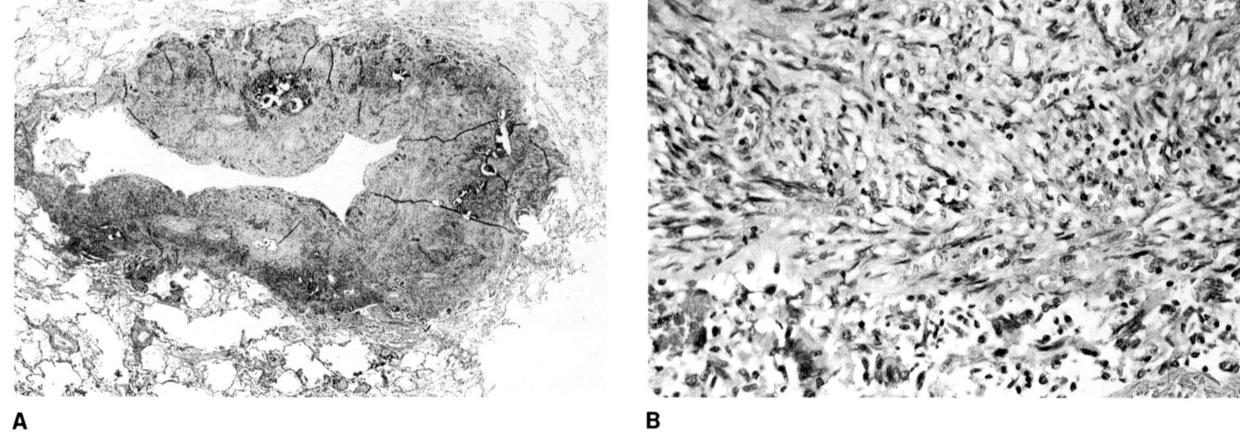

Figure 9–19   *A,* Perivenular Kaposi's sarcoma. *B,* Spindled tumor cells with vascular slits and red cell diapedesis.

although the histologic changes can be subtle and easily overlooked (Purdy et al, 1986).

A premortem diagnosis of pulmonary KS is difficult to establish for the following reasons: (1) the focal nature of involvement (Nash and Fligiel, 1984), (2) the fact that pulmonary KS may have fewer spindle cells than the more classic skin lesions (Garay et al, 1987), and (3) early pulmonary KS lesions are characterized by such a polymorphous inflammatory infiltrate that the atypical spindle cells are hard to discern (Purdy et al, 1986). Extravasated red cells and hemosiderin are helpful features in early lesions like this. From a retrospective comparison of TBB and open lung biopsy in patients with AIDS-related pulmonary KS, Purdy and colleagues (1986) believed that this polymorphous inflammatory lesion was diagnostic of pulmonary KS, and that recognition of it would dramatically increase the yield of TBB.

The most common radiographic finding in Kaposi's sarcoma is the presence of bilateral perihilar infiltrates, seen in approximately 90 percent of patients (Naidich et al, 1989). Other findings may include bilateral nodular densities, a reticular pattern, interstitial and airspace infiltrates, or a normal chest radiograph (Davis et al, 1987; Naidich et al, 1987). These findings are indistinguishable from those in *Pneumocystis* pneumonia. More suggestive of KS are the presence of mediastinal and hilar lymphadenopathy (Fig. 9–20) and uni- or bilateral pleural effusions, which occur in 30 to 50 percent of patients with KS and are rarely seen with *Pneumocystis* infection. Until proved otherwise, the combination of lymphadenopathy and pulmonary infiltrates in a patient with AIDS indicates the presence of KS, lymphoma, or tuberculosis.

Although pulmonary KS is easily confused ra-

diologically with *Pneumocystis carinii* pneumonia, the pulmonary gallium scan is characteristically positive in *Pneumocystis* pneumonia and negative in KS, unless there is concurrent pulmonary infection (Volberding, 1986).

Like lymphangitic carcinomatosis and lymphoma, the distribution of KS along the lymphatics is usually clearly apparent on CT (see Fig. 9–20) (Naidich et al, 1989). Like lymphangitic carcinomatosis and lymphoma, KS leads to uneven nodular thickening of the bronchovascular bundles, interlobular septa, and interlobar fissures. The nodular parenchymal opacities characteristically radiate from the hila to the periphery.

The CT appearance of KS is easily distinguishable from that of *Pneumocystis* pneumonia, which presents mainly with patchy or diffuse airspace opacification in a random distribution and without adenopathy or effusion (Naidich et al, 1989). The pattern and distribution of KS, however, is similar to that of lymphoma.

"BENIGN METASTASIZING LEIOMYOMA"

"Benign metastasizing leiomyoma" (BML) is a rare disorder characterized by multiple nodules of histologically benign smooth muscle in the lung, with variably prominent epithelial-lined clefts. Like lymphangiomyomatosis (LAM) (see Chapter 7), the proliferating cell has the ultrastructural characteristics of smooth muscle (Silverman and Kay, 1976); as in LAM, the disorder is found predominantly in women. However, the clinical, radiologic and pathologic features of the two diseases are otherwise quite different.

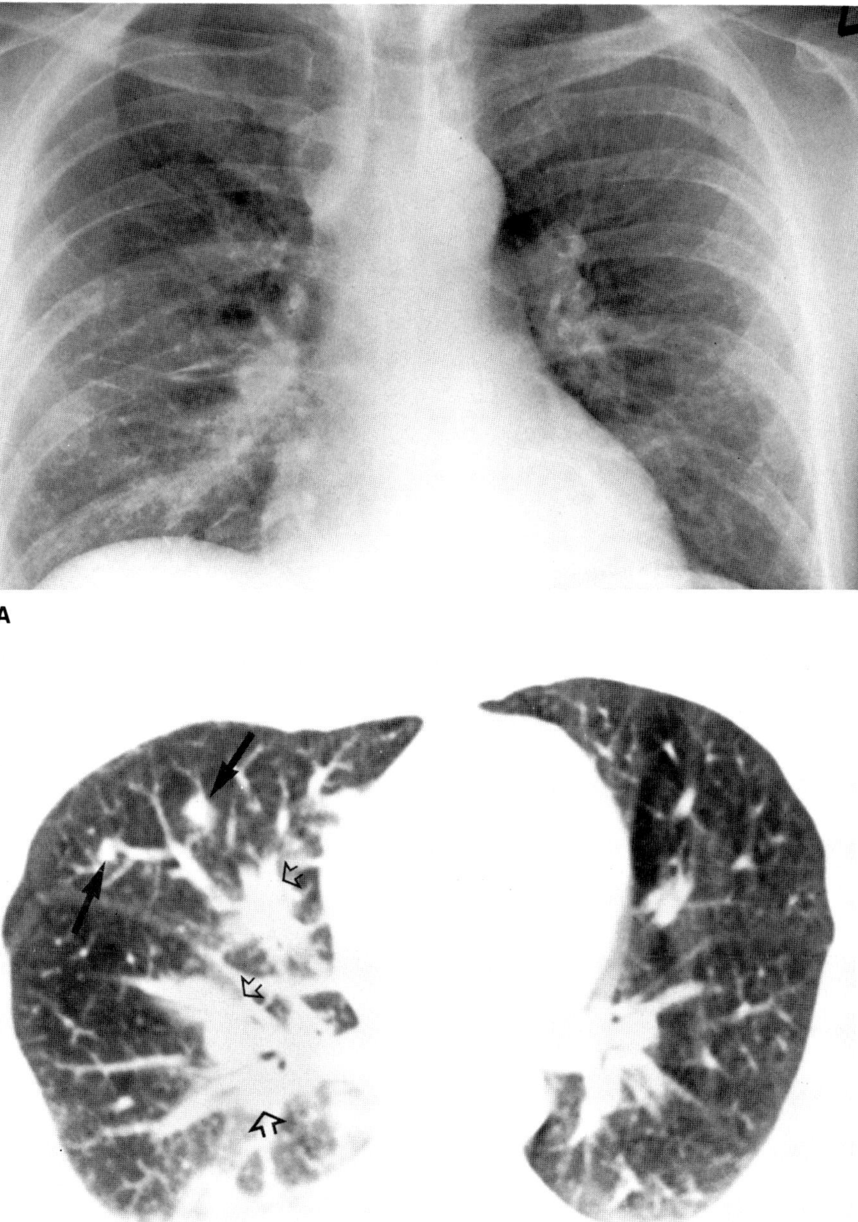

Figure 9–20 Kaposi's sarcoma in a 40-year-old man. *A*, Chest radiograph shows right hilar and paratracheal adenopathy as well as ill-defined increased density in the right lower lung zone. *B*, A 10-mm collimation CT scan through the lower lung zones shows uneven thickening of bronchovascular bundles (*open arrows*) and peribronchovascular nodules (*closed arrows*).

Grossly, the nodules of BML vary from a few millimeters to 5 cm in diameter (Wolff et al, 1979) and are multiple in most cases. Their borders are sharply demarcated, and the lesions seem to "pop out" from the surrounding lung (Fig. 9–21). Interstitial fibrosis and honeycombing are not features of this disease. Microscopically the nodules are composed of well-differentiated smooth muscle cells in interlocking bundles (Fig. 9–22). The nuclei appear benign, necrosis is absent, and mitotic activity is scant. Cysts or clefts lined by benign looking cuboidal or columnar epithelium are usually found.

Several controversies surround this condition. The most important issue is whether these lesions are benign or malignant. The great majority of patients with BML are women who either have, or have undergone surgery for, uterine leiomyomas. At issue is whether these women actually have metastatic low

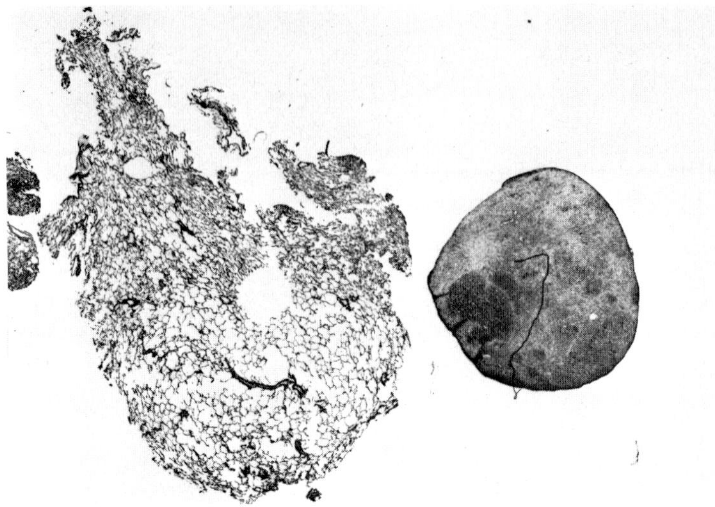

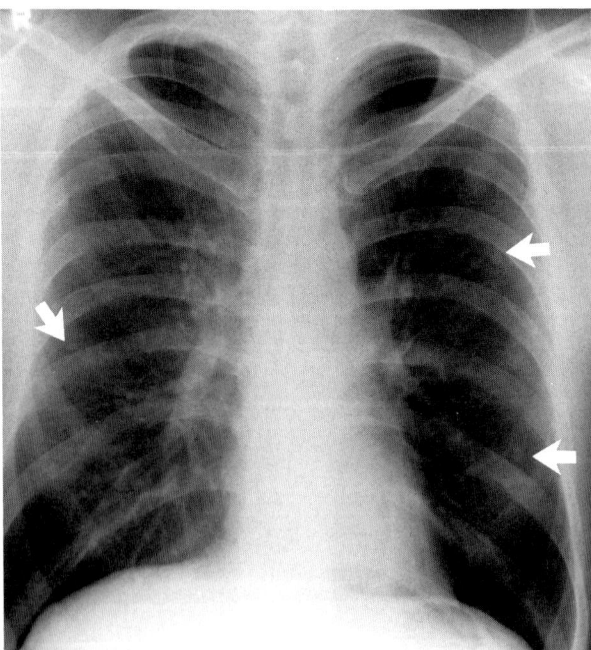

Figure 9–21 Open lung biopsy of benign metastasizing leiomyoma in which nodule "popped out" from adjacent lung.

grade leiomyosarcomas or whether a leiomyoma innocently gained access to a vessel and simply embolized, analogous to benign glandular inclusions in regional lymph nodes (Kheir et al, 1981). BML has an excellent prognosis for long-term survival; however, the lesions have been shown to have minor degrees of mitotic activity (Wolff et al, 1979), to have the potential for indolent but steady growth, and rarely to cause death from respiratory insufficiency. Thus, we view these lesions as metastatic low grade sarcomas, as have others (Wolff et al, 1979).

A related issue is the female predominance in this disease. Three male patients were reported with lesions morphologically indistinguishable from BML (Wolff et al, 1979); all three had leiomyosarcomas of other sites (vein, diaphragm, soft tissue), although in two, the lung lesions preceded detection of the sar-

coma. Presumably, the female predominance is due to the fact that the uterus is so prone to developing smooth muscle tumors. The uterine origin in the majority of cases has therapeutic significance in that enlarging lesions in premenopausal women seem to respond well to hormonal manipulation (Horstmann et al, 1977).

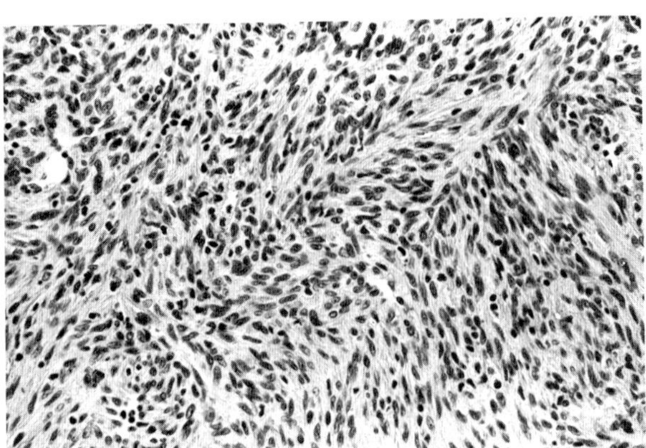

Figure 9–22 Benign-looking smooth muscle cells in benign metastasizing leiomyoma.

Figure 9–23 Chest radiograph in 30-year-old man with benign metastasizing leiomyomas shows a few small bilateral nodules (*arrows*). These did not change appreciably in size over 4 years.

A further controversy is the relationship of BML to lesions referred to as multiple leiomyomatous hamartomas (MLH) primary to the lung (Silverman and Kay, 1976; Wolff et al, 1979). As with BML, virtually all of the patients reported are female and the majority had known uterine smooth muscle tumors. The clinical and pathologic features of MLH and BML are similar. The main reason for separating MLH and BML in the literature seems to have been the belief that the epithelial-lined clefts were an integral part of the tumor rather than entrapped and distorted remnants of lung. Wolff and coworkers (1979) have made a convincing argument that this belief is erroneous and that MLH and BML are the same lesion; we and others (Horstmann et al, 1977) concur. "Metastasizing fibroleiomyoma" (Horstmann et al, 1977) or simply "metastatic leiomyosarcoma of borderline malignant potential" would seem to be terms preferable to "benign metastasizing leiomyoma."

BML is radiologically indistinguishable from metastatic disease except that the lesions tend to grow very slowly (Fig. 9–23).

REFERENCES

Bergin CJ, Müller NL. CT of interstitial lung disease: a diagnostic approach. AJR 1987; 148:8–15.

Blank N, Castellino RA. The intrathoracic manifestations of the malignant lymphomas and the leukemias. Semin Roentgenol 1980; 15:225–245.

Castellino RA. Hodgkin disease: practical concepts for the diagnostic radiologist. Radiology 1986; 159:305–310.

Churg A. Lung biopsy: handling and diagnostic limitations. In Thurlbeck WM, ed. Pathology of the lung. New York: Thieme International, 1988.

Clayton F. Bronchioloalveolar carcinomas: cell types, patterns of growth, and prognostic correlates. Cancer 1986; 57:1555–1564.

Colby TV, Carrington CB. Lymphoreticular tumors and infiltrates of the lung. Pathol Annu 1983a; 18:27–70.

Colby TV, Carrington CB. Pulmonary lymphomas: current concepts. Hum Pathol 1983b; 14:884–887.

Davis SD, Henschke CI, Chamides BK, Westcott JL. Intrathoracic Kaposi sarcoma in AIDS patients: radiographic-pathologic correlation. Radiology 1987; 163:495–500.

Donaldson JC, Kaminsky DB, Elliott RC. Bronchiolar carcinoma: report of 11 cases and review of the literature. Cancer 1978; 41:250-258.

Dugdale DC, Salness TA, Knight L, Charan NB. Endobronchial granulocytic sarcoma causing acute respiratory failure in acute myelogenous leukemia. Am Rev Respir Dis 1987; 136:1248–1250.

Edgerton F, Rao U, Takita H, Vincent RG. Bronchioalveolar carcinoma: a clinical overview and bibliography. Oncology 1981; 38:269–273.

Evans HL. Extranodal small lymphocytic proliferation: a clinicopathologic and immunocytochemical study. Cancer 1982; 49:84–96.

Garay SM, Belenko M, Fazzini E, Schinella R. Pulmonary manifestations of Kaposi's sarcoma. Chest 1987; 91:39–43.

Hamm PG, Judson MA, Aranda CP. Diagnosis of pulmonary Kaposi's sarcoma with fiberoptic bronchoscopy and endobronchial biopsy: a report of five cases. Cancer 1987; 59:807–810.

Hill, CA. Bronchioloalveolar carcinoma: a review. Radiology 1984; 150:15–20.

Horstmann JP, Pietra GG, Harman JA, et al. Spontaneous regression of pulmonary leiomyomas during pregnancy. Cancer 1977; 39:314–321.

Isaacson P, Wright DH. Extranodal malignant lymphoma arising from mucosa-associated lymphoid tissue. Cancer 1984; 53:2515–2524.

Janower ML, Blennerhassett JB. Lymphangitic spread of metastatic cancer to lung: a radiologic-pathologic classification. Radiology 1971; 101:267–273.

Kennedy JL, Nathwani BN, Burke JS, et al. Pulmonary lymphomas and other pulmonary lymphoid lesions: a clinicopathologic and immunologic study of 64 patients. Cancer 1985; 56:539–552.

Kheir SM, Mann WJ, Wilkerson JA. Glandular inclusions in lymph nodes: the problem of extensive involvement and relationship to salpingitis. Am J Surg Pathol 1981; 5:353–359.

Klatte EC, Yardley J, Smith EB, et al. The pulmonary manifestations and complications of leukemia. AJR 1963; 89:598–609.

Koss MN, Hochholzer L, Nichols PW, et al. Primary non-Hodgkin's lymphoma and pseudolymphoma of lung: a study of 161 patients. Hum Pathol 1983; 14:1024–1038.

Kovalski R, Hansen-Flaschen J, Lodato RF, Pietra GG. Localized leukemic pulmonary infiltrates. Chest 1990; 97:674–678.

Maile CW, Moore AV, Ulreich S, Putman CE. Chest radiographic-pathologic correlation in adult leukemia patients. Invest Radiol 1983; 18:495–499.

Manning JT Jr, Spjut HJ, Tschen JA. Bronchioloalveolar carcinoma: the significance of two histopathologic types. Cancer 1984; 54:525–534.

Marchevsky A, Padilla M, Kaneko M, Kleinerman J. Localized lymphoid nodules of lung: a reappraisal of the lymphoma vs. pseudolymphoma dilemma. Cancer 1983; 51:2070-2077.

Mathieson JR, Mayo JR, Staples CA, Müller NL. Chronic diffuse infiltrative lung disease: diagnostic accuracy of computed tomography versus chest radiology. Radiology 1989; 171:111–116.

Miller RR, Nelems B, Evans KG, et al. Glandular neoplasia of the lung: a proposed analogy to colonic tumors. Cancer 1988; 61:1009–1014.

Müller NL, Guerry-Force ML, Lawson L, et al. Clinico-radiologic-pathologic conference: an elderly man with bilateral lung disease. J Can Assoc Radiol 1987; 38:219–221.

Munk PL, Müller NL, Miller RR, Ostrow DN. Pulmonary lymphangitic carcinomatosis: CT and pathologic findings. Radiology 1988; 166:705–709.

Murray JF, Felton CP, Garay SM, et al. Pulmonary complications of the acquired immunodeficiency syndrome. N Engl J Med 1984; 310:1682-1688.

Naidich DP, Garay SM, Leitman BS, McCauley DI. Radiographic manifestations of pulmonary disease in the acquired immunodeficiency syndrome (AIDS). Semin Roentgenol 1987; 22:14-30.

Naidich DP, Tarras M, Garay SM, et al. Kaposi's sarcoma: CT-radiographic correlation. Chest 1989; 96:723-728.

Nash G, Fligiel S. Kaposi's sarcoma presenting as pulmonary disease in the acquired immunodeficiency syndrome: diagnosis by lung biopsy. Hum Pathol 1984; 15:999-1001.

Palosaari DE, Colby TV. Bronchiolocentric chronic lymphocytic leukemia. Cancer 1986; 58:1695-1698.

Peterson H, Snider HL, Yam LT, et al. Primary pulmonary lymphoma: a clinical and immunohistochemical study of six cases. Cancer 1985; 56:805-813.

Purdy LJ, Colby TV, Yousem SA, Battifora H. Pulmonary Kaposi's sarcoma: premortem histologic diagnosis. Am J Surg Pathol 1986; 10:301-311.

Rose RM, Grigas D, Strattemeir E, et al. Endobronchial involvement with non-Hodgkin's lymphoma: a clinical-radiologic analysis. Cancer 1986; 57:1750-1755.

Sahn SA. The pleura. Am Rev Respir Dis 1988; 138:184-234.

Saltstein SL. Pulmonary malignant lymphomas and pseudolymphomas: classification, therapy and prognosis. Cancer 1963; 16:928-955.

Silverman JF, Kay S. Multiple pulmonary leiomyomatous hamartomas: report of a case with ultrastructure examination. Cancer 1976; 38:1199-1204.

Stein MG, Mayo J, Müller NL, et al. Pulmonary lymphangitic spread of carcinoma: appearance on CT scans. Radiology 1987; 162:371-375.

Talavera W, Wasser L, Villamena P, Gould I. Primary pleuropulmonary Kaposi's sarcoma in the acquired immunodeficiency syndrome (Abstract). Am Rev Respir Dis 1988; 137:287.

Tao LC, Delarue NC, Sanders D, Weisbrod G. Bronchioloalveolar carcinoma: a correlative clinical and cytologic study. Cancer 1978; 42:2759-2767.

Trapnell DH. Radiological appearances of lymphangitis carcinomatosa of the lung. Thorax 1964; 19:251-260.

Turner RR, Colby TV, Doggett RS. Well-differentiated lymphocytic lymphoma: a study of 47 patients with primary manifestation in the lung. Cancer 1984; 54:2088-2096.

Volberding PA. Kaposi's sarcoma and the acquired immunodeficiency syndrome. Med Clin North Am 1986; 70:665-675.

Wall CP, Gaensler EA, Carrington CB, Hayes JA. Comparison of transbronchial and open biopsies in chronic infiltrative lung diseases. Am Rev Respir Dis 1981; 123:280-285.

Weiss LM, Yousem SA, Warnke RA. Non-Hodgkin's lymphomas of the lung: a study of 19 cases emphasizing the utility of frozen section immunologic studies in differential diagnosis. Am J Surg Pathol 1985; 9:480-490.

Wolff M, Silva F, Kaye G. Pulmonary metastases (with admixed epithelial elements) from smooth muscle neoplasms: report of nine cases, including three males. Am J Surg Pathol 1979; 3:325-342.

Yousem SA, Colby TV, Carrington CB. Follicular bronchitis/bronchiolitis. Hum Pathol 1985; 16:700-706.

Zibrak JD, Silvestri RC, Costello P, et al. Bronchoscopic and radiologic features of Kaposi's sarcoma involving the respiratory system. Chest 1986; 90:476-479.

CHAPTER 10

Noninfectious Angiitis and Granulomatosis

Five conditions—Wegener's granulomatosis, necrotizing sarcoidal granulomatosis, bronchocentric granulomatosis, lymphomatoid granulomatosis, and allergic angiitis and granulomatosis—are often considered together under the heading of "non-infectious angiitis and granulomatosis." In part this is traditional, since the late Dr. Averill Liebow discussed the first four together in his classic Amberson lecture in 1973. More importantly, the conditions may be hard to diagnose and distinguish from each other histopathologically. The group as a whole is uncommon; apart from Wegener's granulomatosis, these conditions are rare and there is some question as to whether each exists as a separate entity. Two concepts are important: (1) In terms of etiology and pathogenesis, they are very different conditions. (2) They differ in prognosis from benign (necrotizing sarcoidal granulomatosis) to malignant (lymphomatoid granulomatosis).

WEGENER'S GRANULOMATOSIS

Wegener's granulomatosis (WG), the best defined and best understood condition of this group, was first recognized by Klinger in 1931 and defined more clearly by Wegener in 1936. Wegener defined a triad consisting of necrotizing granulomas of the respiratory tract, necrotizing vasculitis, and glomerulonephritis. Since then, WG has become regarded as a morphologic lesion of the lung that may or may not be accompanied by the triad of lesions defined by Wegener.

Clinically, it is more common in males than females and occurs most often in patients between 40 and 60 years of age. Statistically, 95 percent of patients present with lung lesions, most commonly multiple pulmonary nodules, but sometimes may present with diffuse pulmonary hemorrhage (Travis et al, 1987; Myers and Katzenstein, 1987).

The radiographic findings in WG most often consist of mucosal thickening and opacification of the paranasal sinuses as well as bilateral pulmonary nodules or masses (Fauci et al, 1983; Weisbrod, 1989). The nodules usually have ill-defined margins and frequently cavitate (Fig. 10–1); they do not have a lobar predilection. Occasionally, the nodules may be single or may have well-defined margins. The lesions may wax and wane.

Endobronchial involvement occurs in 15 percent of patients and leads to segmental or lobar atelectasis or consolidation (Maguire et al, 1978). Segmental consolidation may also be due to vascular involvement (Fig. 10–2). WG may occasionally cause localized or diffuse tracheal narrowing. Tracheal involvement usually occurs late, but it may infrequently be the presenting feature of WG (Stein et al, 1986). In some patients WG presents as bilateral airspace consolidation because of diffuse pulmonary hemorrhage (Stokes et al, 1982). Pleural effusion occurs in 20 percent of patients.

There may be presenting symptoms referable to the upper respiratory tract, such as epistaxis or deafness, but these are more often recognized only after the lung lesions become apparent. More classically, but less frequently, there may be involvement of the nasopharynx with ulceration or even destruction of the nasal septum with resulting "saddle nose." Renal abnormalities such as renal failure, proteinuria, and hematuria are presenting symptoms in 85 percent of patients. In a small percentage of cases, renal lesions may only be recognized by biopsy. Other signs and symptoms include ocular lesions (keratoconjunctivitis, granulomatous sclerouveitis), polyarthralgia, and skin lesions with ulceration due to vasculitis. Less commonly there may be peripheral neuritis, cranial nerve neuritis, or coronary vasculitis. Circulating immune complexes have been described with complex-like deposits in glomerular lesions. Hepatitis B antigen is not recorded.

The lesions in the lung consist of well-defined yellowish-gray nodules, described by Liebow (1973) as "white infarcts" with the implication that they were always the result of vasculitis. This has been disputed (Fienberg, 1981; Mark et al, 1988) and an

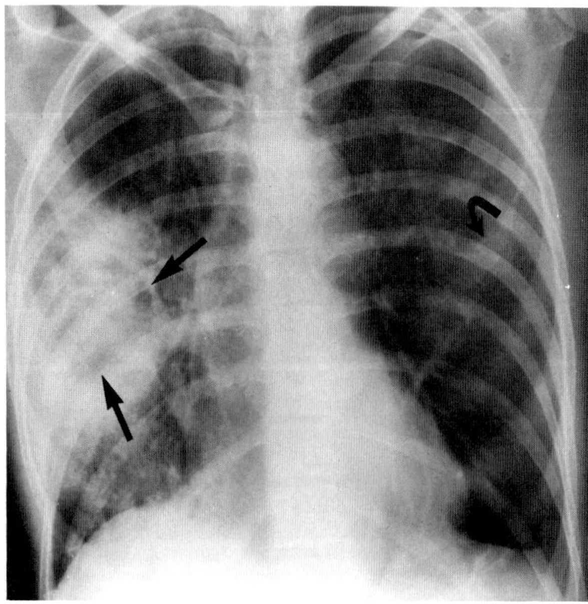

Figure 10–1   Wegener's granulomatosis in a 51-year-old patient. A large area of consolidation with early cavitation (*straight arrows*) is present in the right lung. A 2-cm diameter cavitating nodule (*curved arrow*) is present in the left lung.

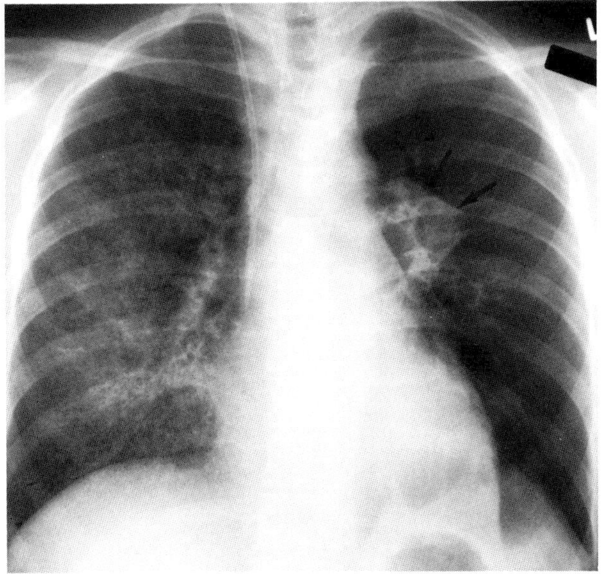

A

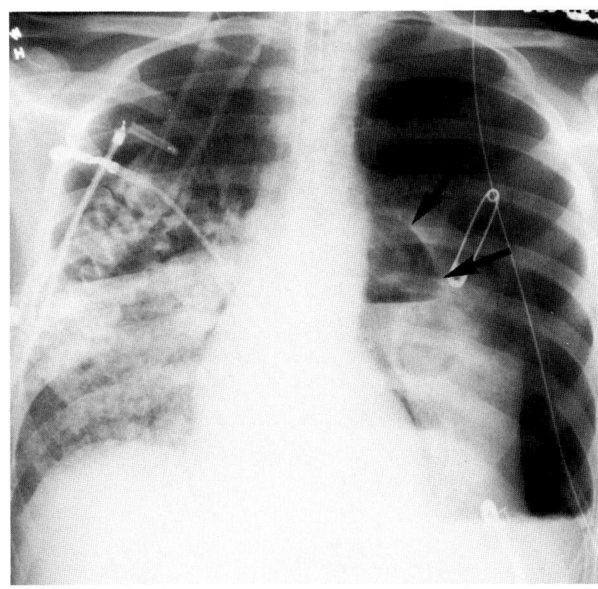

B

Figure 10–2   Wegener's granulomatosis in a 16-year-old male patient who presented initially with pulmonary hemorrhage. *A*, Mixed reticulonodular and airspace patterns are present in the right lung related to recurrent hemorrhage. Dense consolidation of the superior segment of the left lower lobe is shown (*arrows*). *B*, Three weeks later, a large cavity has replaced the entire superior segment (*arrows*). Infarction of the superior segment resulted in a bronchopleural fistula, and the development of the tension left hemopneumothorax.

alternative hypothesis advanced that WG is due to pathergic necrosis of collagen in vascular and extravascular sites. Microscopically the lesion shows central necrosis and the margins of the necrotic areas are serpiginous ("geographic necrosis") (Fig. 10–3). Palisaded histiocytes with multinuclear giant cells appear at the margins (see Fig. 10–3). A key feature is the presence of necrotizing vasculitis outside of the necrosis, and the vasculitis is often at least partly granulomatous (Fig. 10–4). The distribution and severity of the vasculitis can be highlighted by elastin stains, and these are strongly recommended in cases of possible WG (see Fig. 10–4). Palisading granulomas, sometimes seen in the adjacent lung parenchyma, may create confusion with necrotizing sarcoidal granulomatosis (NSG), and several of Liebow's cases of NSG were originally included as examples of Wegener's granulomatosis. Granulomatous bronchitis and chondritis are occasionally seen, creating potential confusion with bronchocentric granulomatosis (Fig. 10–5). A variety of inflammatory cells may be seen, including polymorphonuclear leukocytes, eosinophils, and sometimes rather atypical mononuclear cells. The presence of dramatic tissue eosinophilia may raise the question of allergic angiitis and granulomatosis (Yousem and Lombard, 1988). Atypical lymphoid cells require that the diagnosis of

lymphomatoid granulomatosis (LYG) be considered. (Again, examples of LYG were included in the original series of WG.) Systemic necrotizing vasculitis was considered an integral part of the syndrome by Wegener but is not always recognized. The renal lesions of WG are typically segmental glomerular necrosis and crescent formation, although it should be noted that these are not pathognomonic.

In 1966 Carrington and Liebow described "limited Wegener's granulomatosis." Until then, Wegener's granulomatosis had been considered a uniformly fatal condition, with consistent renal involvement. Carrington and Liebow pointed out that the lung lesions could occur in the absence of renal lesions or necrotizing vasculitis and that, under these circumstances, the prognosis might be good. Carrington and Liebow include the presence of skin and upper respiratory tract lesions in this "limited" category, a concept that has been modified since then. It has become apparent that patients with limited WG may have occult renal lesions, as shown by renal biopsy, and that the subsequent occurrence or absence of the classic triad is unpredictable. A further modification has become necessary, as the complete syndrome is now eminently treatable with cytotoxic drugs, resulting in a 5-year survival rate of 90 to 95 percent. A more rational approach is the Mayo Clinic

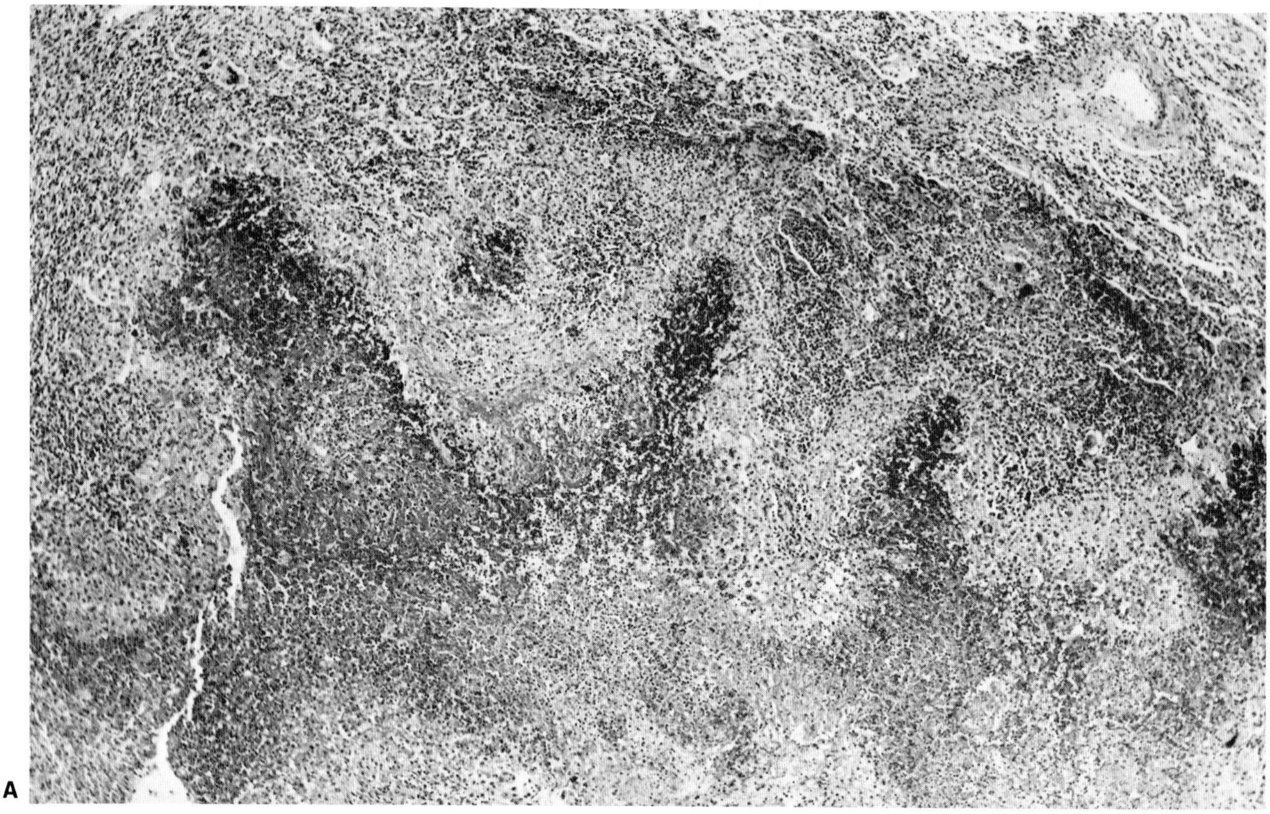

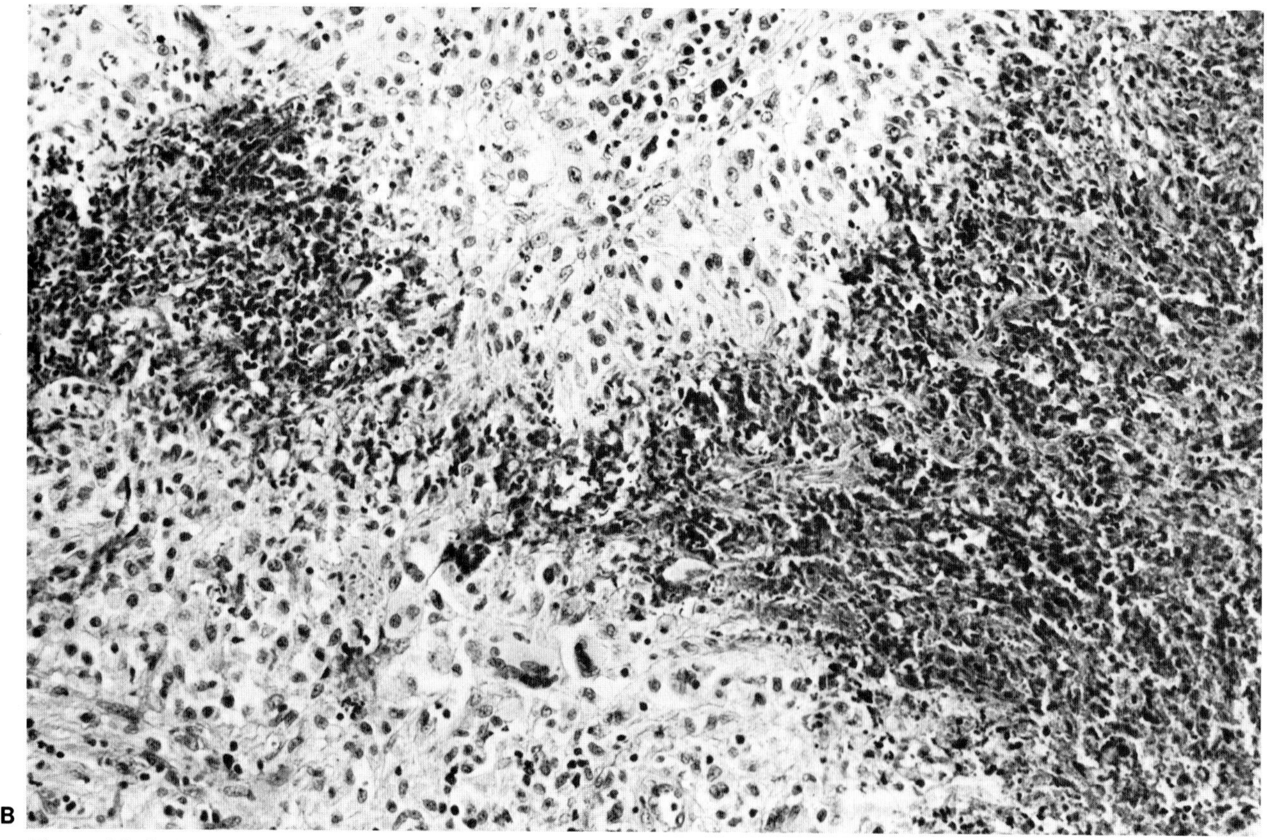

Figure 10–3 Wegener's granulomatosis. *A*, Typical "geographic necrosis". *B*, Palisading histiocytes and multinucleated cells at the edge of the necrotic zone.

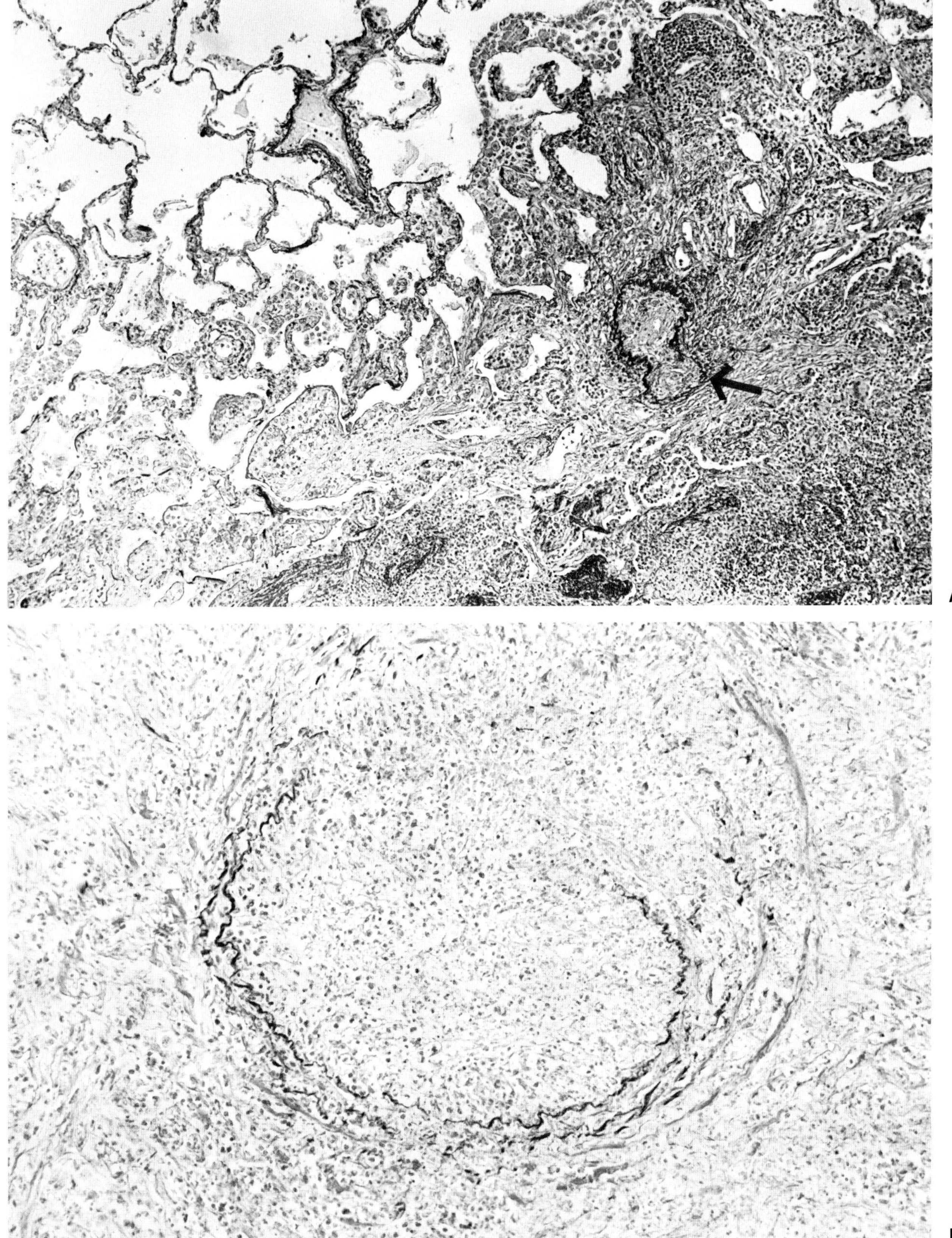

Figure 10–4 Wegener's granulomatosis. *A*, Granulomatous vasculitis at edge. *B*, Enhancement of vascular involvement by elastin stains.

ELK system, which, in effect, is a staging system. This describes the extent of disease on presentation: *E* for ear, nose, and throat; *L* for lung; and *K* for kidney (DeRemee et al, 1976, 1978).

Infections, particularly tuberculosis and histoplasmosis, may closely mimic WG. In a survey of cases diagnosed as WG at a major teaching hospital, Katzenstein and coworkers (Katzenstein, 1980; Ulbright and Katzenstein, 1980) emphasized that granulomatous vasculitis is a common finding in infectious granulomas. It is now conventional wisdom that infections should be carefully considered and excluded in all cases of suspected WG, particularly in "limited WG" and especially in cases with a solitary lesion. To add to the confusion, DeRemee and colleagues (1985) and others have demonstrated reversal of some cases of WG with the antimicrobrial sulfamethoxazole-trimethoprim (Israel, 1988; Fukuda et al, 1989).

Serologic detection of circulating antibodies to neutrophil cytoplasmic antigens may prove to be a valuable tool in the diagnosis of WG (Vander Woude et al, 1985), analogous to the detection of anti-DNA antibodies in systemic lupus erythematosus. The sensitivity and specificity of this test depends on the pattern and strength of the reaction accepted as a "positive" result, and there are occasional false-positive results, particularly in patients with other vasculitides (Harrison et al, 1989). Nevertheless, this test has considerable potential value in diagnosis, assessment of disease activity, and early detection of relapses in patients with WG (Nolle et al, 1989; Tervaert et al, 1989).

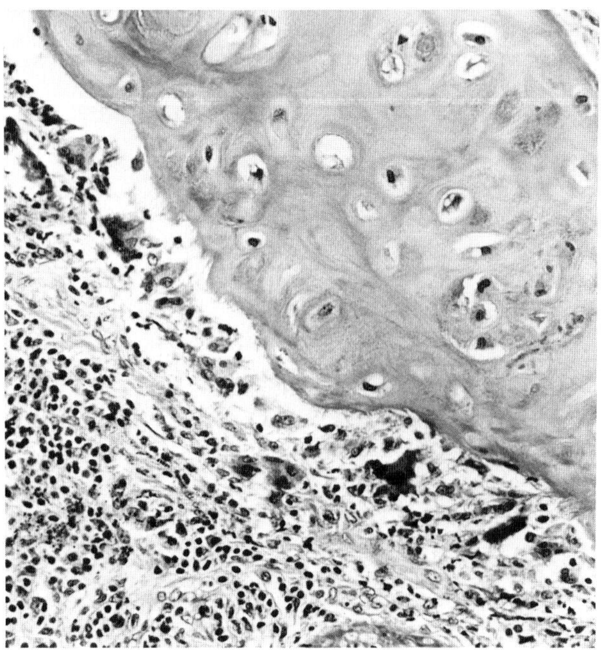

Figure 10–5 Wegener's granulomatosis with granulomatous chondritis.

ALLERGIC ANGIITIS AND GRANULOMATOSIS (CHURG-STRAUSS SYNDROME)

In 1951 Churg and Strauss described a group of patients who had asthma and died but who also had angiitis and phlebitis; the great majority (93 percent) also had lung infiltrates, which in retrospect appears to be what is now referred to as chronic eosinophilic pneumonia (see Chapter 7). Necrotizing granulomas were present in the lungs and elsewhere, and an eosinophilic infiltrate was a prominent feature in the vasculitis. In 1957 Rose and Spencer reported on a large series of patients with polyarteritis nodosa and divided them into those with and those without pulmonary symptoms. Those with pulmonary symptoms corresponded closely both clinically and pathologically with the cases described by Churg and Strauss. Since then a few large series of the Churg-Strauss syndrome have been reported. In one, by definition, all patients had asthma (Chumbley et al, 1977). Among the other cases reported, the great majority of patients had asthma before or at presentation (Rosenberg et al, 1975; Koss et al, 1981).

Churg-Strauss disease is rare. The Mayo Clinic series had only 30 cases so classified, and among these only four underwent lung biopsies. Lung biopsy or autopsy material was described in 4 cases from the Armed Forces Institute of Pathology series (Koss et al, 1981). We have only seen one case (Kus et al, 1985). The histologic features in the lung consist of eosinophilic pneumonia, vasculitis with palisading giant cells involving medium-sized pulmonary arteries, and occasionally arteritis of the bronchial arteries. Fibrinoid necrosis of the pulmonary arteries occurs in about 40 percent of cases. An important feature is the numerous extravascular granulomas with central necrosis. There is a dense eosinophilic infiltrate at the margins of the granuloma and also in the vessels.

There is considerable overlap between the lesions of Churg-Strauss and eosinophilic pneumonia. The main distinguishing features are the extravascular granulomas and the granulomatous nature of the vasculitis in the former. In eosinophilic pneumonia, "eosinophilic abscesses" are frequently present, but these occur within airspaces. Vasculitis can be found by careful search in about two-thirds of patients with eosinophilic pneumonia, but phlebitis and small vessel involvement (microangiitis) are much more common than arteritis. The nature of the vasculitis of eosinophilic pneumonia is typically a perivascular cuff of lymphocytes and eosinophils with relatively few cells in the vessel wall itself. One major clinical distinction between Churg-Strauss disease and eosinophilic pneumonia is prognosis. In Churg-Strauss disease, by definition (since they were originally described from autopsies) the disease was uniformly fatal; eosinophilic pneumonia responds dramatically to steroids. Newer information suggests that the present 5-year survival of Churg-Strauss syndrome is about 60 percent. Another important clinical difference between the two entities is the high frequency of extrapulmonary involvement in Churg-Strauss syndrome. Skin lesions (purpura or nodules) occur in two-thirds of patients and peripheral neuropathy in about the same proportion. About one-half of patients have hypertension. Glomerulonephritis in Churg-Strauss disease is relatively uncommon and rarely leads to renal failure.

Eosinophils are usually present but not particularly numerous in the lung lesions of WG. Yousem and Lombard (1988) described four cases of WG in which pulmonary tissue eosinophilia was dramatic; in such cases the differential diagnosis between WG and Churg-Strauss syndrome may be difficult. Clinical findings (asthma, peripheral eosinophilia, extrapulmonary sites of involvement), radiologic findings, and the more destructive tissue reaction in WG are useful differentiating features.

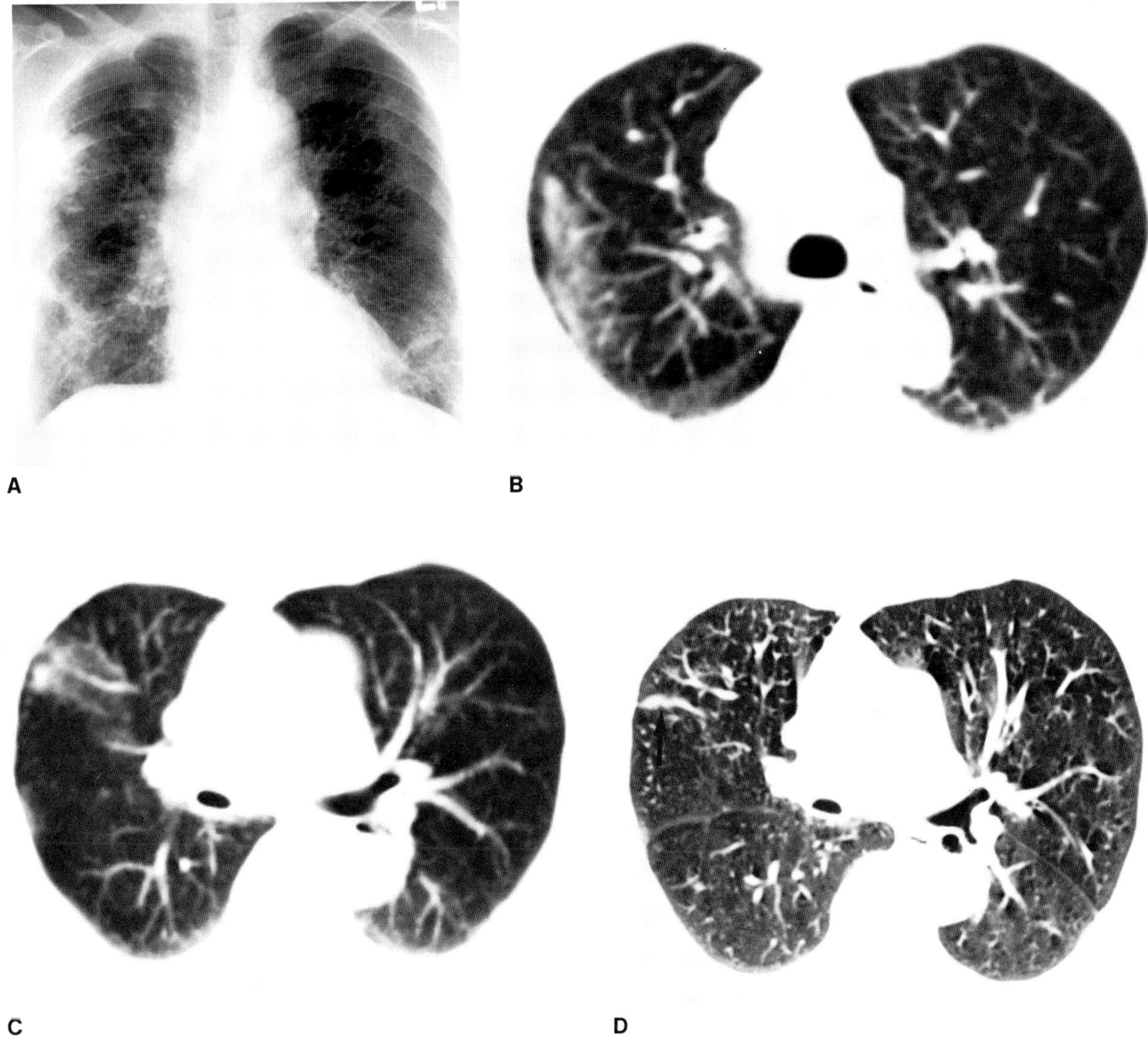

Figure 10–6 Churg-Strauss syndrome in a 71–year-old woman. *A*, Chest radiograph shows peripheral airspace consolidation. CT scan at level of carina (*B*) and right middle lobe (*C*) shows patchy consolidation. *D*, CT scan 3 years later shows mild residual scarring (*arrow*) in right middle lobe.

Radiologically the majority of patients with Churg-Strauss have fleeting nonsegmental pulmonary infiltrates. These infiltrates often have a peripheral distribution similar to that of chronic eosinophilic pneumonia (Churg, 1983). Long-term follow-up in one patient with Churg-Strauss showed residual parenchymal scarring in the areas that previously had pulmonary infiltrates (Fig. 10–6). Less commonly, nodular infiltrates similar to the other granulomatoses, cavitating lesions, and pleural effusions may be seen.

NECROTIZING SARCOIDAL GRANULOMATOSIS

Necrotizing sarcoidal granulomatosis (NSG) is characterized by the presence of numerous sarcoid-like granulomas in the lung, *plus* the presence of necrosis involving large areas of the lung, *plus* vasculitis, of which three varieties were described by Liebow in 1973. The first was a curious granulomatous vasculitis, in which granulomas extended around the vessel wall, involving the external elastic lamina, which Liebow contrasted to temporal arteritis that involves the internal elastic lamina. The second was a mononuclear infiltrate that involved the entire vessel wall and may lead to occlusion. The third was extensive sarcoid-like granulomas that extended through the vascular walls and might occlude them.

Clinically, there is a female preponderance in most series and a wide age range. Nonspecific pulmonary symptoms such as cough, chest pain, and shortness of breath are common. About one-fourth of patients have no symptoms. Occasional patients have extrapulmonary disease, including uveitis and central nervous system involvement; most have the systemic symptoms of fever, sweats, and malaise.

Radiologically, NSG presents most commonly with multiple pulmonary nodules that may cavitate (Romer 1977; Churg et al, 1979). Other manifestations include solitary nodules or ill-defined nodular

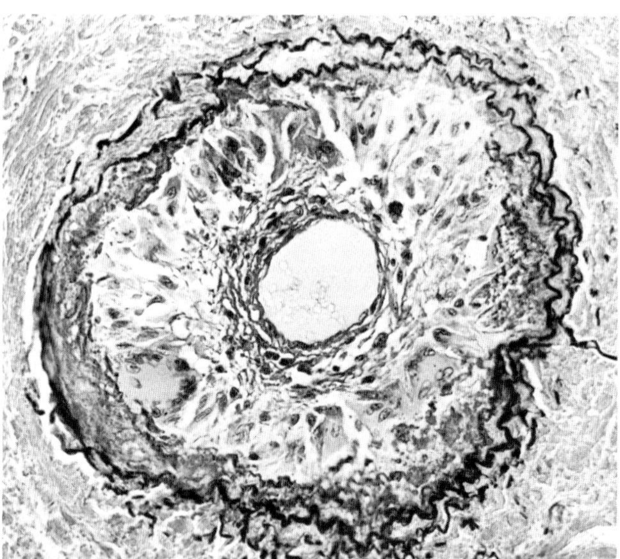

B

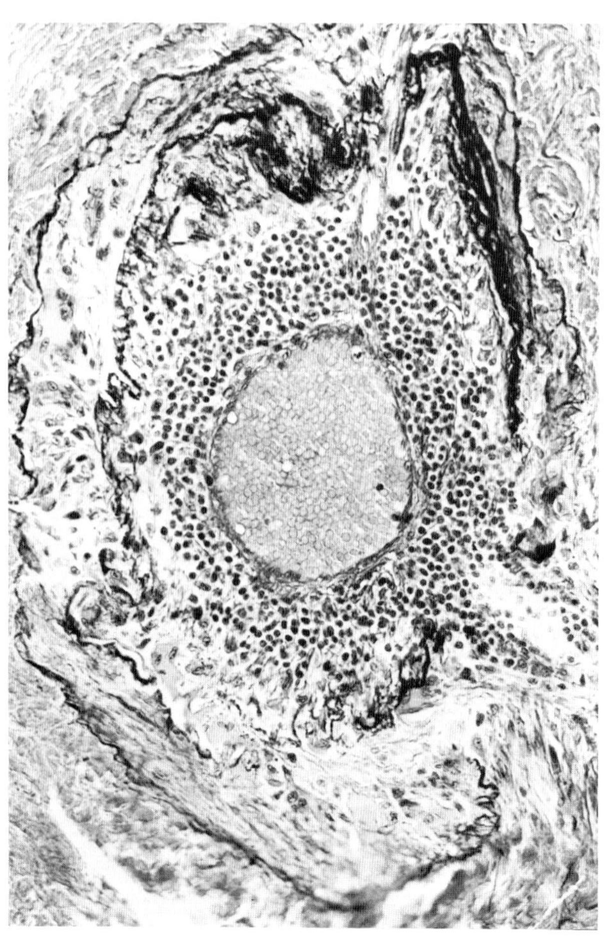

A

Figure 10–7 Necrotizing sarcoidal granulomatosis. *A*, Mononuclear cell vasculitis with giant cells involving the external elastic lamina. *B*, Variant of vasculitis characterized by sarcoid granuloma of vessel wall.

infiltrates. Hilar adenopathy was unusual in two series (Liebow, 1973; Koss et al, 1980), but it was described in approximately 50 percent in another (Churg et al, 1979).

The basic pathologic diagnostic criteria include a combination of sarcoid-like granulomas, necrosis, and the types of vasculitis described by Liebow (Fig. 10-7). The confluent areas of necrosis may be caseous, fibrinous, infarct-like, or apparently healed with extensive fibrosis (Churg et al, 1979). Punctate necrosis within individual sarcoid-like granulomas is also common (Fig. 10-8).

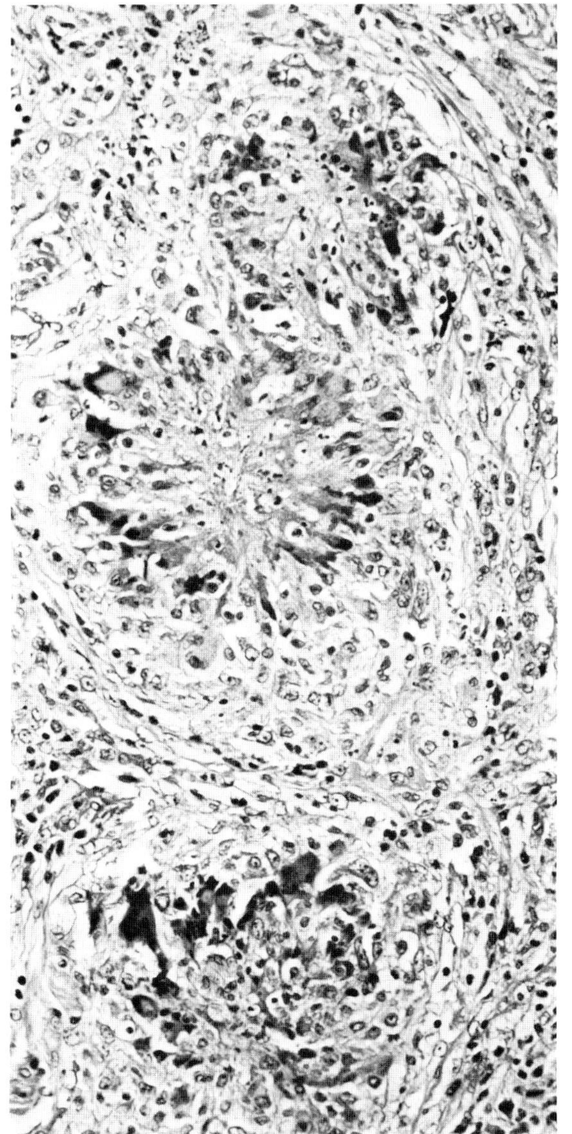

Figure 10–8 Punctate necrosis in granulomas of necrotizing sarcoidal granulomatosis.

The relationship between classic sarcoidosis and NSG is controversial, and the overlap depends to a great extent on the diagnostic criteria used to include or exclude NSG. For example, Churg (1983) implied that "numerous sarcoid-like granulomas, which are not present in any other form of angiitis and granulomatosis," would be virtually diagnostic of NSG in the proper context and that central "hyalinization but no necrosis" is still consistent with NSG. Using these criteria, some of the patients with NSG in the study by Churg and coworkers (1979) had clinical features of sarcoidosis. Carrington (1976) observed that vascular involvement and especially venulitis was found in over half of cases of sarcoidosis. An additional bit of evidence suggesting a relationship between sarcoidosis and NSG is the common finding of noncaseating granulomas in the typical juxtalymphatic distribution quite distant from the necrotic nodule(s) in cases of NSG (Fig. 10-9). Koss and coworkers (1980) reviewed 13 cases of NSG and found *Aspergillus* antigen in the granulomas in one case, leading them to speculate that NSG may be a variant of allergic alveolitis rather than sarcoidosis.

The prognosis in cases of NSG is excellent. Bilateral or diffuse infiltrates and multiple nodules respond well to steroid therapy. Isolated nodules are often excised for diagnostic purposes, and such localized lesions seldom recur following surgery.

LYMPHOMATOID GRANULOMATOSIS

Lymphomatoid granulomatosis (LYG) was first described by Liebow and colleagues (1972) as a subset of cases of angiitis and granulomatosis. The 40 cases of that original article were distinguished on the basis of an angioinvasive, angiodestructive infiltrate of atypical mononuclear cells. In that original series, and in an updated version that included 152 cases (Katzenstein et al, 1979), the clinical features were characterized. It was twice as common in males than females, and most cases occurred in the age range of 30 to 60 years. The characteristic presentation was of systemic complaints such as fever, malaise, weight loss, and chest complaints such as cough and dyspnea. In 45 percent of patients there was skin involvement with small nodules and a vasocentric atypical lymphoid infiltrate histologically resembling that in the lung. At autopsy 45 percent of patients had renal involvement in the form of mass lesions, but clinically evident renal symptoms were uncommon. The next most common site of involvement was the nervous system (20 percent), with central nervous system manifestations or peripheral neuritis. The pulmonary infiltrates in lymphomatoid granulomatosis most often consist of bilateral nod-

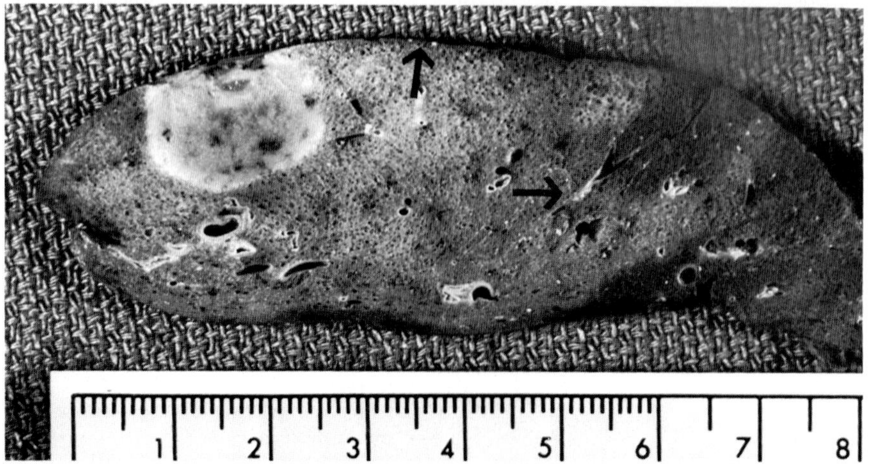

Figure 10–9 Dominant nodule in necrotizing sarcoidal granulomatosis with sarcoid-like granulomas in perilymphatic distribution (*arrows*) away from the nodule.

ules or nodular infiltrates, 1 to 8 cm in diameter, usually with ill-defined and irregular margins; the nodules sometimes cavitate (Wechsler et al, 1984), and may simulate metastatic carcinoma (Liebow et al, 1972; Katzenstein et al, 1979). Less commonly LYG may present with patchy bilateral segmental consolidation (Fig. 10–10). The consolidation may be due to pulmonary infarction or hemorrhage (Wechsler et al, 1984; Dee et al, 1982). Small pleural effusions are often present. In 20 percent of patients with lymphomatoid granulomatosis, reticulonodular densities are present (Wechsler et al, 1984).

From the time of the original description, the relationship of LYG to lymphoma has been debated. In the original series (Liebow et al, 1972) and its extension (Katzenstein et al, 1979), it was noted that while lymph nodes, bone marrow, and spleen often showed lymphoid hyperplasia and/or scattered atypical lymphoid cells, they did not appear overtly lymphomatous at presentation (virtually by definition). Furthermore, the polymorphic but cytologically benign infiltrate accompanying the atypical elements excluded any of the known lymphomas in the classification schemes available at that time. "The difficulty of comparison, or contrast, of lymphomatoid granulomatosis with lymphomas as it involves the lung is that there are great uncertainties in the definition of the latter. Thus, the 'baseline' itself is not well established" (Liebow et al, 1972). The original investigators used the status of the nodes, marrow, and/or spleen as a major criterion to distinguish LYG from lymphoma at presentation. In these two series, progression from LYG to lymphoma so defined was documented in 12 percent of cases.

Since then, some light and much heat has been generated in the LYG-lymphoma controversy. Be-

cause of the diagnostic sophistication achieved in the study of lymphomas, it has become apparent that organ involvement without nodal involvement is not uncommon. Colby and Carrington (1982) used "identification of monomorphous foci of atypical lymphoid cells" as the diagnostic point separating LYG (which lacked such foci) from vasoinvasive lymphoma (which contained such foci). They were able to classify such vasoinvasive lymphomas into one of the accepted large cell lymphoma categories in the great majority of cases, although in some instances it required examination of many blocks to find the monomorphic focus within the polymorphic background. Lymphoid marker studies have shown that many cases diagnosed as LYG are proliferations of T cells and especially helper T cells (Nichols et al, 1982). It has been suggested that in the event of loss of one or more pan-T markers, the lesion should be viewed as T-cell lymphoma, and without such antigenic loss, the lesions should be viewed as LYG (Weiss et al, 1985; Donner et al, 1990). Myers (1990) recommended that all cases of LYG be viewed as part of the family of peripheral T-cell lymphomas. Alternatively, Pisani and DeRemee (1990) suggested that LYG is an immunologic reaction to such diverse disease processes as cancer, autoimmunity, and viral infections. Another approach has been to include LYG under the grouping of "lymphoproliferative disorders of the lung" (Gibbs and Seal, 1978). This broad category includes lymphoid interstitial pneumonia (see chapter 7), Sjögren's syndrome, diffuse lymphocytic lymphoma, other lymphomas and LYG, since it regards them all as part of a continuum. However convenient this latter concept may be, it has little value in understanding immunophenotypic data, in predicting prognosis, or in directing therapy. The dilemma in distinguishing between nonlympho-

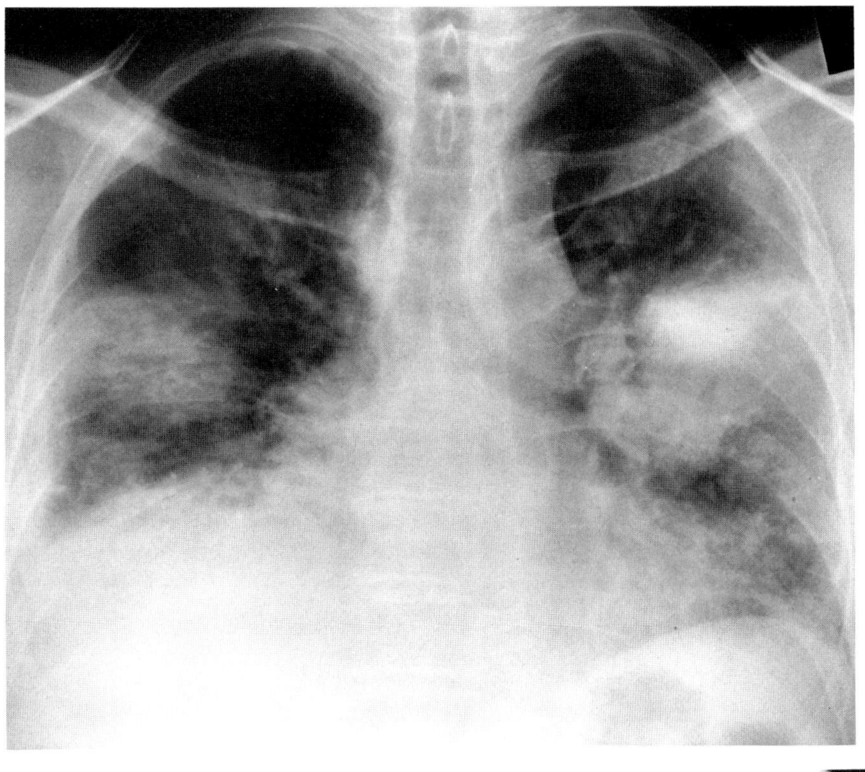

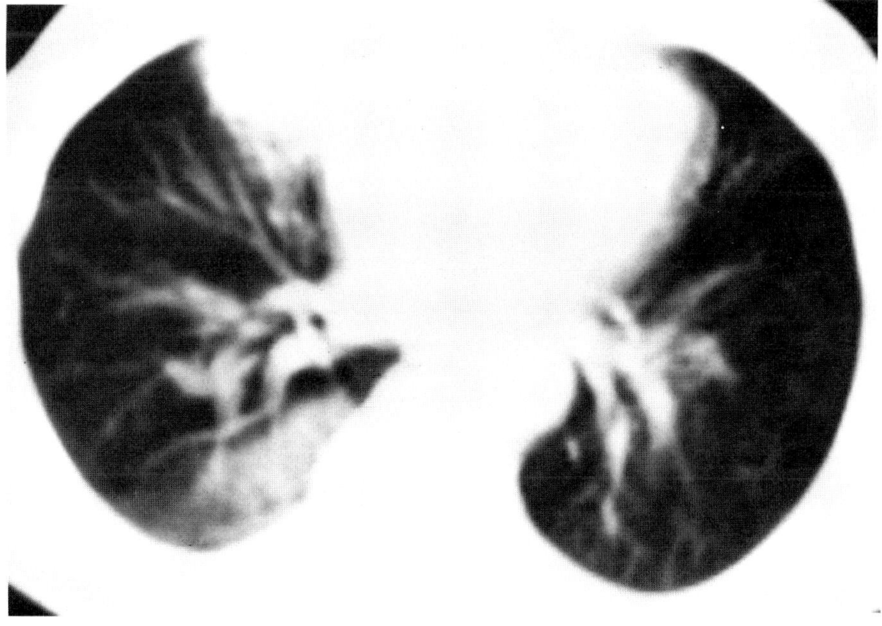

Figure 10–10 Lymphomatoid granulomatosis in a 66-year-old man. *A*, Chest radiograph shows bilateral areas of consolidation and right pleural effusion. *B*, CT scan 2 years later shows segmental consolidation in the right middle and lower lobes.

proliferative angiitis and granulomatosis, LYG, and vasocentric lymphoma has its analog in the upper airways and paranasal sinuses. "Lethal midline granuloma" is now viewed as a syndrome, some cases being due to WG, some to "frank" (cytologically obvious) lymphoma, and some to "polymorphic reticulosis" (DeRemee et al, 1978) which are primarily T-cell polymorphous vasocentric lymphoid proliferations.

The criteria for histologic diagnosis of LYG are not precise. The features originally described (Liebow et al, 1972) stipulate that there be "granulomatosis" as reflected by necrosis (Fig. 10–11), although well-defined necrotizing or non-necrotizing granulomas are distinctly uncommon. The infiltrate was described as "variegated, a characteristic that served to distinguish it from that of the usual lymphoma" and included small lymphocytes, transformed "atypical" lymphocytes, "atypical" immunoblasts, plasma cells, occasional polymorphonuclear leukocytes, and rare eosinophils (Fig. 10–12). Finally, the infiltrate displayed a predilection to invade blood vessel walls with variable elastin disruption (see Fig. 10–12).

Secondary findings included bronchiolar infiltration, obstructive pneumonia, granulation tissue, and fibrosis. Colby and Carrington's (1982) later recommendation is that foci of monomorphic cells are a feature of lymphoma rather than of LYG, a recommendation that if applied retrospectively would change the diagnosis in some of the original cases. If T-cell subset studies on frozen tissue are available, the results may further affect the final diagnostic impression. The finding of lymphoid "tracking" along lymphatic routes is typically seen in lymphoma, although there are no data to suggest that tracking excludes a diagnosis of LYG. Our view is that the majority of cases diagnosed as LYG are non-Hodgkin's lymphoma with dominant vasocentricity. When such cases can be classified within one of the conventional classifications of lymphoma, LYG should not be the diagnosis. Some cases remain which do not easily fit into these classifications and are characterized by a polymorphous infiltrate of cells that include lymphocytes with varying degrees of differentiation, plasma cells, and large mononuclear cells with abundant amphophilic

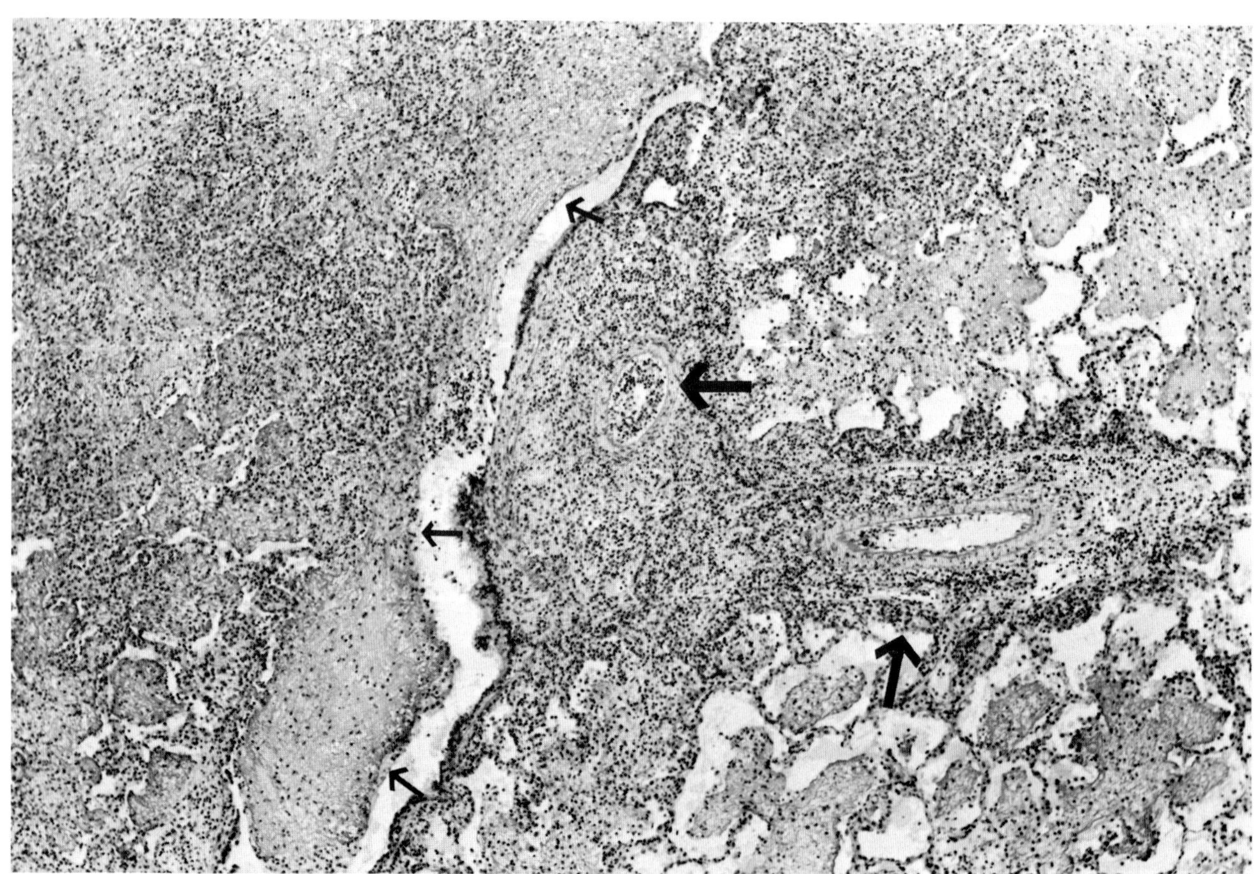

Figure 10–11 Lymphomatoid granulomatosis with zone of necrosis (*small arrows*), cellular rim, and vasocentric mononuclear infiltrate (*large arrows*).

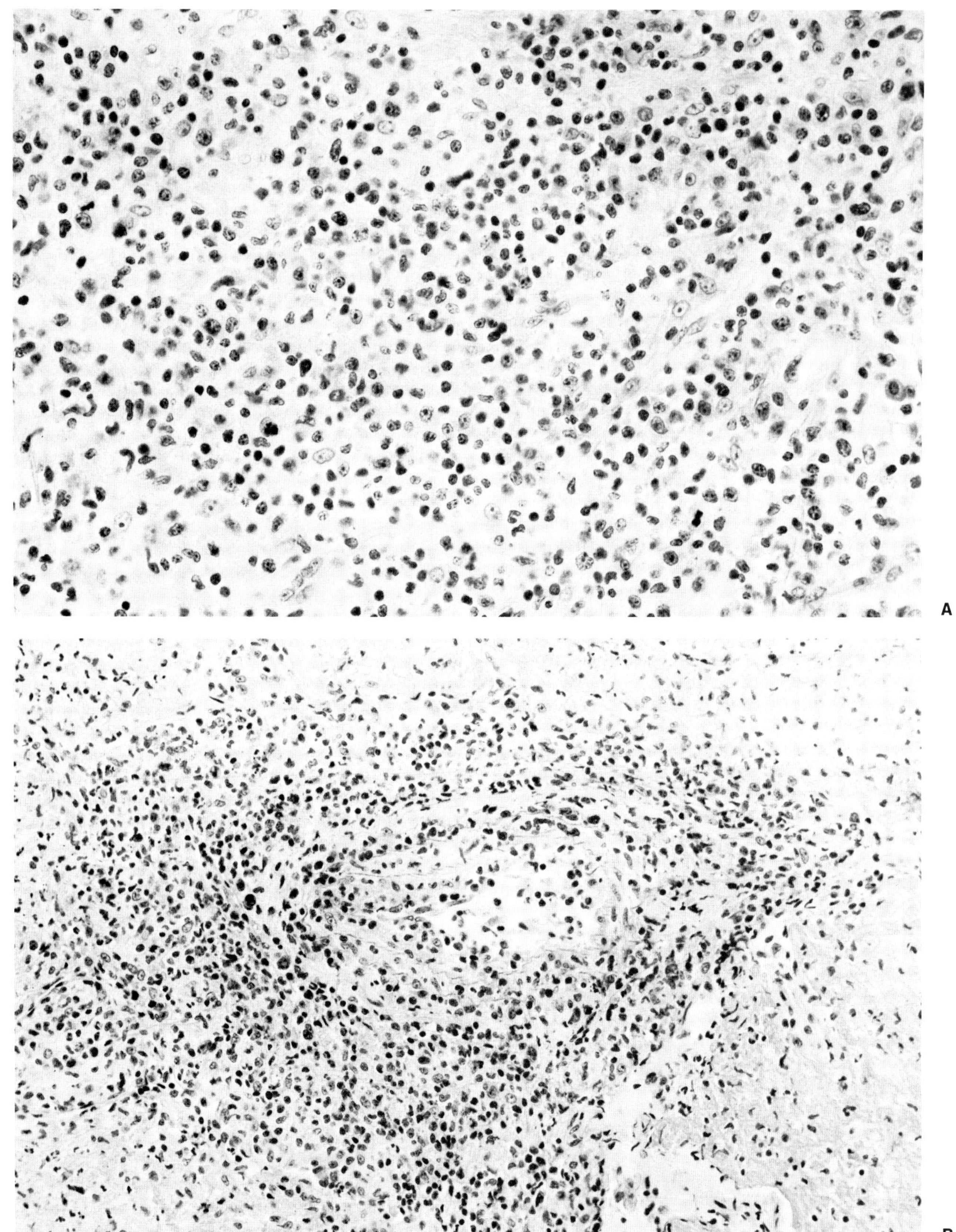

Figure 10–12   Variegated infiltrate with atypical cells (*A*) and vasocentricity (*B*) in lymphomatoid granulomatosis.

cytoplasm, eccentric nuclei, and prominent nucleoli. The diagnosis of LYG is justified in such cases.

Other diagnostic possibilities are usually not so difficult to exclude as lymphoma. Confusion with NSG may occur because both NSG and LYG have necrosis and both have an infiltrative mononuclear vasculitis. However, well-formed noncaseating granulomas are sparse or absent in LYG and prominent in NSG, the various types of vasculitis seen in NSG are not present in LYG, and the mononuclear cells in NSG are not atypical. The cellular infiltrate in Wegener's granulomatosis is occasionally quite pleomorphic. The most important features that separate them are the serpiginous margins in WG, the presence of multinucleated giant cells at the margins, and necrotizing vasculitis away from the lesion with cells that cannot be classified as malignant. Saldana and coworkers (1977) coined the term "benign lymphocytic angiitis and granulomatosis" (BLAG) to describe a lesion with a dense entirely benign-looking lymphoid infiltrate, vasocentricity without elastin destruction, and variable degrees of necrosis. They contrasted BLAG to their idea of LYG, which included a cytologically malignant-looking lymphoid infiltrate. Our understanding is that the latter would now be viewed as lymphoma, and BLAG would now be viewed as LYG with particularly benign cytology.

When LYG was originally described, the prognosis was dismal. Median survival was only 14 months, with the usual cause of death being disease progression in the chest or in the central nervous system. Katzenstein and colleagues (1979) noted that patients with fewer atypical cells had a better prognosis than those with many atypical cells, the implication possibly being that patients with lesions that would now be viewed as large cell lymphoma have a worse prognosis than patients with lesions that would be viewed as LYG. In Saldana's series, patients with BLAG (or low-grade LYG) did extraordinarily well with chemotherapy. Fauci and coworkers (1982) were highly successful in treating patients with LYG with steroids and cyclophosphamide but were unsuccessful in treating patients in whom overt lymphoma had developed from LYG.

The early series stated that 10 to 15 percent of patients with LYG develop nodal lymphoma by the time of death. With our current understanding (or lack thereof), the question "What proportion of patients with LYG develop lymphoma?" is more difficult to answer, since there is no universally accepted criteria for what constitutes LYG, what constitutes lymphoma, and how one distinguishes evolution of LYG to lymphoma from lymphoma that is diagnosed at its outset.

BRONCHOCENTRIC GRANULOMATOSIS, ALLERGIC BRONCHOPULMONARY ASPERGILLOSIS, AND MUCOID IMPACTION OF BRONCHI

Bronchocentric granulomatosis (BCG), allergic bronchopulmonary aspergillosis (ABPA), and mucoid impaction of bronchi (MIB) are grouped together because of their tendency to occur together (Katzenstein et al, 1975; Boskin et al, 1988). BCG is characterized by the replacement of walls of bronchi and bronchioles by granulomatous inflammation. ABPA is defined as the syndrome of pulmonary infiltrates, eosinophilia, asthma, and serologic evidence of al-

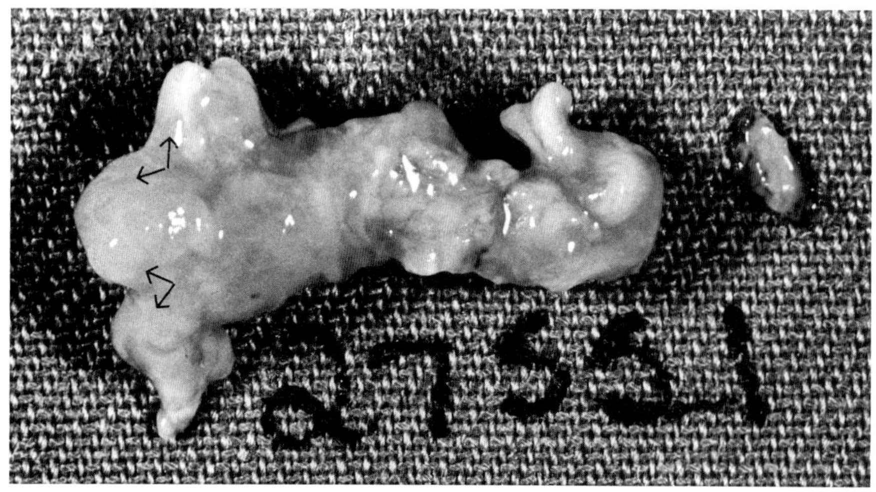

A

Figure 10–13   *A,* Mucus plug in mucoid impaction of bronchi due to allergic bronchopulmonary aspergillosis. Note branching (*arrows*) conforming to bronchus.

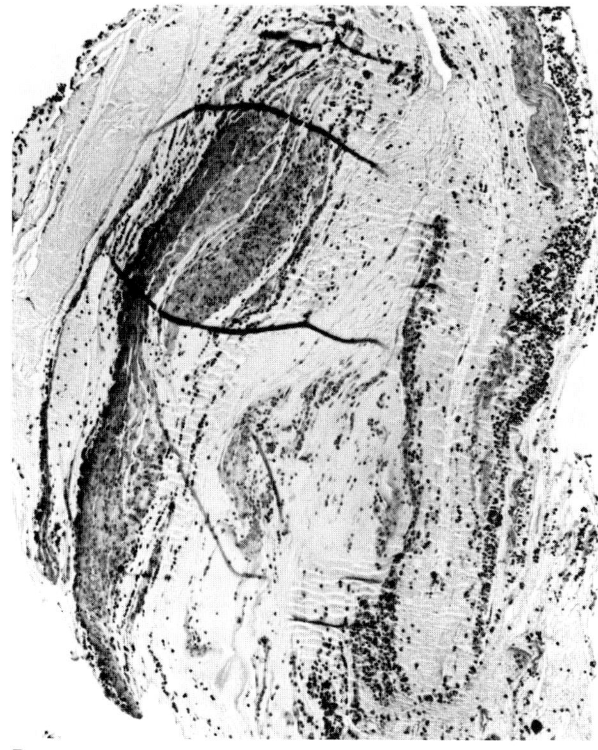

B

Figure 10–13, cont'd *B*, Laminated "allergic mucin" in mucoid impaction of bronchi.

lergy to *Aspergillus*. MIB is defined as the obstruction of a proximal bronchi by plugs of thick mucus. When seen in association with BCG or ABPA, MIB usually has the histologic features of "allergic mucin": laminated arrangement of basophilic neutral mucin alternating with eosinophils, eosinophilic debris, and Charcot-Leyden crystals (Fig. 10–13).

BCG was first described by Liebow (1973) and amplified by Katzenstein and colleagues (1975). In contrast to the diseases previously discussed in this chapter, the lesions of BCG are primarily related to bronchi. Confusion with the other noninfectious granulomas and vasculitic diseases arises in cases in which the peribronchial inflammatory process is associated with vasculitis in the contiguous pulmonary artery. In the earliest stage, there is ulceration of airway epithelium and replacement by palisaded histiocytes. The airways are filled with necrotic debris (Fig. 10–14). Subsequently, the lumen of the involved airway fills with granulomatous exudate, resulting in an apparently spherical granuloma (see Fig. 4–12). The apparently circular granulomas can be recognized to be in an intra-airway position by identifying the accompanying artery. Another feature of BCG is the presence of varying degrees of eosinophilia in the peribron-

chiolar infiltrate. The distinction between BCG and the vasocentric processes described previously in this chapter becomes difficult only when there is dramatic contiguous involvement of arteries (Fig. 10–15). Helpful distinguishing features are as follows: arteritis is not found in company with a normal bronchus in BCG; veins are spared in BCG; and necrosis involves the airways rather than the parenchyma in BCG.

In the description by Katzenstein and coworkers (1975), about half of the patients had asthma and these patients were young (average age, 20 years) and had severe systemic symptoms; 90 percent had peripheral eosinophilia, and fungi were seen within the necrotic bronchial contents in 90 percent of cases histologically. This group of patients commonly demonstrated the overlap of BCG, ABPA, and MIB. The patients diagnosed as BCG without asthma were older (average age, 50 years) and had milder symptoms, but peripheral eosinophilia was still common (50 percent). These patients were much less likely to have MIB or demonstrable intraluminal fungi. In another large series of cases (Koss et al, 1981) asthma and/or tissue eosinophilia were seen in one third of patients, but identifiable fungi were rarely found, even in the asthmatic patients. An uncommon variant has been described in which *Aspergillus* hyphae were identified in BCG not associated with asthma, eosinophilia, or MIB (Nagata et al, 1990); we have seen a similar case.

Bronchocentric granulomatosis usually is unilateral and involves the upper lobes. One to three nodular densities ranging from 2 to 6 cm in diameter are present in 60 percent of patients (Robinson et al, 1982). The nodules usually have ill-defined irregular margins. In contrast to WG and LYG, the nodules rarely cavitate. Unilateral or bilateral airspace consolidation, usually in the upper lobes, is seen in 30 percent of patients. The infiltrates may have a peripheral distribution similar to that of chronic eosinophilic pneumonia. Asthmatic patients with bronchocentric granulomatosis may have mucoid impaction with "glove-finger" branching shadows and central bronchiectasis.

Clinically, ABPA is fairly distinctive, with the previously mentioned constellation of asthma, eosinophilia, pulmonary infiltrates, and hypersensitivity to *Aspergillus*. Patients may have chest pain and usually have constitutional symptoms. The majority of patients cough up mucus plugs (probably MIB), in which *Aspergillus* may be demonstrated either histologically or by culture. The pathology of ABPA is less well defined since these patients seldom require biopsy or resection for diagnosis or treatment. Pathologic features were first described by Hinson and coworkers in 1952, who noted bronchial dilatation and tissue eosinophilia but not granulomatous bron-

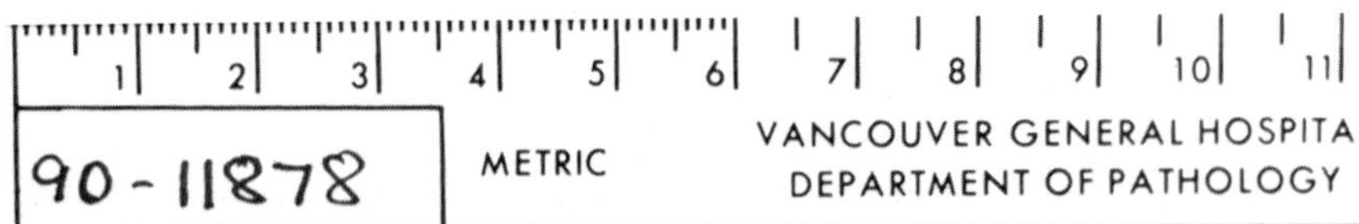

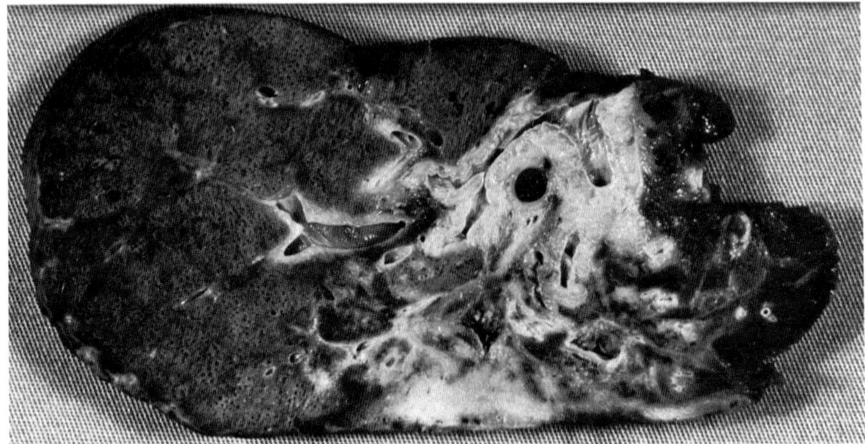

A

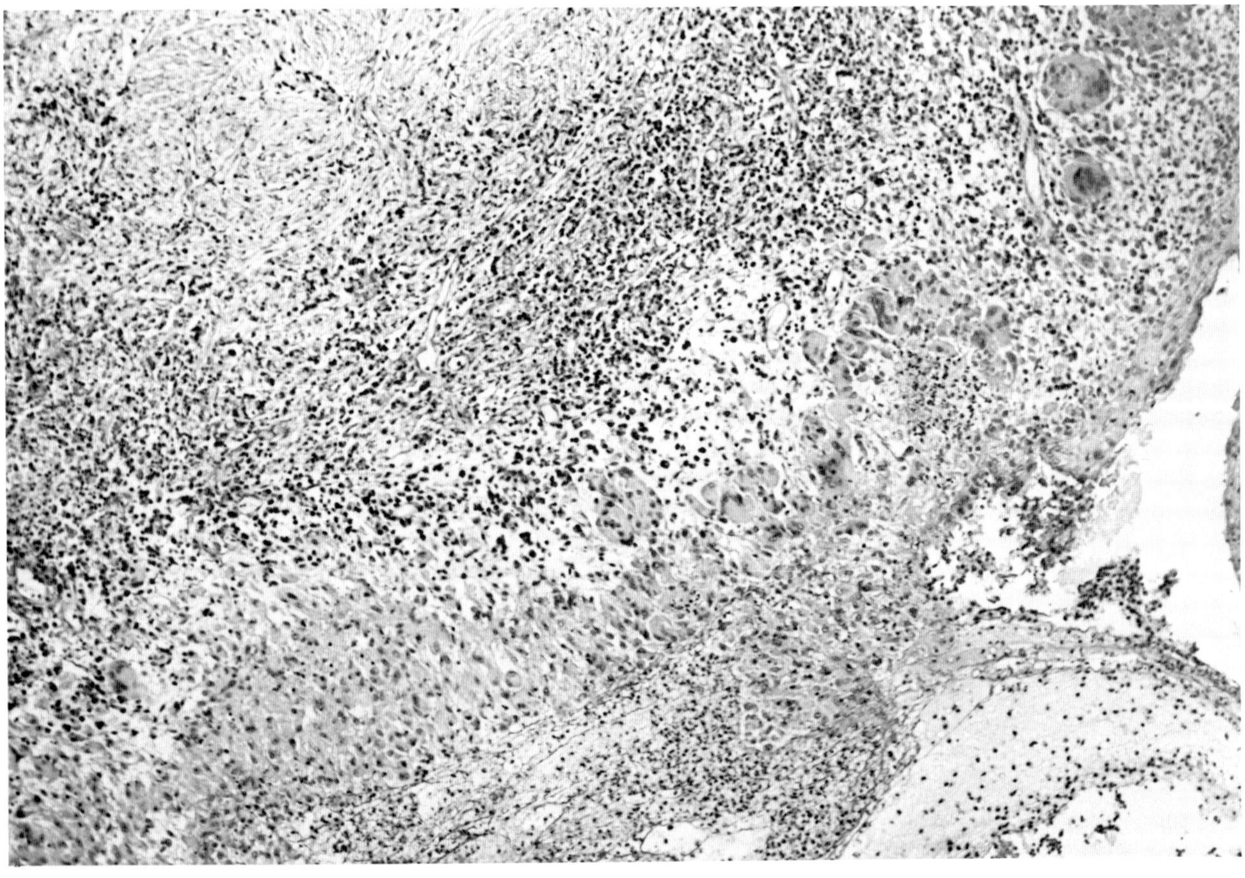

B

Figure 10–14   *A*, Bronchocentric granulomatosis. *B*, Bronchial mucosa is partly eroded and replaced by palisading histiocytes.

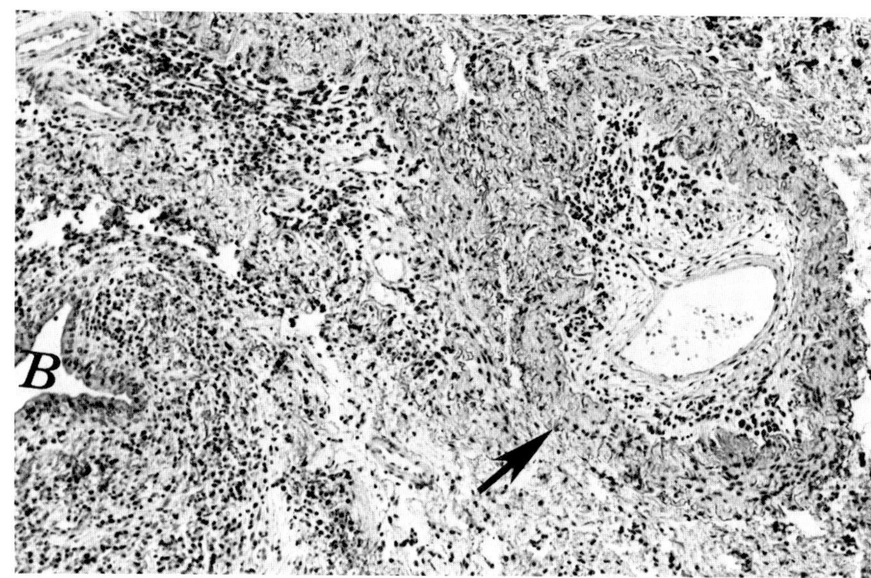

Figure 10–15 Adjacent secondary arteritis in bronchocentric granulomatosis (*arrow;* B = bronchus).

chial disruption or secondary vasculitis. Boskin and colleagues (1988) described the findings in resection specimens in 18 cases of ABPA: bronchial/bronchiolar granulomatous disruption (BCG) occurred in 15 cases, MIB with allergic mucin in 11, and fungal fragments within airway lumens in 14 cases; eosinophilic pneumonia and obstructive pneumonia were also common.

Radiologically, allergic bronchopulmonary aspergillosis may present as transient or recurrent infiltrates and often extensive unilateral or bilateral airspace consolidation (Fisher et al, 1984). It tends to involve mainly the upper lobes. The features may resemble chronic eosinophilic pneumonia. Mucoid impaction is seen as gloved-finger branching shadows, which represent dilated bronchi filled with secretions (Fig. 10-16*A*). Mucoid impaction in damaged dilated bronchi may lead to massive unilateral or bilateral airspace consolidation. The bronchographic or CT findings are diagnostic. Proximal bronchi (second- to fifth-order beyond segmental bronchi) show bronchiectasis, whereas the more distal bronchi are normal in size (Fig. 10-16*B*).

MIB, defined as the obstruction of proximal bronchi by plugs of thick mucus (Boskin et al, 1988), may be seen in various nonhypersensitivity settings such as cystic fibrosis, distal to a tumor, and chronic bronchitis. In these settings, the lamination typical of allergic mucin is not present, and there is neutrophilic rather than eosinophilic debris in the mucin. MIB with allergic mucin is very suggestive of ABPA, and fungal fragments can be demonstrated in many such cases. As in the cases of BCG and

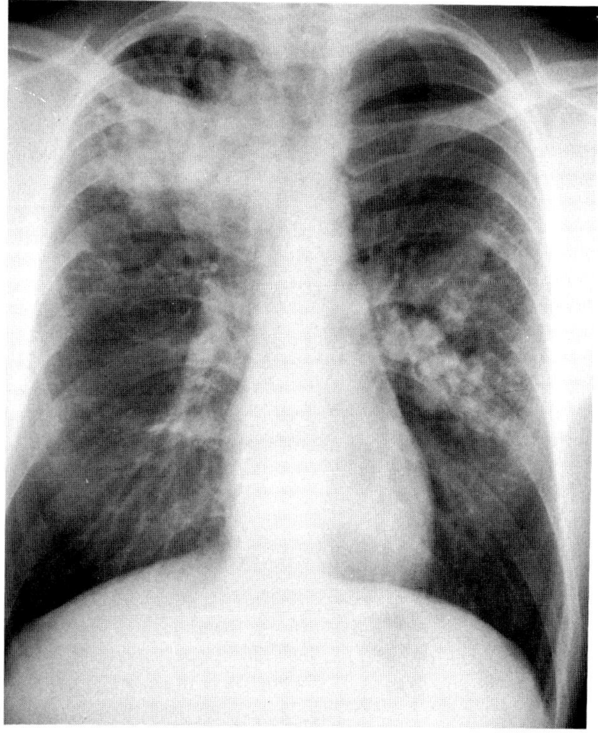

A

Figure 10–16 *A,* Chest radiograph in 70-year-old asthmatic man shows characteristic gloved-finger branching shadows of allergic bronchopulmonary aspergillosis with mucoid impaction. *Continued.*

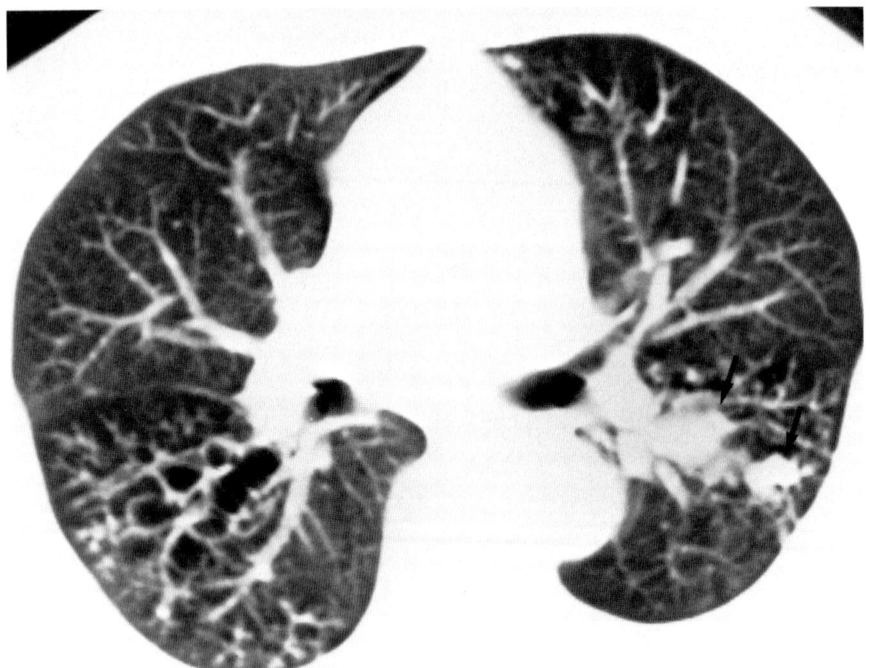

Figure 10–16, cont'd *B,* A 10-mm collimation CT scan through lower lung zones in another patient shows varicose bronchiectasis in right lower lobe and mucoid impaction in left lower lobe (*arrows*).

B

ABPA, tissue invasion by the fungi is not a feature of MIB.

Lesions identical to the noneosinophilic variant of BCG have been shown with endobronchial infection by mycobacteria, histoplasma, and blastomycetes (Myers and Katzenstein, 1986). Tazelaar and coworkers (1989) described three immunocompromised patients in whom aspergillosis (in two) and mucormycosis (in one) produced a morphologic reaction of noneosinophilic BCG, with the important reminder that with immunocompromise, the fungi may become invasive.

REFERENCES

Boskin CH, Myers JL, Greenberger PA, Katzenstein ALA. Pathologic features of allergic bronchopulmonary aspergillosis. Am J Surg Pathol 1988; 12:216–222.

Carrington CB. Structure and function in sarcoidosis. NY Acad Sci 1976; 278:265–283.

Carrington CB, Liebow AA Limited form of angiitis and granulomatosis of Wegener's type. Am J Med 1966; 41:497–527.

Chumbley LC, Harrison EG Jr, DeRemee RA. Allergic angiitis and granulomatosis (Churg-Strauss syndrome): report and analysis of 30 cases. Mayo Clin Proc 1977; 52:477–484.

Churg A. Pulmonary angiitis and granulomatosis revisited. Hum Pathol 1983; 14:868–883.

Churg A, Carrington CB, Gupta R. Necrotizing sarcoid granulomatosis. Chest 1979; 76:406–413.

Churg J, Strauss L. Allergic granulomatosis, allergic angiitis and periarteritis nodosa. Am J Pathol 1951; 27:277.

Colby TV, Carrington CB. Pulmonary lymphomas simulating lymphomatoid granulomatosis. Am J Surg Pathol 1982; 6:19–32.

Crissman J. Midline malignant reticulosis and lymphomatoid granulomatosis. Arch Pathol Lab Med 1979; 103:561.

Dee PM, Arora NS, Innes DJ Jr. The pulmonary manifestations of lymphomatoid granulomatosis. Radiology 1982; 143:613–618.

DeRemee RA, McDonald TJ, Harrison EG, Coles DT. Wegener's granulomatosis. Mayo Clin Proc 1976; 51:777–781.

DeRemee RA, McDonald TJ, Weiland LH. Wegener's granulomatosis: Observations on treatment with antimicrobial agents. Mayo Clin Proc 1985; 60:27–32.

DeRemee RA, Welland L, McDonald T. Polymorphic reticulosis, lymphomatoid granulomatosis. Two entities or one? Mayo Clin Proc 1978; 53:634.

Donner LR, Dobin S, Harrington D, et al. Angiocentric immunoproliferative lesion (lymphomatoid granulomatosis). Cancer 1990; 65:249–254.

Fauci A, Haynes B, Costa J, et al. Lymphomatoid granulomatosis: prospective clinical and therapeutic experience over 10 years. N Engl J Med 1982; 306:68–74.

Fauci AS, Haynes BF, Katz P, Wolff SM. Wegener's granulomatosis: prospective clinical and therapeutic experience with 85 patients for 21 years. Ann Intern Med 1983; 98:76–85.

Fienberg R. The protracted superficial phenomenon in pathergic (Wegener's) granulomatosis. Hum Pathol 1981; 12:458–467.

Fisher MR, Mendelson EB, Mintzer RA. Allergic bronchopulmonary aspergillosis: a pictorial essay. Radiographics 1984; 4:445–463.

Fukuda K, Yuasa K, Uchizano A, et al. Three cases of Wegener's granulomatosis treated with an antimicrobial agent. Arch Otolaryngol Head Neck Surg 1989; 115:515–518.

Gibbs AR, Seal RME. Primary lymphoproliferative conditions of the lung. Thorax 1978; 33:140-152.

Glimp RA, Bayer AS. Fungal pneumonias. Part 3. Allergic bronchopulmonary aspergillosis. Chest 1981; 80:85–94.

Harrison DJ, Simpson R, Kharbanda R, et al. Antibodies to neutrophil cytoplasmic antigens in Wegener's granulomatosis and other conditions. Thorax 1989; 44: 373–377.

Hinson KF, Moon AJ, Plummer NS. Bronchopulmonary aspergillosis: a review and a report of eight new cases. Thorax 1952; 7:317–333.

Israel HI. Sulfamethoxazole-trimethoprim therapy for Wegener's granulomatosis. Arch Intern Med 1988; 148:2293–2295.

Katzenstein ALA. Necrotizing granulomas of the lung. Hum Pathol 1980; 11:596–597.

Katzenstein AL, Carrington CB, Liebow AA. Lymphomatoid granulomatosis. Cancer 1979; 43:360–373.

Katzenstein AL, Liebow AA, Friedman PJ. Bronchocentric granulomatosis, mucoid impaction and hypersensitivity reactions to fungi. Am Rev Respir Dis 1975; 111:497–537.

Klinger H, Frankfurt Z. Grenzformen der periarteritis nodosa. Pathology 1931; 42:455.

Koss M, Antomovych T, Hochholzer L. Allergic granulomatosis (Churg-Strauss syndrome): pulmonary and renal morphologic findings. Am J Surg Pathol 1981; 5:21–28.

Koss MN, Hochholzer L, Feigin DW, et al. Necrotizing sarcoid-like granulomatosis: clinical, pathologic and immunopathologic features. Hum Pathol 1980; 11: 510–519.

Koss MN, Robinson G, Hochholzer L. Bronchocentric granulomatosis. Hum. Pathol 1981; 12:632–638.

Kus J, Bergin C, Miller R, et al. Lymphocyte subpopulations in allergic granulomatosis and angiitis (Churg-Strauss syndrome). Chest 1985; 87:826–827.

Leavitt RY, Fauci AS. Pulmonary vasculitis. Am Rev Respir Dis 1986; 134:149–166.

Liebow AA. The J. Burns Amberson lecture. Pulmonary angiitis and granulomatosis. Am Rev Respir Dis 1973; 108:1–18.

Liebow AA, Carrington CB, Friedman PJ. Lymphomatoid granulomatosis. Hum Pathol 1972; 3:457–558.

Maguire R, Fauci AS, Doppman JL, Wolff SM. Unusual radiographic features of Wegener's granulomatosis. AJR 1978; 130:233–238.

Mark EJ, Matsubara O, Tan-Liu NS, Fienberg R. The pulmonary biopsy in the early diagnosis of Wegener's (pathergic) granulomatosis. Hum Pathol 1988; 19: 1065–1071.

Myers JL. Lymphomatoid granulomatosis: past, present,… future? Mayo Clin Proc 1990; 65:274–277.

Myers JL, Katzenstein ALA. Granulomatous infection mimicking bronchocentric granulomatosis. Am J Surg Pathol 1986; 10:317–322.

Myers JL, Katzenstein ALA. Wegener's granulomatosis presenting with massive pulmonary hemorrhage and capillaritis. Am J Surg Pathol 1987; 11:895–898.

Nagata N, Sueishi K, Tanaka K, Iwata Y. Pulmonary aspergillosis with bronchocentric granulomas. Am J Surg Pathol 1990; 14:485–488.

Nichols PW, Koss M, Levine AM, Lukes RJ. Lymphomatoid granulomatosis: a T-cell disorder? Am J Med 1982; 72:467–471.

Nolle B, Specks V, Ludemann J, et al. Anticytoplasmic autoantibodies: their immunodiagnostic value in Wegener granulomatosis. Ann Intern Med 1989; 111: 28–40.

Pisani RJ, DeRemee RA. Clinical implications of the histopathologic diagnosis of pulmonary lymphomatoid granulomatosis. Mayo Clin Proc 1990; 65:151–163.

Robinson RG, Wehunt WD, Tsou E, et al. Bronchocentric granulomatosis: roentgenographic manifestations. Am Rev Respir Dis 1982; 125:751–756.

Romer FK. Sarcoidosis with large nodular lesions simulating pulmonary metastases. Scand J Respir Dis 1977; 58:11.

Rose GA, Spencer H. Polyarteritis nodosa. QJ Med 1957; 26:43–81.

Rosenberg T, Medsger T Jr, De Cicco F, Fireman P. Allergic angiitis and granulomatosis (Churg-Strauss syndrome). J Allergy Clin Immunol 1975; 55;56.

Saldana MJ, Patchefsky AS, Israel HI, Atkinson GW. Pulmonary angiitis and granulomatosis. Hum Pathol 1977; 8:391–409.

Stamenkovic I, Toccanier M, Kapanci Y. Polymorphic reticulosis (lethal midline granuloma) and lymphomatoid granulomatosis. Identical or distinct entities? Virchows Arch |A| 1981; 390:81–91.

Stein MG, Gamsu G, Webb WR, Stulbarg MS. Computed tomography of diffuse tracheal stenosis in Wegener granulomatosis. J Comput Assist Tomogr 1986; 10: 868–870.

Stephens M, Reynolds S, Gibbs AR, Davies B. Allergic bronchopulmonary aspergillosis progressing to allergic granulomatosis and angiitis (Churg-Strauss syndrome). Am Rev Respir Dis 1988; 137:1226–1228.

Stokes TC, McCann BG, Rees RT, et al. Acute fulminating intrapulmonary hemorrhage in Wegener's. Thorax 1982; 37:315–326.

Tazelaar HD, Baird AM, Mill M, et al. Bronchocentric mycosis occurring in transplant recipients. Chest 1989; 96:92–95.

Tellis CJ, Putman JS. Cavitation in large multinodular pulmonary disease: a rare manifestation of sarcoidosis. Chest 1977; 71:792–793.

Tervaert JWC, Vander Woude FJ, Fauci AS, et al. Association between active Wegener's granulomatosis and anticytoplasmic antibodies. Arch Intern Med 1989; 149:2461–2465.

Travis WD, Carpenter HA, Lie JT. Diffuse pulmonary hemorrhage: an uncommon manifestation of Wegener's granulomatosis. Am J Surg Pathol 1987; 11:702–708.

Ulbright TM, Katzenstein ALA. Solitary necrotizing granulomas of the lung: differentiating features and etiology. Am J Surg Pathol 1980; 4:13–28.

Vander Woude FJ, Rasmussen N, Lobatto S, et al. Autoantibodies against neutrophils and monocytes: tool for diagnosis and marker of disease activity in Wegener's granulomatosis. Lancet 1985; 1:425–429.

Wechsler RJ, Steiner RM, Israel HL, Patchefsky AS. Chest radiograph in lymphomatoid granulomatosis: comparison with Wegener granulomatosis. AJR 1984; 142:79–83.

Wegener F. Uber generalisierte, septishe Gefaberkrangungen. Verh Dtsch Ges Pathol 1936; 29:202–210.

Weisbrod GL. Pulmonary angiitis and granulomatosis: a review. J Can Assoc Radiol 1989; 40:127–134.

Weiss LM, Yousem SA, Warnke RA. Non-Hodgkin's lymphoma of the lung. Am J Surg Pathol 1985; 9:480–490.

Yousem SA, Lombard CM. The eosinophilic variant of Wegener's granulomatosis. Hum Pathol 1988; 19:682–688.

CHAPTER 11

PNEUMOCONIOSIS

The term "pneumoconiosis," defined by its Greek roots, means dust in the lung. Organic or nonmineral dusts cause a variety of lung lesions, usually immunologically mediated, and have been discussed earlier (see extrinsic allergic alveolitis in Chapter 7). The reaction of the lung to inorganic dust depends on several factors. The composition of the minerals is important because of individual solubilities and toxic reactions. The size of the particles determines the site of deposition within the respiratory tract, whereas their concentration determines load (Becklake, 1976). Particles greater than 5 μm in aerodynamic diameter (a description of how they behave rather than their actual diameter) lodge in the nose and large airways. Particles from 1 to 5 μm in aerodynamic diameter lodge in the acinus. Particles less than 1 μm in diameter behave like gases and thus are also breathed out, but many lodge in airspaces. The ability of the respiratory system to clear or to isolate particles and the respiratory system's competence in repairing damage, determine the nature of lesions. Finally, individual susceptibility is a variable that prevents one person from acquiring disease, while an identically exposed individual develops significant lesions.

In assessing patients with pneumoconiosis, the clinical history, pulmonary function tests, radiologic findings, and histopathology must be taken into consideration. In a study of 52 patients, morphologic lesions were found to predate functional or radiologic changes, which became apparent at various times depending on the disease (Gaensler, 1972). Identification of the injurious dust in tissue samples may be essential; methods of determining dusts within the lung, such as electron probe microanalysis, are discussed in detail in a recent monograph, which also provides a comprehensive review of occupational lung disease (Churg and Green, 1988).

Only inorganic dusts that are encountered reasonably frequently at biopsy will be discussed here; complete data are available in recent monographs and chapters on occupational lung disease (Churg and Green, 1988; Parkes, 1982; Morgan and Seaton, 1984; Heppleston, 1988).

ASBESTOSIS

Asbestosis is pneumoconiosis caused by inhalation of a group of fibrous silicates that have varying combinations of magnesium, iron, aluminum, calcium, and sodium (Becklake, 1976). Asbestos is found in many industries and in many forms, and occupational and other exposures are legion. Two main types exist, serpentine and amphibole (Mossman and Gee, 1989). Chrysotile is the only example of the serpentine form, but many subtypes of the amphibole type exist, crocidolite (Cape Blue asbestos) and amosite being the best known. Amphibole asbestos has a higher pathogenicity than does serpentine asbestos, at least partly because the straighter fiber configuration of amphibole asbestos allows deeper penetration into the lung periphery.

The insidious development of shortness of breath is the first clinical symptom of asbestosis. Inspiratory crackles initially are heard in the bases of the lung but become widespread as the disease advances. Finger clubbing is present in about 75 percent of the patients, but the severity is not proportional to the radiologic extent of disease. Pulmonary function tests classically show a restrictive pattern, but there is also evidence of airflow obstruction in many patients who have been exposed to asbestos (Becklake, 1976).

Pathologically, asbestosis is basically a fibrosing lung disease similar in many ways to usual interstitial pneumonia (UIP). Like UIP, the process is usually worse subpleurally and in the basal zones. In some instances, there is diffuse fine fibrosis of the alveolar walls with relative retention of alveolar structure; in other instances coarser "honeycomb" fibrosis develops. At the light microscopic level, the characteristic feature used to distinguish asbestosis from UIP is the presence of asbestos bodies, which are composed of a central core of asbestos, encrusted with iron. Characteristically they have knobs at each end and the body appears beaded (Fig. 11–1). In addition to the classic asbestos body, a variety of other iron-encrusted bodies of various shapes and sizes may be seen (Fig. 11–2). Crouch and Churg (1984) believe

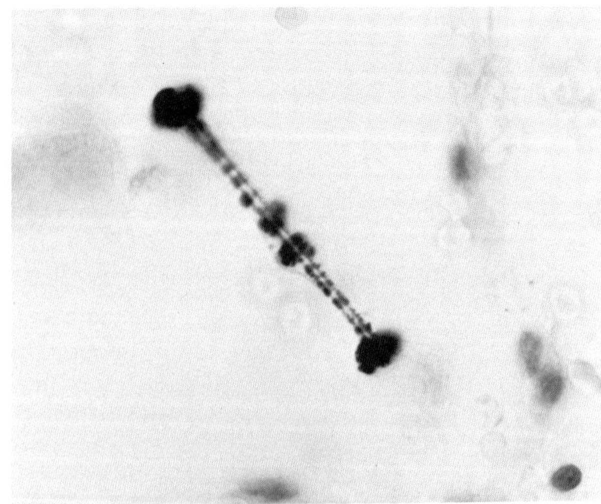

Figure 11–1   Classic asbestos body with clear core and beaded iron coating (iron-stain, × 1,000).

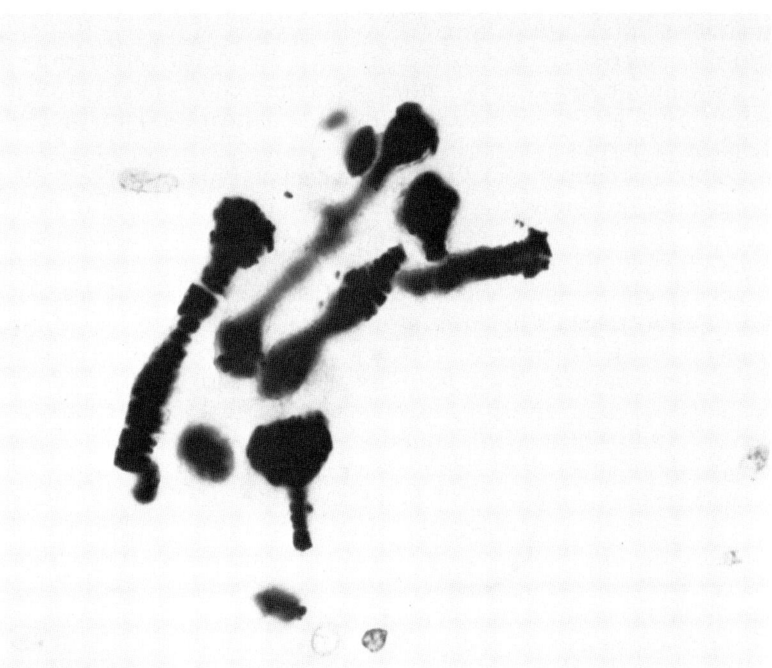

Figure 11–2 Ferruginous bodies of various shapes not diagnostic of asbestos (iron-stain, × 1,000).

that these atypical ferruginous bodies also can be identified as asbestos, provided that they have an optically clear core. Other substances may produce iron-coated bodies including diatomaceous earth, aluminum silicate, fiberglass, and various minerals, but these substances do not give rise to the classic beaded appearance or the clear fiber core (Crouch and Churg, 1984). Asbestos fibers are found both free and surrounded by macrophages and are not doubly refractile. Without the iron coating, asbestos fibers cannot be visualized by light microscopy. The iron coating is most likely derived from phagocytosed red cells and is transferred to the fiber while it is enclosed within phagolysosomes. Tissue analysis has shown that only a few asbestos fibers have an iron coating that is sufficiently thick to be visualized with light microscopy, and thus numbers of asbestos bodies markedly underestimate total asbestos fiber load (Churg, 1982). For that reason, the finding of even one or two asbestos bodies in a tissue section indicates significant exposure to asbestos (although not necessarily asbestos-induced disease). Kuhn and Kuo (1973) described cytoplasmic hyaline inclusions resembling Mallory bodies in alveolar epithelium in several cases of asbestosis. Similar inclusions have also been found in UIP, radiation pneumonitis, and organizing pneumonia and are believed to be a nonspecific reaction to injury (Warnock et al, 1980). Giant cells containing asteroid bodies are also fairly frequently encountered in lungs with asbestos-related fibrosis.

In experimental asbestosis, there are exudative, proliferative, and fibrotic lesions of respiratory bronchioles and alveolar ducts. Studies on the airway lesions in human asbestos disease (Churg and Wright, 1983; Wright and Churg, 1984) have shown a type of fibrosis with pigment deposition in respiratory bronchioles and alveolar ducts which those investigators believe is quite distinct from tobacco-related injury. It is possible that such lesions are responsible for the obstructive functional defect noted in some asbestosis patients, although some investigators believe that exposure to asbestos independent of tobacco smoking does not cause clinically important small airway dysfunction (Mossman and Gee, 1989).

Animal studies as well as epidemiologic studies have shown a dose-response relationship between asbestos exposure and lung fibrosis, although the correlation is weak (Becklake, 1976; Churg, 1982). One problem in dose-response studies is the difficulty in determining inhaled and retained dose. Another problem is variability in fibrogenicity; for example, amphibole asbestos is probably more fibrogenic than serpentine, uncoated fibers are probably more fibrogenic than iron-coated ones, and long fibers are more fibrogenic than short ones. Ashcroft and Heppleston (1973) measured the asbestos content of lungs with varying degrees of fibrosis and found poor correlation between the concentration of fibers and the degree of fibrosis. The implication of these observations is that there are probably some cases of asbestosis with very few asbestos bodies which cannot be distinguished from UIP on the basis of light microscopy.

In addition to asbestosis, other pulmonary consequences of asbestos exposure include conglomerate massive fibrosis, pleural effusion, pleural fibrosis, pleural plaque, mesothelioma, and lung cancer. Progressive massive fibrosis (nodular lesions more than 1 cm in diameter) may occur throughout the lung fields (Gough, 1965), but this complication is rare unless exposure to silica is also present. Pleural effusions due to asbestos are usually unilateral bloody exudates and resolve slowly (Gaensler and Kaplan, 1971). In a review of 22 patients with benign asbestosis-related effusion, Robinson and Musk (1981) found that this complication occurred an average of 16 years after first exposure and spontaneously resolved within 4 to 5 months. In approximately one-third of patients, the effusion recurs a second time, but multiple recurrences are unusual. There were no findings in the fluid or in pleural biopsies that were diagnostic of asbestos etiology. There is no definite association between pleural plaques and pleural effusion, and the development of pleural plaques is unexplained, but they tend to be bilateral and involve only the parietal pleura. Common sites are over the ribs, at the lung bases, and the aponeurotic areas of the diaphragm. Grossly, they are lobulated, white thickenings of the pleura. Microscopically, a plaque is formed of acellular hyaline fibrous tissue with interlacing bands of collagen, producing a basket-weave pattern. Asbestos bodies are rarely seen in them, although uncoated fibers are often demonstrable with special techniques (Becklake, 1976). Pleural plaques are indicative only of asbestos exposure and are not apparently a predisposing factor to the development of other complications. Diffuse pleural fibrosis is the least common asbestos-related benign pleural disease. Histologically the process is similar to pleural plaques, but the visceral pleura is involved in diffuse pleural fibrosis. If underlying lung is entrapped by the process, a tumorlike radiologic abnormality, so-called "round atelectasis," may be produced.

Malignant mesothelioma of pleura (and peritoneum) has a confirmed association with exposure to amphibole asbestos but probably not exposure to chrysotile asbestos. Smokers exposed to asbestos, and particularly amphibole asbestos, have a 50- to 100-fold risk of developing lung cancer over the normal nonsmoking population. Nonsmokers with high asbestos exposure are at minimal, if any, increased risk of developing lung cancer. An association between asbestos exposure and gastrointestinal, ovarian, laryngeal, and hematologic malignancies has been suggested, but such an association is questionable (Mossman and Gee, 1989).

Radiologically the earliest changes of asbestosis are seen in the region of the costophrenic angle and consist of irregular opacities giving a fine reticular pattern. As fibrosis progresses the reticulation becomes more prominent and coarser and may extend to the mid and upper lung zones.

In the appropriate occupational setting, the chest radiograph has generally been accepted as sufficient evidence of the presence of asbestosis without histologic proof (American Thoracic Society, 1986). However, the chest radiograph as an indicator of disease has several limitations. Considerable observer error is seen, particularly in patients with a normal or near-normal chest radiograph (Weill, 1987). Some studies have an incidence of histologic evidence of parenchymal fibrosis with a normal chest radiograph that ranges from 10 to 20 percent (Gaensler, 1972; Kipen et al, 1987).

Studies using conventional computed tomography (CT) yielded conflicting results. Early trials in subjects who were exposed to asbestos found that conventional CT was significantly more sensitive than chest radiographs in detecting pleural thickening and parenchymal fibrosis (Katz and Kreel, 1979). In those CT studies, interstitial fibrosis appeared as areas of coarse honeycombing. Begin and colleagues (1984) analyzed the usefulness of conventional CT scans relative to posteroanterior and four-view radiographs of the chest for detecting asbestos-related pleural and parenchymal fibrosis in 127 workers. They found that CT scans were not helpful in identifying asbestosis in 19 percent of 53 subjects in whom chest radiographs were abnormal (ILO profusion greater than or equal to 1/0).

Aberle and coworkers (1988a) compared high-resolution CT (HRCT) with conventional CT in 29 subjects with occupational exposure to asbestos. All of the individuals studied had evidence of mild to severe abnormalities consistent with asbestosis on standard chest radiographs. They demonstrated that HRCT was considerably more sensitive than conventional CT in the detection of both pleural plaques and parenchymal fibrosis. Several studies have shown that high-resolution CT may demonstrate pleural and parenchymal abnormalities even in patients with normal radiographs (Aberle, 1988b; Friedman, 1988). Staples and colleagues (1989) reviewed 169 asbestos-exposed subjects with no evidence of asbestosis on chest radiographs (ILO profusion less than 1/0) and found that 57 (34 percent) had HRCT features consistent with asbestosis. They found a significant difference between the pulmonary function profiles of asbestos-exposed workers who had HRCT findings consistent with asbestosis and profiles of workers with normal or near-normal HRCT findings. The abnormal group had lower

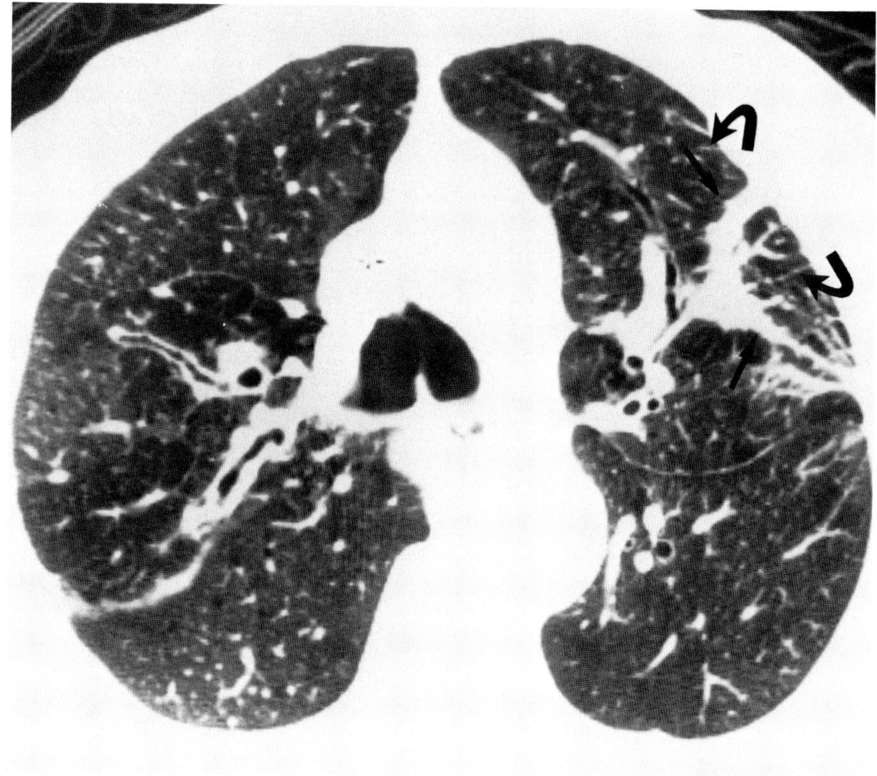

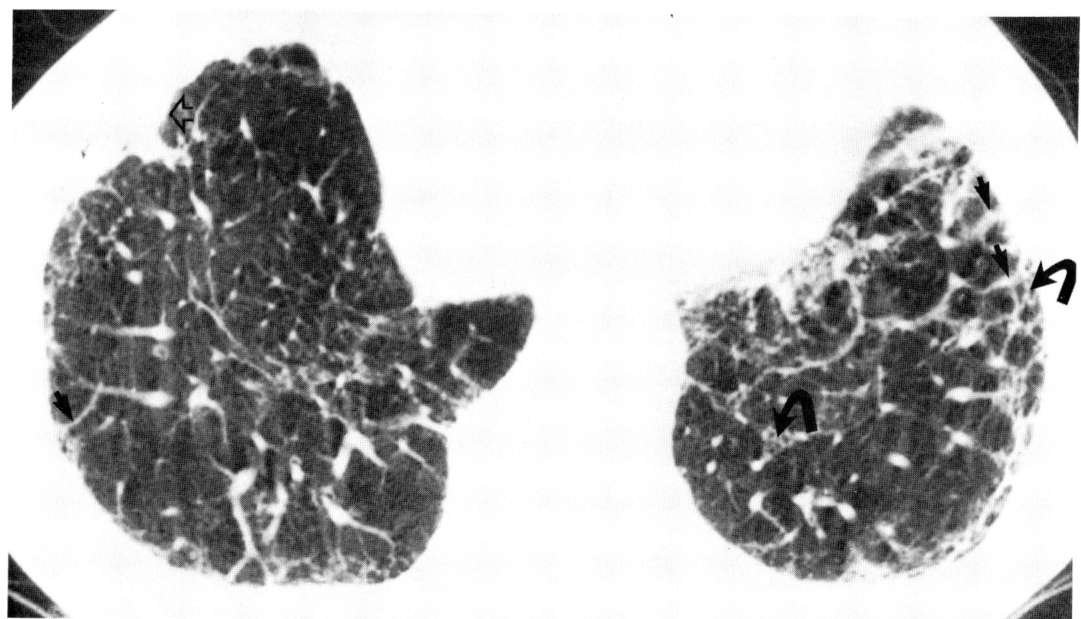

Figure 11–3   High-resolution CT (HRCT) in patient with asbestosis. *A*, HRCT at level of tracheal carina shows broad linear bands extending to the pleura (*straight arrows*) and thickening of interlobular septa (*curved arrows*) anterolaterally in the left lung. *B*, HRCT through the lung bases in another patient demonstrates thickened interlobular septa (*straight arrows*) and intralobular structures (*curved arrows*), giving a reticular pattern predominantly in the subpleural lung regions. A pleural plaque is present anterolaterally on the right side (*open arrow*).

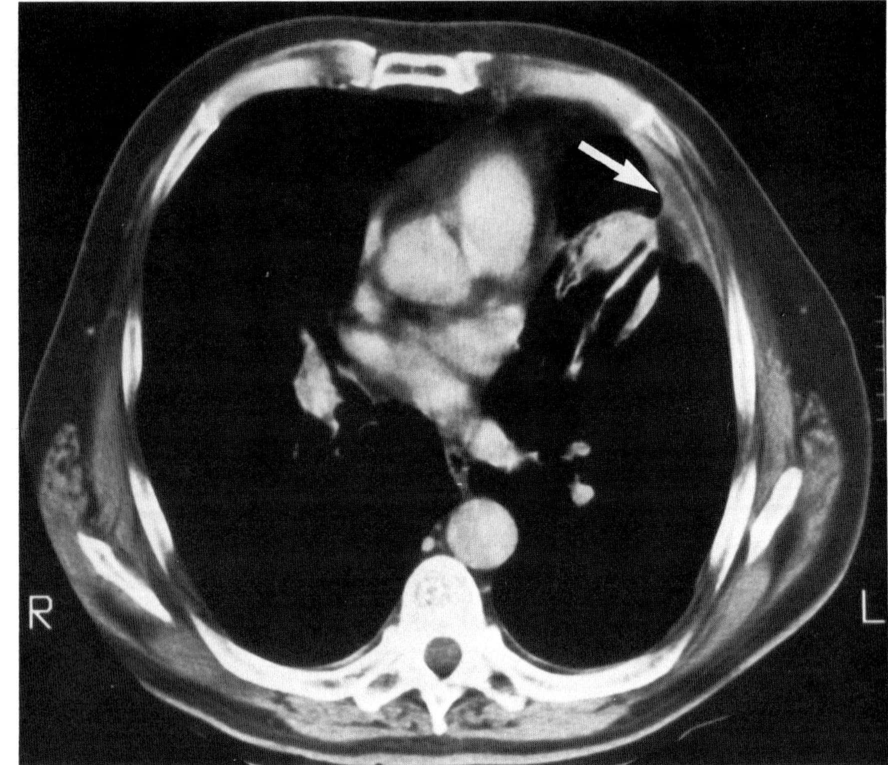

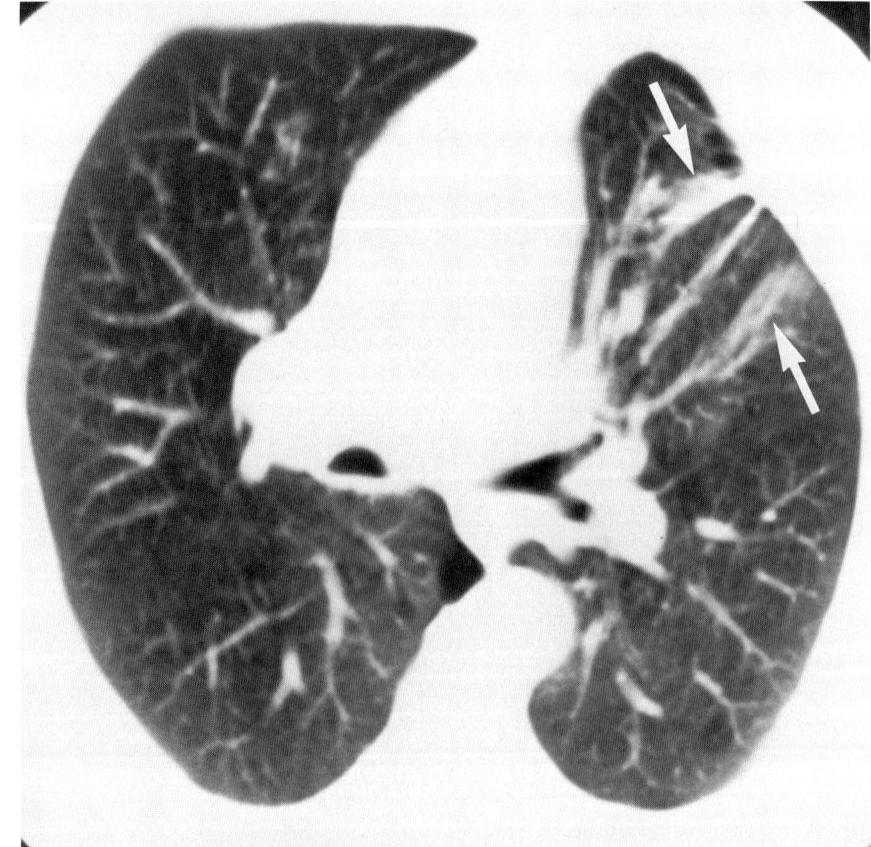

Figure 11–4 A 64-year-old man with a long history of exposure to asbestos. *A*, CT scans on soft tissue windows show mass-like lesion in the lingula extending to a localized area of pleural thickening (*arrow*). *B*, CT scans slightly above the level of the "mass," on lung windows, show pulmonary vessels curving toward the area of pleural thickening (*arrows*), a feature characteristic of rounded atelectasis.

mean values of vital capacity, as well as higher mean dyspnea scores.

HRCT findings characteristic of asbestosis include (1) linear densities of variable length within 1 cm and parallel to the pleura; (2) linear densities 2 to 5 cm in length running through and extending to a pleural surface (Fig. 11-3); (3) thickened interlobular septal lines and thickening of structures within the secondary pulmonary lobule; and (4) honeycombing (Aberle et al, 1988a and b). On CT, the parenchymal changes may be indistinguishable from those associated with UIP.

As pointed out by McLoud (1989), it is controversial whether the small irregular opacities seen in an exposed population, particularly if they are of low profusion or severity, really indicate asbestosis. Irregular opacities in exposed individuals may be related to age or smoking, although this relationship also is controversial. The lack of such pathologic proof raises questions regarding the specificity of the described HRCT findings. However, although the information available is limited, it seems unlikely that the HRCT findings of asbestosis could in any way be related to cigarette smoking (Blanc and Gamsu, 1988).

CT can also be helpful in the diagnosis of round atelectasis, which may mimic a lung tumor on the chest radiograph. Round atelectasis characteristically abuts an area of pleural thickening, and the associated loss of volume on CT can be clearly identified as the vessels and bronchi curve toward the area of pleural thickening (Fig. 11-4) (Carvalho and Carr, 1990). Round atelectasis may occur with any resolving benign pleural effusion, but the great majority are seen in patients exposed to asbestos (Hillerdal, 1989). The most common sites of round atelectasis are the lingula, right middle lobe, and lower lobes.

SILICOSIS

Silicosis is a chronic fibrosing pulmonary disease resulting from prolonged exposure to free silica. Silicon dioxide occurs naturally in three crystalline forms: quartz, cristobalite, and tridymite. Quartz is the most common and is found in many rocks. Siliceous minerals are ubiquitous and thus exposure may occur in many industries and occupations. Particles that range from 0.5 to 5 μm in diameter are most

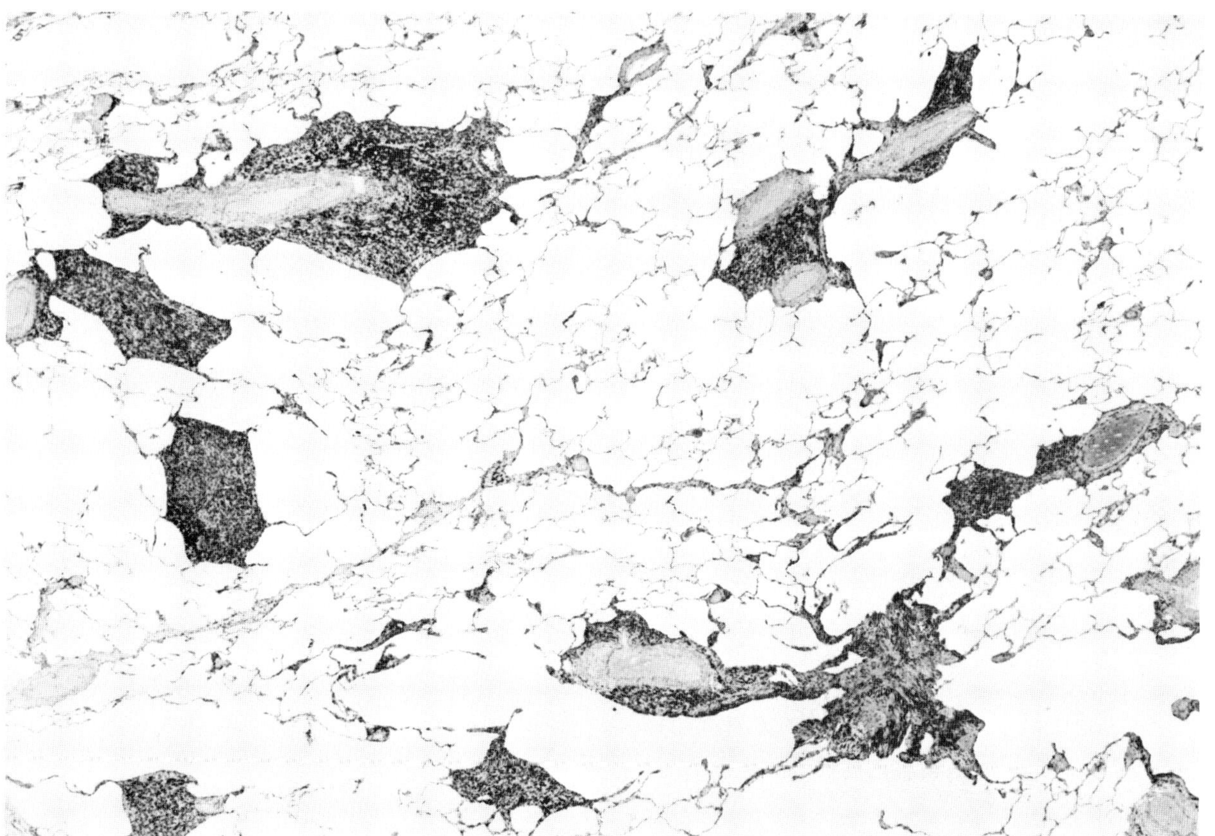

Figure 11-5 Early lesions of silicosis with nodules of dust (1 to 2 mm) beside distal respiratory bronchioles.

likely to cause disease. The concentration and size of the particles are factors that predict the likelihood of one's developing silicosis (Parkes, 1982).

Silicosis begins with phagocytosis of the inhaled particles by alveolar macrophages (Ziskind et al, 1976). The silica is initially contained in a phagolysosome. Owing to an unknown toxic effect, possibly to reactive silanol groups, the lysosomal membrane breaks down and releases acid hydrolases into the cell. This results in death of the macrophage and liberation of silica so the cycle is repeated. The nonlipid material released from the macrophage stimulates fibroblasts, and fibrogenesis is initiated. The fibrosis is not confined to the lung but is also present in the lymph nodes to which the macrophages migrate. An immunologic mechanism has been implicated because of increased serum levels of gamma globulin, the presence of autoantibodies in the serum, and the presence of gamma globulins in the silicotic lesions in many patients. Nevertheless, the immunologic component does not appear to participate in macrophage killing or fibrogenesis, and its role in the pathogenesis of silicosis is of secondary importance.

Three morphologic types of silicosis are described: simple nodular silicosis, conglomerate sili-cosis (progressive massive fibrosis), and acute silicosis. In the nodular form the lung parenchyma is characterized by gray-black, well-circumscribed nodules with a diameter of 0.5 to 5 mm. If tuberculosis is present, these nodules may be cavitated. The hilar lymph nodes are frequently enlarged and may be calcified, typically at the rim of the node ("egg-shell calcification"). Microscopically, the diagnostic lesion is the silicotic nodule, or islet, which usually is located beside a respiratory bronchiole (Fig. 11–5). The islet contains a central hyalinized whorled mass of acellular collagen, and peripheral to this are layers of macrophages and plasma cells (Fig. 11–6). Variable quantities of dust can be identified morphologically; if high in quartz and small in particle size, very little dust can produce severe fibrosis. It should be noted that silica is poorly refractile; the highly refractile, usually abundant, material often seen is due to associated silicates. Continuing exposure to dust increases the number and size of existing nodules, but even after exposure ceases, the nodules may continue to enlarge owing to the migration of macrophages peripherally and continued fibrogenesis.

Conglomerate silicosis (progressive massive fibrosis) has the same general features as nodular silicosis, but larger nodules are formed that coalesce to

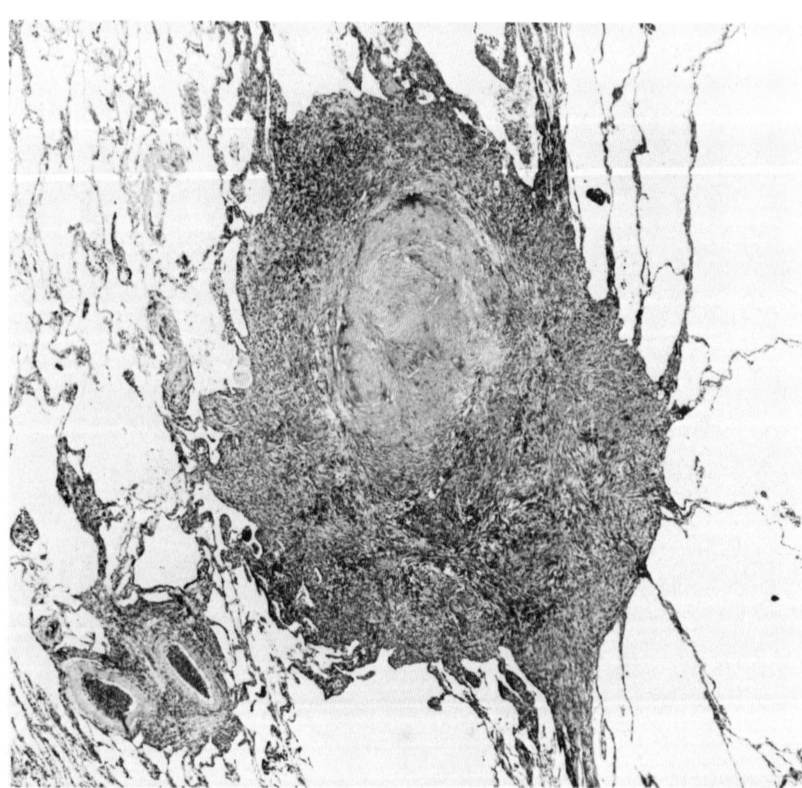

Figure 11–6 Silicotic islet.

form masses greater than 1 cm in diameter (Fig. 11-7). The conglomerate lesions tend to be located in the upper lobes, and the lung around these lesions often shows irregular emphysema with bullae. Pleural fibrosis and adhesions are more common and more severe in conglomerate silicosis than in nodular silicosis. Microscopically, the conglomerate masses consist of coalescent islets in a hyalinized fibrous background. Vascular thrombosis or obliterative endarteritis is common. Necrosis and cavitation may occur because of either ischemia or superimposed tuberculosis.

There appears to be synergism in the injurious effects of silicosis and tuberculosis. This synergism apparently is due, at least in part, to an inhibiting effect that silica produces on the ability of macrophages to contain the growth of mycobacteria. Conventional pulmonary tuberculosis is an important cause of morbidity in patients with silicosis, who also have a high incidence of tuberculosis (Snider, 1978), although this complication is becoming less frequent. Tuberculosis has been implicated in the progression of conglomerate silicosis even in the absence of cavitation, insofar as mycobacterial infection is known to increase, perpetuate, and make cellular reactions to dust particles progressive. Both *Mycobacterium tuberculosis* and nontuberculous mycobacteria have this untoward synergism with silicosis. Tuberculosis in the setting of silicosis may have unusual radiologic features, and biopsy or thoracotomy may

be required to rule out a lung neoplasm (Fig. 11-8).

Acute silicosis is a rare but rapidly developing lesion that results from an overwhelming exposure to free silica. The particles involved are small, usually from 1 to 2 μm in diameter, and have a high quartz concentration. These conditions are found particularly during sandblasting, which is the usual method of exposure leading to acute silicosis. Nodules are sparse, and instead the lungs have a gray consolidated appearance with diffusely increased interstitial markings. Microscopically, alveoli are filled by an eosinophilic foamy exudate that contains many macrophages. There is prominent type-II cell hyperplasia with interstitial fibrosis. The histologic features may resemble those of alveolar proteinosis or desquamative interstitial pneumonia (see Chapter 7). The exact mechanism of the production of the acute lesion is not known.

Clinically, the main symptoms of simple nodular silicosis develop late. Cough is accompanied by progressive shortness of breath. Infections with mycobacteria or fungi may result in weight loss and other constitutional symptoms and signs. Nodular silicosis runs a protracted course and is usually only associated with minor symptoms and pulmonary function abnormalities. Conglomerate silicosis progresses over a period of years and is associated with major functional abnormalities. Pulmonary function tests are not specific and may be normal early in the disease, or may show either an obstructive or a

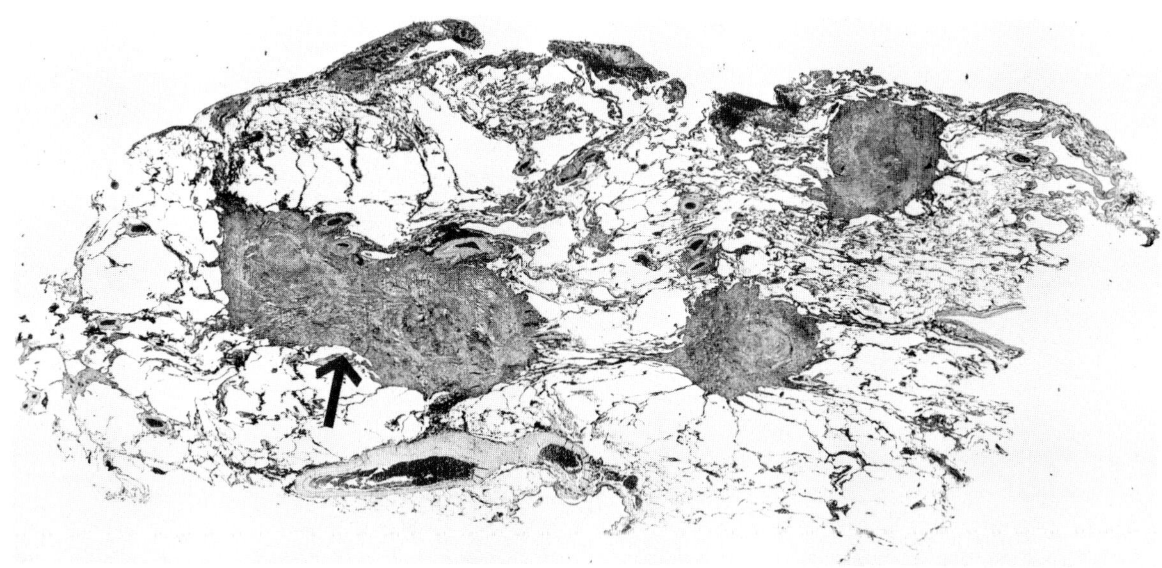

Figure 11-7   Coalescence of islets (*arrow*) to form a lesion over 1 cm in size. Note irregular emphysema at the edge of nodules.

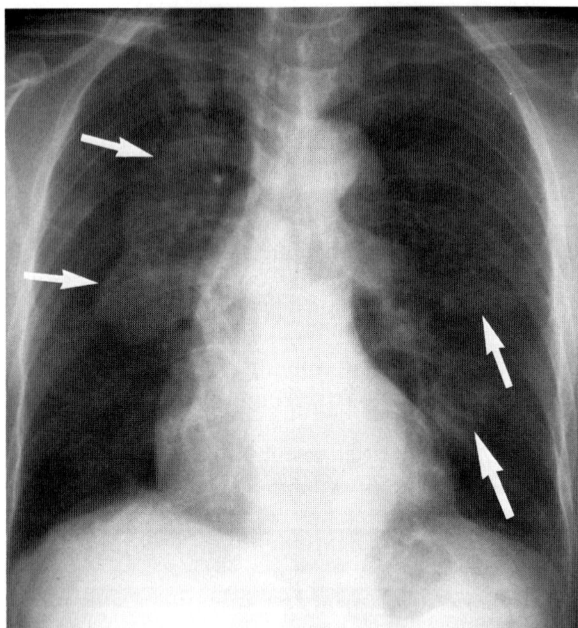

Figure 11–8   A 75-year-old man presented with fever and lung masses. Chest radiograph shows conglomerate lobulated mass in right hilar region (*arrows*) and two ill-defined nodules in left lung (*arrows*). The patient also had subcarinal lymphadenopathy. On open lung biopsy of right upper lobe, he was found to have silicotuberculosis.

restrictive defect, or both. Diffusing capacity is decreased, and exercise-induced hypoxia can be observed late in the course. Patients with acute silicosis may develop symptoms within 6 months after exposure, followed by progressive deterioration and intractable hypoxia, and may have a severe restrictive defect.

The characteristic radiologic pattern of silicosis consists of well-circumscribed nodules usually measuring 2 to 5 mm in diameter and involving mainly the upper lung zones. Confluence of nodules may result in large opacities of conglomerate silicosis. These conglomerate masses tend to develop in the midportion or periphery of the upper lung zones and migrate toward the hila, leaving overinflated emphysematous spaces between the conglomerate mass and the pleura (Pendergrass, 1958).

Hilar lymphadenopathy is present in many patients. The nodes are often calcified. A characteristic peripheral "egg-shell" calcification is seen in approximately 5 percent of cases and is virtually pathognomonic of silicosis.

On CT, as on the radiograph, the most characteristic feature is the presence of nodules (Bergin et al, 1986). In patients with mild silicosis, these nodules may be seen only in the upper lobes. They vary in size but usually measure 2 to 5 mm in diameter. A posterior predominance of nodules is often seen on CT (Fig. 11–9). More severe silicosis is characterized on CT by an increase in the number and size of nodules. CT is not superior to the standard chest radiograph for early detection of small opacities in workers exposed to silica. Indeed, mild disease is easier to detect on the radiograph than on CT (Begin et al, 1987). However, CT provides significant additional information on the stage of the disease, since it detects coalescence of nodules that may not be apparent on the radiograph. Early recognition of coalescence of silicotic lesions is important because such coalescence is associated with the appearance of respiratory symptoms, the deterioration of lung function, and the progression of nodular to conglomerate silicosis.

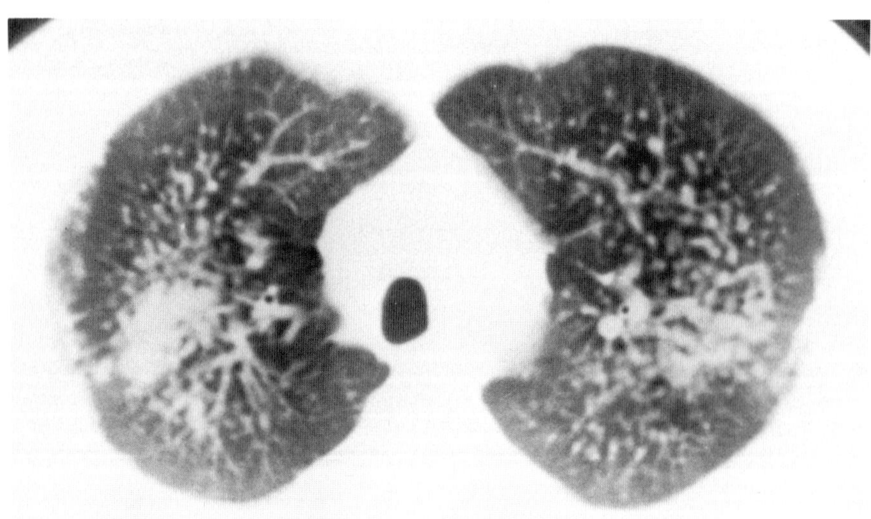

Figure 11–9   Conventional 10-mm collimation CT in a patient with silicosis demonstrates nodules situated mainly in the posterior one-half of the lungs. Early coalescence of nodules is present on the right side.

Kinsella and colleagues (1990) reviewed pulmonary function tests and chest CT scans in 30 subjects with silicosis. Eighteen of them were either current smokers or former smokers, and 12 were nonsmokers. The extent of emphysema was the strongest independent predictor of pulmonary function impairment; extent of silicosis was also an independent predictor, albeit a weaker one. In those subjects who did not have evidence of progressive massive fibrosis, smokers had worse emphysema than did nonsmokers. In progressive massive fibrosis, the severity of emphysema in smokers and nonsmokers was not statistically different. These data indicate that silicosis in the absence of progressive massive fibrosis does not cause significant emphysema and that it is primarily the degree of emphysema rather than silicotic nodules that determines the level of pulmonary dysfunction in these patients.

BERYLLIOSIS

Beryllium aluminum silicate was first recognized as an occupational hazard in fluorescent-lamp workers. Its use in this industry was discontinued, but because of its structural characteristics, beryllium is used in metallic, alloy, and oxide forms in numerous industries including the fields of nuclear weapons and nuclear energy (Kriebel et al, 1988).

Berylliosis may be an acute or a chronic disease. The acute variety is thought to be due to a direct cytotoxic effect analogous to other direct irritants and is characterized by edema or diffuse alveolar damage. The chronic form, which is apparently at least partly related to cell-mediated immunity, is a multiorgan disease in which the lung is most severely involved. The histologic appearance is that of noncaseating granulomatous inflammation indistinguishable from sarcoidosis. Radiologically, chronic berylliosis is also similar to sarcoidosis insofar as the usual findings are diffuse nodular or nodular and linear infiltrates. Hilar adenopathy is said to be present in 40 percent of cases (Kriebel et al, 1988). The criteria for diagnosis of chronic berylliosis requires either historical evidence of significant exposure to beryllium or the presence of beryllium in tissue as assessed by mineral analysis.

OTHER DUSTS

A variety of other dusts may be encountered in the lung; some of these dusts are fibrogenic, others are not (Table 11-1). These disorders are reviewed in

TABLE 11-1

LESS COMMON PNEUMOCONIOSES

DUST	INDUSTRY	PRESENCE OF FIBROSIS	CHARACTERISTIC FEATURES
Aluminum	Metal refining	Idiosyncratic, interstitial fibrosis	Occasional granulomata, black interstitial dust
Antimony	Mining alloy	No	Dust-bearing macrophages
Coal (anthracosis)	Coal workers	No	Black dust in peribronchial aggregates
Barium (baritosis)	Miners, grinders, aspiration	Minimal	Macrophages containing granules of dust
Fiberglass	Manufacturing	No	Particle as negative space
Iron (siderosis)	Welders' oxyacetylene, silver finishers	No	Iron dusts
Magnesium silicate (talcosis)	Talc inhalation	Lower-lobe fibrosis, granulomas	Doubly refractive particles, often needle-shaped
Tin dioxide (stannosis)	Tin smelting, mining, refining	No	Macrophage aggregates in small nodules
Titanium	Dye	No	Particles within macrophages

detail elsewhere (Heppleston, 1988) and only the two more common fibrogenic dusts will be specifically mentioned here.

Aluminosis

Aluminum has been associated with diffuse interstitial fibrosis with black dust and occasional giant cells seen histologically. This complication is quite uncommon and appears to be associated with heavy exposure to fine-flake aluminum as used in the explosives industry. Several other unusual patterns of lung disease associated with aluminum exposure have been described, including foreign body granulomatosis (Chen et al, 1978), sarcoid-like granulomatosis (deVuyst et al, 1987), alveolar proteinosis (Miller et al, 1984), and desquamative interstitial pneumonia (Herbert et al, 1982).

Pulmonary Talcosis

Talc inhalation has been associated with occupationally acquired fibrosing lung disease. This fibrogenic potential of talc is apparently independent of fibrous asbestos or silica that commonly contaminates the material. The severity of talcosis is dose related so that disabling disease generally requires many years of occupational exposure to develop (Vallyathan and Craighead, 1981). The early lesions consist of fibrohistiocytic nodules in a peribronchiolar or perivascular location, containing many strongly birefringent talc particles. With more prolonged exposure, diffuse subpleural fibrosis develops, possibly owing to confluence of nodules. The diffuse form also contains multinucleated giant cells, with birefringent crystals. The type of talcosis related to intravenous drug abuse, described in Chapter 13, is quite different from occupational talcosis.

REFERENCES

Aberle DR, Gamsu G, Ray CS, Feuerstein IM. Asbestos-related pleural and parenchymal fibrosis: detection with high-resolution CT. Radiology 1988a; 166:729–734.

Aberle DR, Gamsu G, Ray CS. High-resolution CT of benign asbestos-related diseases: clinical and radiographic correlation. AJR 1988b; 151:883–891.

American Thoracic Society. Statement on diagnosis of nonmalignant diseases related to asbestos. Am Rev Respir Dis 1986; 134:363–368.

Ashcroft T, Heppleston AG. The optical and electron microscopic determination of pulmonary asbestos fibre concentration and its relations to the human pathological reaction. J Clin Pathol 1973; 26:224–234.

Becklake M. Asbestos-related diseases of the lung and other organs: their epidemiology and implications for clinical practice. Am Rev Respir Dis 1976; 114:187–227.

Begin R, Bergeron D, Samson L, et al. CT assessment of silicosis in exposed workers. AJR 1987; 148:509–514.

Begin R, Boctor M, Bergeron D, et al. Radiographic assessment of pleuropulmonary disease in asbestos workers: posteroanterior, four view films, and computed tomograms of the thorax. Br J Ind Med 1984; 41:373–383.

Bergin CJ, Müller NL, Vedal S, Chan-Yeung M. CT in silicosis: correlation with plain films and pulmonary function tests. AJR 1986; 146:477–483.

Blanc PD, Gamsu G. The effect of cigarette smoking on the detection of small radiographic opacities in inorganic dust disease. J Thorac Imag 1988; 3:51–56.

Carvalho PM, Carr DH. Computed tomography of folded lung. Clin Radiol 1990; 41:86–91.

Chen W, Monnat RJ Jr, Chen M, Mottet NK. Aluminum-induced pulmonary granulomatosis. Hum Pathol 1978; 9:705–711.

Churg A. Fiber counting and analysis in the diagnosis of asbestos-related disease. Hum Pathol 1982; 13:381–392.

Churg A, Green FHY, eds. Pathology of occupational lung disease. New York: Igaku-Shoin, 1988.

Churg A, Wright JL. Small airways disease and mineral dust exposure. Pathol Annu 1983; 18:233–251.

Crouch A, Churg A. Ferruginous bodies and the histologic evaluation of dust exposure. Am J Surg Pathol 1984; 8:109–116.

deVuyst P, Dumortier P, Schandene L, et al. Sarcoid-like lung granulomatosis induced by aluminum dusts. Am Rev Respir Dis 1987; 135:493–497.

Friedman AC, Fiel SB, Fisher MS, et al. Asbestos-related pleural disease and asbestosis: a comparison of CT and chest radiography. AJR 1988; 150:269–275.

Gaensler EA. Pathological, physiological and radiological correlations in the pneumoconioses. Ann NY Acad Sci 1972; 200:574.

Gaensler EA, Kaplan AI. Asbestos pleural effusion. Ann Intern Med 1971; 74:178.

Gough J. Differential diagnosis in the pathology of asbestosis. Ann NY Acad Sci 1965; 132:368.

Heppleston AG. Environmental lung disease (chapter 23). In: Thurlbeck WM, ed. Pathology of the Lung. New York: Thieme International, 1988.

Herbert A, Sterling G, Abraham J, Corrin B. Desquamative interstitial pneumonia in an aluminum welder. Hum Pathol 1982; 13:694–699.

Hillerdal G. Rounded atelectasis: clinical experience with 74 patients. Chest 1989; 95:836–841.

Katz D, Kreel L. Computed tomography in pulmonary asbestosis. Clin Radiol 1979; 30:207–213.

Kinsella N, Müller NL, Vedal S, et al. Emphysema in silicosis: a comparison of smokers with nonsmokers using pulmonary function testing and computed tomography. Am Rev Respir Dis 1990; 141:1497–1500.

Kipen HM, Lilis R, Suzuki Y, et al. Pulmonary fibrosis in asbestos insulation workers with lung cancer: a radiological and histopathological evaluation. Br J Ind Med 1987; 44:96-100.

Kriebel D, Brain JD, Sprince NL, Kazemi H. The pulmonary toxicity of beryllium. Am Rev Respir Dis 1988; 137:464-473.

Kuhn C III, Kuo TT. Cytoplasmic hyaline in asbestosis: a reaction of injured alveolar epithelium. Arch Pathol Lab Med 1973; 95:190-194.

McLoud TC. Critical review. Invest Radiol 1989; 24:636-637.

Miller RR, Churg AM, Hutcheon M, Lam S. Pulmonary alveolar proteinosis and aluminum dust exposure. Am Rev Respir Dis 1984; 130:312-315.

Morgan WKC, Seaton A. Occupational lung diseases. 2nd ed. Philadelphia: WB Saunders, 1984.

Mossman BT, Gee JB. Asbestos-related diseases. N Engl J Med 1989; 320:1721-1730.

Parkes WR. Occupational lung disorders. 2nd ed. London: Butterworth, 1982.

Pendergrass EP. Caldwell Lecture 1957. Silicosis and a few of the other pneumonoconioses: observations of certain aspects of the problem, with emphasis on the role of the radiologist. AJR 1958; 80:1-41.

Robinson BW, Musk AW. Benign asbestos pleural effusion: diagnosis and course. Thorax 1981; 36:896-900.

Snider DE. The relationship between tuberculosis and silicosis. Am Rev Respir Dis 1978; 118:455-460.

Staples CA, Gamsu G, Ray CS, Webb WR. High resolution computed tomography and lung function in asbestos-exposed workers with normal chest radiographs. Am Rev Respir Dis 1989; 139:1502-1508.

Vallyathan NV, Craighead JE. Pulmonary pathology in workers exposed to nonasbestiform talc. Hum Pathol 1981; 12:28-35.

Warnock WL, Press M, Churg A. Further observations on cytoplasmic hyaline in the lung. Hum Pathol 1980; 11:59-65.

Weill H. Diagnosis of asbestos-related disease. Chest 1987; 91:802-803.

Wright JL, Churg A. Morphology of small-airway lesions in patients with asbestos exposure. Hum Pathol 1984; 15:68-74.

Ziskind M, Jones RN, Weill H. Silicosis. Am Rev Respir Dis 1976; 113:643-665.

CHAPTER 12

CHRONIC AIRFLOW OBSTRUCTION

THE CONCEPT OF FLOW OBSTRUCTION

Lung biopsy is rarely indicated in patients with chronic airflow obstruction and thus is seldom done. The exception is in patients with unexplained airflow obstruction, i.e., not associated with smoking, chronic bronchitis and emphysema. It may also be done when an incorrect clinical diagnosis of chronic infiltrative disease has been made (Macklem et al, 1971; Myers et al, 1987).

There are fairly well-defined clinical and pathologic criteria for the diagnosis of chronic bronchitis, asthma, and emphysema, and the volume of information is large (Thurlbeck, 1976). The content of this section will therefore be limited to (1) a brief consideration of the concept of chronic airflow obstruction (since this is common knowledge expected of every physician), (2) an abbreviated survey of the pathology of emphysema, and (3) a consideration of those few medical conditions in which biopsies may be performed. Bronchiolitis obliterans with organizing pneumonia (BOOP), perhaps more properly termed cryptogenic organizing pneumonia (COP), is dealt with in Chapter 7, as it is in reality an intra-alveolar filling process with primarily a restrictive functional defect.

Chronic obstructive lung disease, better referred to as chronic airflow obstruction (CAO) or chronic airflow limitation, is a syndrome with many different causes. It is recognized clinically by abnormalities of tests of expiratory flow, and the patient's dysfunction is determined by the degree to which flow is diminished. Flow is determined by two factors: the force that is applied to the airways and the resistance to flow within the lungs. The former is determined by the elastic recoil of the lung. Emphysema is thought to be associated with loss of elastic recoil so that flow limitation may occur in emphysematous lungs even if the airways are normal. Increased resistance to flow may be caused by a wide variety of lesions in the airways including intraluminal mucus, narrowing of the lumen of airways, and inflammation of the airways.

An important concept is that the peripheral airways, defined as conducting (i.e., nonalveolated) airways less than 2 mm in internal diameter, contribute only about 20 percent of the total resistance to flow in the respiratory system (Hogg et al, 1968). Therefore, significant obstruction can occur in the peripheral airways without markedly increasing airflow resistance. For example, if every other peripheral airway was destroyed, then peripheral airway resistance would double. However, this would only increase *total* airway resistance by 20 percent, a change that is difficult to detect. Thus, tests of expiratory

function thought to reflect mainly total airway resistance, such as the FEV_1, might be normal. The low proportion that peripheral airways contribute to total airway resistance has been challenged (Kappos et al, 1981; Van Brabandt et al, 1983). Further, the FEV_1 has been described as abnormal in the presence of mild bronchiolar abnormalities (Berend et al, 1979), refuting the idea that this lung function test is insensitive. However, lesions in the peripheral airways are the usual cause of obstruction in patients with significant airflow obstruction. As indicated, biopsy specimens in this setting are rarely obtained, but the problem of chronic airflow obstruction does arise from time to time. Should it be necessary, for whatever reason, to quantitate peripheral airway lesions (for example, in lung resection specimens in this setting), the details of a grading system have been published (Wright et al, 1985), and a panel of grading pictures can be obtained from Dr. J. C. Hogg (Pulmonary Research Laboratory, St. Paul's Hospital, Burrard Street, Vancouver, B.C., V6Z 1Y5, Canada).

EMPHYSEMA

The definition of emphysema is more than 25 years old. Both the World Health Organization (1963) and the American Thoracic Society (1962) adopted essentially the same definition: "Emphysema defines a condition of the lung characterized by abnormal, permanent enlargement of airspaces distal to the terminal bronchiole, accompanied by destruction of their walls." This definition differed from the original one of a Ciba Foundation Symposium (1959), which included enlargement of the acinus (the airspaces distal to the terminal bronchiole) without destruction. The World Health Organization and American Thoracic Society committees did not define "destruction," and a National Institutes of Health Committee met to decide what was meant by emphysema and to review previous definitions (Snider et al, 1985).

This meeting resulted in a three-step decision. First, the condition of respiratory airspace enlargement was recognized: "Respiratory airspace enlargement is defined as an increase in airspace size as compared with the airspace (size) of normal lungs. The term applies to airspace enlargement distal to the terminal bronchiole, whether occurring with or without fibrosis or destruction."

Three major categories of airspace enlargement were recognized (Table 12-1). The first was simple airspace enlargement, of which there were two categories: congenital and acquired. The best example of the congenital form is Down's syndrome, which beyond the first few years of life is characterized by alveoli and alveolar ducts that are too large and too few (Cooney and Thurlbeck, 1982; Cooney et al, 1988). A more important condition is congenital lobar emphysema, which is described further below. The category of airspace enlargement with fibrosis includes increased airspace size in association with infiltrative lung disease. A typical example of acquired simple airspace enlargement would be the compensatory increase in size consequent upon atelectasis or pneumonectomy.

The second step was a redefinition of emphysema: "Emphysema is a condition of the lung characterized by abnormal, permanent enlargement of airspaces distal to the terminal bronchiole accompanied by the destruction of their walls, and without obvious fibrosis." This definition implied that emphysema is not accompanied by fibrosis, a notion that has not been adequately investigated. It also implies that postinflammatory fibrosis is not involved in the pathogenesis of emphysema, a view that has been challenged recently (Snider et al, 1988). Finally, irregular or paracicatricial emphysema (Thurlbeck, 1976) was excluded from the definition, which has bearing on the lung in idiopathic spontaneous pneumothorax, as discussed further below.

The third step was the definition of destruction: "Destruction in emphysema is defined as nonuniformity of the pattern of respiratory airspace enlargement so that the orderly appearance of the acinus and its components is disturbed and may be lost." This did little but formalize the subjective assessment of emphysema—i.e., the involved portion of the lung somehow looks different from adjacent normal lung or from normal lungs in other patients.

Centriacinar Emphysema

In centriacinar emphysema the proximal part of the acinus, the respiratory bronchiole, is selectively or dominantly enlarged and destroyed. The term "proximal acinar emphysema" is an alternative term that is more precise. Two forms of centriacinar emphysema are recognized.

Centrilobular Emphysema

Centrilobular emphysema (CLE) is typically associated with cigarette smoking and chronic bronchitis. The lesion is more common and more severe in the upper zones of the lung. It varies in severity from lobule to lobule and within the same lobule (Fig. 12–1). Because of its association with cigarette smoking it is usually present in lungs or lobes resected for lung cancer. Occasionally, it may be important to quantitate the emphysema. The panel grading method (Thurlbeck et al, 1970) has been widely used for this purpose and even on slices of

TABLE 12–1

RESPIRATORY AIRSPACE ENLARGEMENT

Simple airspace enlargement
   Congenital
   Acquired

Emphysema
   Centriacinar emphysema
   Panacinar emphysema
   Distal acinar emphysema

Airspace enlargement with fibrosis

fixed distended lungs (Wright et al, 1986) It was, however, devised for rapid estimation of emphysema in paper-mounted whole-lung sections for epidemiologic purposes.

Dust Pneumoconiosis

Accumulation of nonfibrogenic, or only mildly fibrogenic, dust or atmospheric soot has been thought to result in dilatation of the respiratory bronchioles. The National Institute of Health definition of emphysema would include these lesions under the heading of emphysema, and the best studied example is due to inhalation of coal, so-called simple pneumoconiosis of coal workers or focal emphysema (Heppleston, 1955).

Panacinar Emphysema

In panacinar emphysema, the acinus is more or less uniformly enlarged (Fig. 12–2) and destroyed. It occurs in the following different clinical situations (Table 12–2) (Thurlbeck, 1976).

Familial Emphysema Associated with Alpha-1-Antitrypsin (Proteinase Inhibitor) Deficiency

Alpha-1-globulin has long been known to be associated with an ability to inactivate trypsin. Subsequent studies showed that the amount and type of alpha-1-antitrypsin are determined by a pair of codominant alleles and that alpha-1-antitrypsin is a highly effective antielastase. This is of significance because elastolysis is the primary lesion in experimental, and probably human, emphysema (Janoff, 1985). Some 28 alleles have been found and are designated by upper-case letters. In addition a null allele is recognized, described as 0. The phenotype is designated as a superscript following "Pi" (proteinase inhibitor). The common normal allele is M, and this

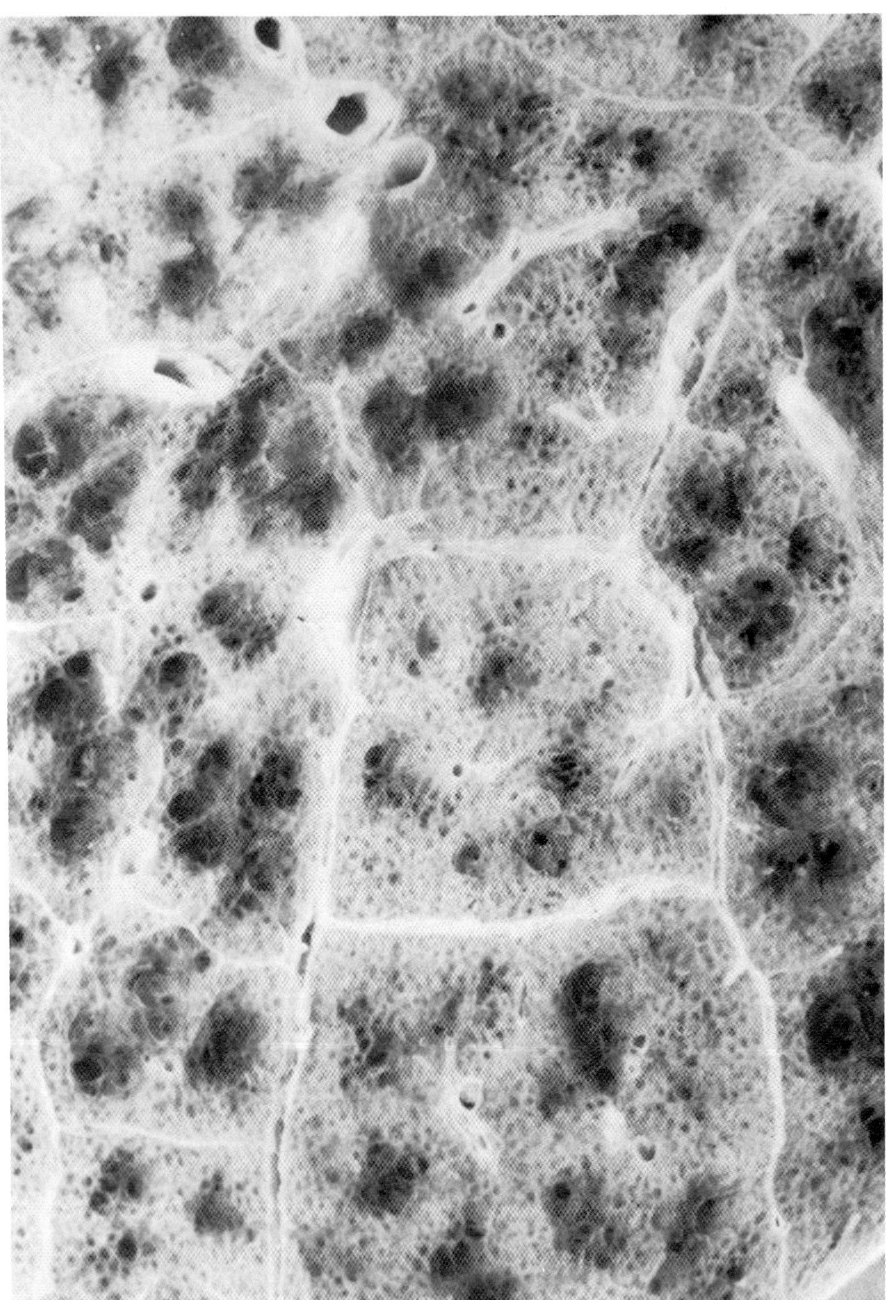

Figure 12–1 Centrilobular emphysema. Note the obvious lesions near the center of the lobules. The emphysematous spaces vary quite considerably in size, and there are variations within the lobules. (Reproduced with permission from Thurlbeck WM. Chronic airflow obstruction in lung disease. Philadelphia: WB Saunders, 1976).

is designated Pi^{MM} if both alleles can be identified. However, this often cannot be done and generally the designation is Pi^{M}. The most significant allele associated with proteinase insufficiency is Z. The phenotype, depending on the circumstances, may be designated as Pi^{Z} or Pi^{ZZ}. Much attention has been paid to Pi^{MZ} since this is relatively frequent, affecting approximately 3 percent of the North American white population. (Pi^{ZZ} is found in fewer than 1 in 1,000 whites and is virtually unknown in blacks and Asians.) The question has arisen of whether or not emphysema is increased in severity in patients with Pi^{MZ}, but the evidence is now that it is not (Idell and Cohen, 1983). Pi^{ZZ} is associated with a greatly increased frequency of emphysema and is the most common form of emphysema in patients under the

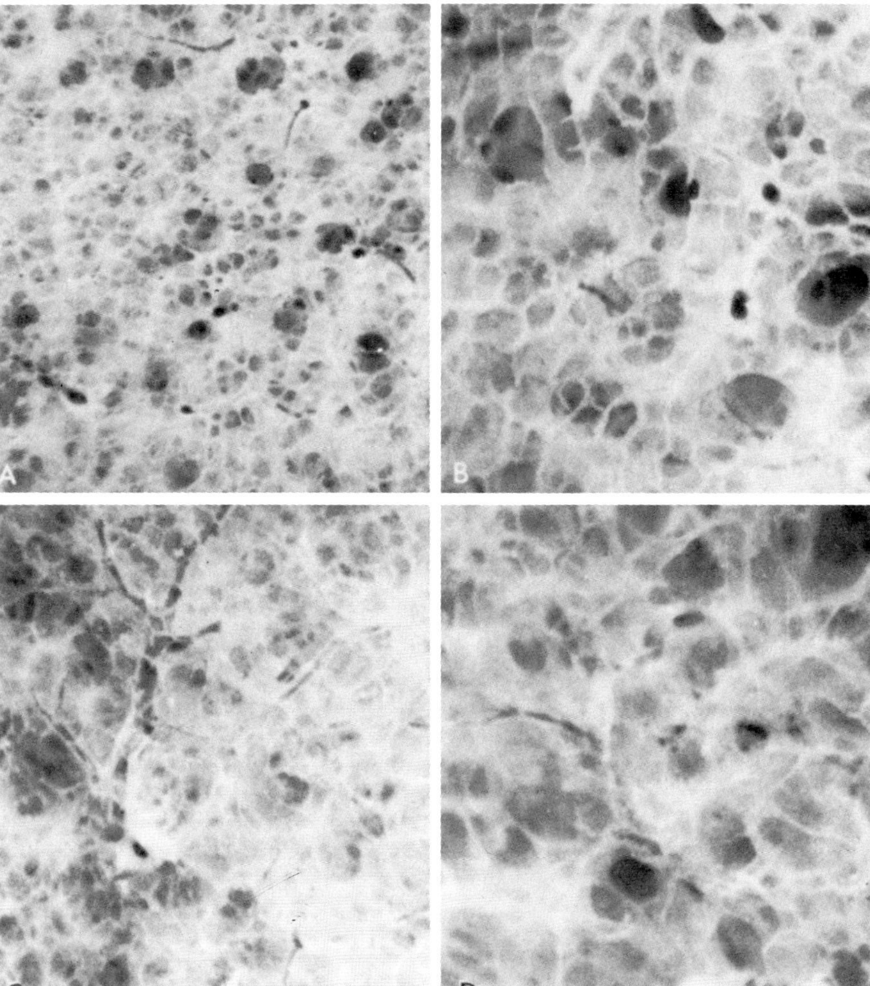

Figure 12–2   Panacinar emphysema (*C, D*) is compared with normal lung (*A, B*) at magnifications of 13× (*A, C*) and 26× (*B, D*). Note the diffuse loss of parenchyma approximately uniform through the acinus. (*A* and *B* from Thurlbeck WM. Pulmonary emphysema. Am J Med Sci 1963; 246:110–131. *C* and *D* from Thurlbeck WM. Chronic airflow obstruction in lung disease. Philadelphia: WB Saunders, 1976).

age of 40. Panacinar emphysema is the type of emphysema that occurs and it is characteristically symmetric and worst in the lower zones of the lungs.

Emphysema in Young Subjects

Familial emphysema may occur with normal Pi levels. This is a poorly investigated subject, but emphysema similar in type to Pi^Z has been described in young people (Martelli et al, 1974); however, the epidemiologic data were insufficient to investigate its familial properties.

Lower Zonal Panacinar Emphysema Associated with Upper Zonal CLE

Perhaps the most classic lesion encountered in patients with clinically evident emphysema and

chronic airflow obstruction is a combination of CLE in the upper zones of the lungs and panacinar emphysema in the lower zones. The association with cigarette smoking and chronic productive cough is

---

TABLE 12–2

PANACINAR (PANLOBULAR) EMPHYSEMA

Alpha-1-antitrypsin deficiency

Emphysema in young adults

In association with centrilobular emphysema and chronic airflow obstruction

Age associated

Associated with bronchial and bronchiolar obstruction

---

the same as for CLE. It is uncertain whether the lower zonal lesions represent progression of CLE. We have taken the pragmatic approach that since the emphysema is panacinar in type, it should be so designated.

Panacinar Emphysema Associated with Age

Panacinar emphysema may be noted in some 10 to 20 percent of autopsied patients over 70 years of age. It is then most commonly found in the lower zone of the lungs, usually in subpleural regions. It is not particularly associated with cigarette smoking and is asymptomatic (Thurlbeck, 1976).

Panacinar Emphysema Associated with Bronchial and Bronchiolar Obliteration

Why emphysema should occur distal to bronchial and bronchiolar obliteration is unclear. The process may be focal, but of interest is the occasional occurrence of widespread bronchial and bronchiolar obliteration, mainly on one side. This leads to unilateral pulmonary transradiancy (emphysema) or the Swyer-James (or MacLeod) syndrome (Thurlbeck, 1976). Clinically, patients have a unilateral hyperlucent lung as seen radiologically (Fig. 12–3). There is diminished blood flow to the affected side, and the opposite lung often appears to have increased

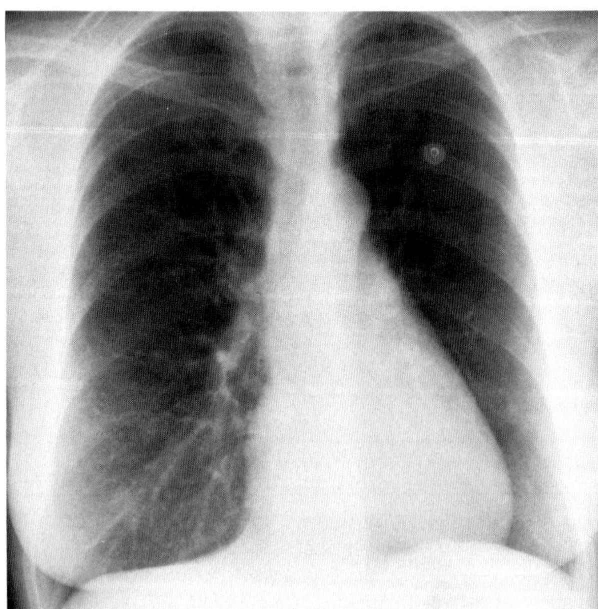

Figure 12–3   A 45-year-old woman with Swyer-James syndrome. The chest radiograph shows characteristic hyperlucency of the left lung with decreased vascularity and a small hilum. The lung volume is slightly decreased.

markings because of increased blood flow. The expiratory radiograph is diagnostic: the affected lung traps air on expiration and thus appears much larger than the contralateral lung, and the mediastinum shifts to the unaffected side. Surgery is not usually indicated, but when done such emphysema as is present is panacinar in type. The airways are dilated, and the syndrome has also been described as "bronchiectasis without atelectasis." It should be noted that the airflow obstruction is due not to emphysema, but to airway obliteration. The former is a consequence of the latter.

Marti-Bonmati and colleagues (1989) described the CT findings in nine patients with Swyer-James syndrome. On computed tomography (CT), the affected lung demonstrated diminished attenuation in eight patients, with one lung being very small but with normal attenuation. On full inspiration, lung volume was smaller in the affected side in six patients and normal in three. One patient showed normal lung density on chest radiographs but decreased density on CT. All nine patients had findings of bronchiectasis on CT scans.

Congenital Lobar Emphysema

This condition is most commonly found in the neonatal period but infrequently can present later in childhood. It is categorized clinically by respiratory embarrassment and radiologically by gross overinflation of a lobe. The mediastinum is shifted to the opposite side, and the remaining lung becomes compressed. Frequently there is an associated cardiac anomaly. The majority of cases are due to intrinsic or extrinsic bronchial compression such as by adjacent vessels or flap valves within the bronchi or defects in bronchial cartilage (Case Records, 1990). It has been suggested that some cases may be nonobstructive and due to "polyalveolar lobe" (Hislop and Reid, 1970). These cases are not different clinically from other forms of congenital emphysema.

Distal Acinar Emphysema

In distal acinar emphysema the distal or peripheral part of the acinus—the alveolar ducts and alveolar sacs—is selectively involved. Two associations have been described (Edge et al, 1966): idiopathic spontaneous pneumothorax of young adults and the curious syndrome of "bullous disease of the lung" (Laurenzi et al, 1962). In this syndrome, which was described in patients of about 30 years of age, multiple bullae were seen radiologically. Only minimal airflow obstruction was present except when there was superimposed infection. One of the cases described by Edge and coworkers (1966) with widespread distal acinar emphysema corresponded closely to this description.

Bullae

A bulla was defined as an emphysematous space greater than 1 cm in diameter in the inflated state (Ciba Symposium, 1959). Whereas bullae are fairly frequently seen radiologically, pathologically they seldom are true bullae in that they contain remnants of lung tissue. Those that occur in the upper zones of the lung are usually centilobular emphysematous spaces, and those in the lower zone of the lung represent greatly attenuated lung tissue in panacinar emphysema, bordered by lobular septa (Thurlbeck and Simon, 1978).

Large bullae may occasionally be resected, allowing normal but compressed lung to re-expand. The usual classification is that of Reid (1967).

Type-I Bullae: These have a narrow neck; the walls and deep surfaces are mainly pleura and connective tissue; and the bullae contain only air or a few flimsy strands of lung. Type-I bullae are most commonly seen near the apex of the lung.

Type-II Bullae: These have a broad base and are superficial. The walls are formed by pleura, and the deep surface is a region of emphysematous lung. The bullae usually contain emphysematous lung and they are located superficially; blood vessels can usually be seen crossing them. Type-II bullae may occur anywhere in the lung.

Type-III Bullae: These are similar to type-II bullae but lie within the lung substance. As such, the walls are formed by emphysematous lung tissue and contain emphysematous lung. Type-III bullae may also be found in any part of the lung.

Standard chest radiography and pulmonary function tests have been shown to be poorly sensitive in the diagnosis of emphysema (Thurlbeck and Simon, 1978), and attention has turned to the possible role of CT (Foster et al, 1986; Bergin et al, 1986; Miller et al, 1989). Recent technical improvements in CT of the chest have brought considerable enhancement of its spatial resolution, allowing detection of small abnormalities in the pulmonary parenchyma. High-resolution CT (HRCT) allows direct demonstration of the areas of lung destruction and is undoubtedly superior to the chest radiograph in detecting the presence of emphysema. HRCT also allows assessment of the extent and severity of em-

physema. CT has a high specificity for emphysema, emphysema being rarely overcalled in normal individuals or in patients with severe hyperinflation due to other causes (Kinsella et al, 1988).

On CT, emphysema is characterized by the presence of areas of abnormally low attenuation (Fig. 12–4). Mild to moderate proximal acinar (centriacinar) emphysema is characterized on HRCT by the presence of small round areas of abnormally low attenuation near the center of the secondary pulmonary lobule (Murata et al, 1989). This centrilobular distribution cannot be appreciated on conventional CT. These areas of abnormally low attenuation correspond to well-circumscribed holes seen pathologically within the secondary pulmonary lobule (Hruban et al, 1987). With more severe emphysema the holes become confluent, and the centrilobular distribution is no longer recognizable either on HRCT or pathologically. HRCT may demonstrate areas of centriacinar emphysema not apparent on conventional CT and allows a better assessment of the extent and severity of involvement (Miller et al, 1989).

Using HRCT and a state-of-the-art scanner, Hruban and colleagues (1987) were able to identify even mild centriacinar emphysema when they scanned 20 postmortem lung specimens. The

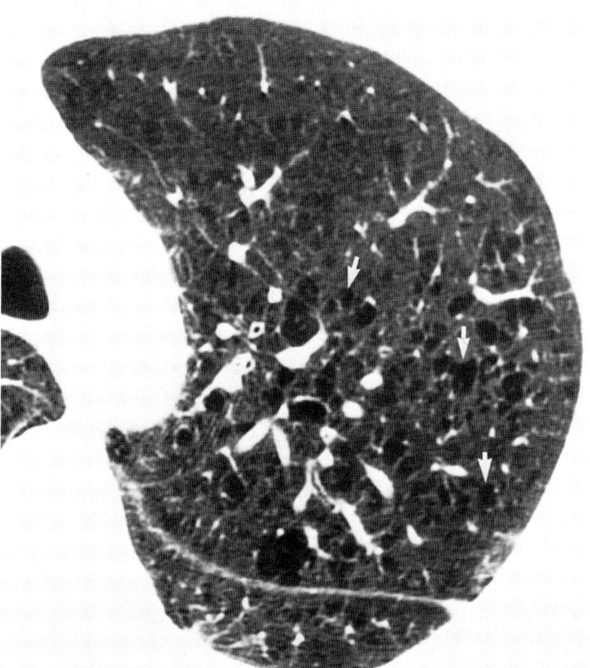

Figure 12–4 A 59-year-old smoker. High-resolution CT through the left upper lobe shows characteristic areas (0.5 to 1 cm diameter) of abnormally low attenuation representing centrilobular emphysema (*arrows*).

correlation between the in-vitro CT emphysema score and the pathologic grade was r = 0.91. The ability of HRCT of lung specimens to demonstrate accurately the location and degree of emphysema was also shown by Webb and coworkers (1988). These results indicate that CT has the potential to identify accurately the presence and severity of centriacinar emphysema. Although it may be possible to obtain a correlation of close to one-to-one between CT and the pathologic specimen in vitro, it is not possible at the present time to obtain such a good correlation in vivo. Using a GE 9800 scanner, we obtained a CT-pathologic correlation of 0.81 when using 10-mm collimation scans and 0.85 when using 1.5-mm collimation scans (Miller et al, 1989). In this series, 33 of 38 patients had emphysema. Of these, four patients with mild centriacinar emphysema were thought to have no emphysema on CT.

Although mild emphysema may be missed on HRCT, it is clearly the best technique to diagnose emphysema in vivo. With careful analysis, even mild emphysema can usually be detected. In 42 patients with mild to moderate centrilobular emphysema, Kuwano et al (1990) found no significant difference between HRCT and the pathology scores.

While relatively mild centrilobular emphysema may often be detectable on CT, this is not the case with panacinar emphysema. Panacinar emphysema leads to a "diffuse simplification" of the lung structure with progressive loss of tissue until little remains but the supporting framework of vessels, septa, and bronchi (Thurlbeck, 1976). Holes less than 1 cm in diameter, characteristically present in mild and moderate centriacinar emphysema, are usually not seen in panacinar emphysema. In severe panacinar emphysema, the "simplification of the lung parenchyma" leads to the widespread areas of low attenuation with a paucity of vascular markings, allowing distinction between panacinar emphysema and normal lung parenchyma (Fig. 12–5). However, mild and moderately severe panacinar emphysema are often impossible to distinguish from

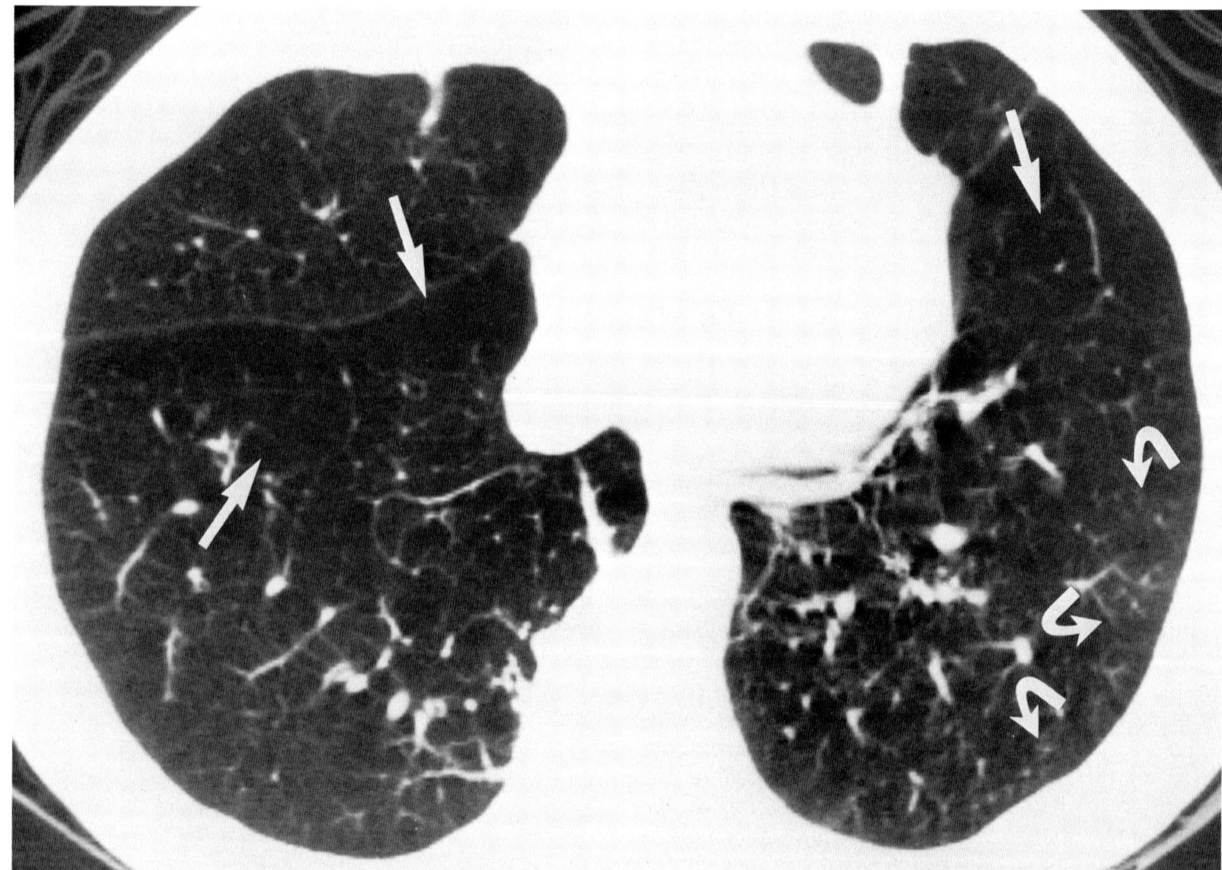

Figure 12–5   High-resolution CT through the lung bases in a 49-year-old woman with alpha-1-antitrypsin deficiency. Areas of severe panacinar emphysema are seen as widespread areas of abnormally low attenuation. These can be identified throughout most of the right lung and anterior aspect of the visualized left lung (*straight arrows*). Relatively normal parenchyma can be seen posteriorly in the left lower lobe (*curved arrows*).

adjacent normal parenchyma on CT (Miller et al, 1989).

Distal acinar emphysema is characterized by involvement of the distal part of the acinus and is therefore most striking adjacent to the pleura and interlobular septa (Fig. 12–6). Even mild distal acinar emphysema is easily detected by HRCT (Miller et al, 1989).

CT assessment of emphysema has a number of potential limitations. It is influenced by scanner type, collimation, window level, window width, and inter- and intra-observer variability. The results of the various recent studies can be summarized as showing a high sensitivity and specificity for CT in the detection of emphysema and a good correlation between the CT and the pathologic emphysema panel scores.

It should be noted, however, that mild emphysema may be missed on CT. Furthermore, in patients with more severe emphysema, the extent of emphysema is underestimated on CT because localized areas of destruction less than 0.5 cm in diameter are usually missed (Miller et al, 1989). Thus, while CT is presently undoubtedly the most sensitive method for diagnosing emphysema in vivo, it does not detect the earliest stages of emphysema and cannot be used definitively to rule out the diagnosis. In clinical practice, HRCT rarely is used to diagnose emphysema, except in the preoperative assessment of patients un-

dergoing bullectomy (Fig. 12–7). The majority of patients referred for bullectomy have well-demarcated bullae and varying degrees of emphysema (Gaensler et al, 1986). CT allows for an assessment not only of the extent of bullous disease but also the degree of compression and the severity of emphysema in the remaining lung parenchyma (Morgan and Strickland, 1984; Carr and Pride, 1984).

BRONCHIOLITIS OR SMALL AIRWAY DISEASE

Biopsies may be performed in patients with airflow obstruction due to peripheral airway disease under a number of circumstances. Sometimes this may occur because of a mistaken diagnosis of infiltrative lung disease. A broad classification of bronchiolitis is given in Table 12–3.

Lesions in Bronchioles in Smokers

Bronchiolitis is an integral part of the lesions found in smokers with chronic bronchitis and varying degrees of pulmonary dysfunction. As indicated, these are of limited concern in terms of biopsy. It is important to recognize that the lesions in patients with mild CAO may be both qualitatively and quantitatively different from those in patients with severe CAO. In mild CAO, bronchiolar inflammation plays the most important role; in severe CAO, narrowing and tortuosity of the bronchioles are the dominant lesions (Nagai et al, 1985). In both mild and severe CAO goblet cell metaplasia is important. These

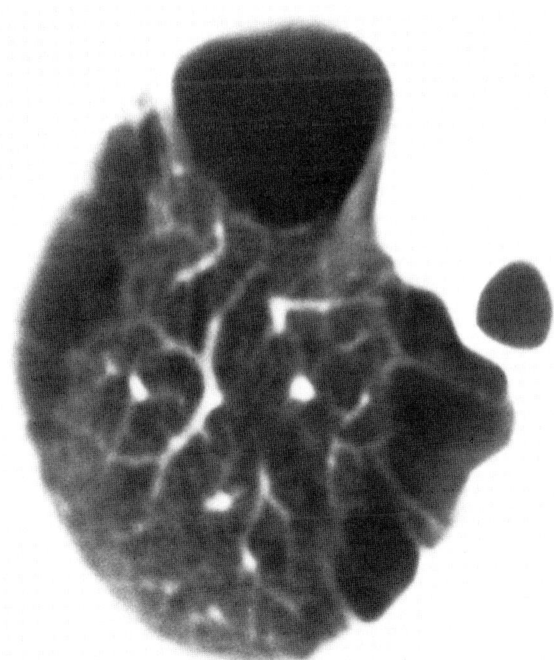

Figure 12–6 In this patient with distal acinar emphysema, the areas of abnormally low attenuation are situated in the subpleural lung regions.

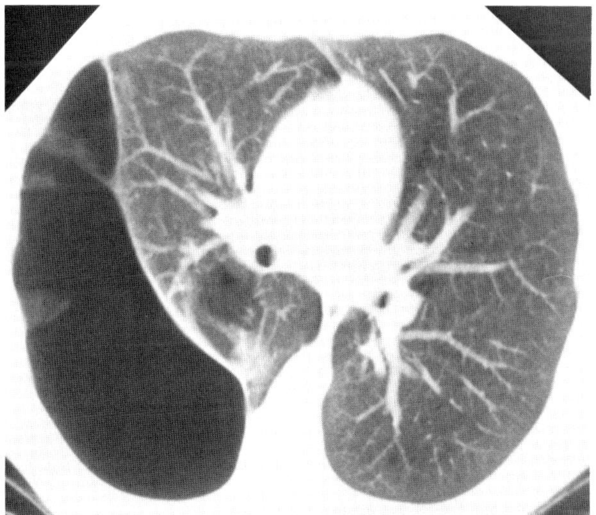

Figure 12–7 A 34-year-old man with extensive bullous disease of the right lung. Only mild emphysema is identified on the left side.

TABLE 12–3

BRONCHIOLITIS

Associated with cigarette smoking

Special forms of bronchiolitis
- Irritants and viral infections
- Rheumatoid bronchiolitis
- Diffuse panbronchiolitis
- Graft-versus-host disease
- Heart-lung transplant
- Follicular bronchitis/bronchiolitis
- Respiratory bronchiolitis
- Mineral dust airways disease
- L-tryptophan bronchiolitis
- Cryptogenic bronchiolitis

lesions and their functional correlations have been reviewed in detail elsewhere (Thurlbeck, 1985, 1988, 1990). Tobacco-associated respiratory bronchiolitis is dealt with separately in another section.

Lesions in Bronchioles in Patients with Unusual Forms of CAO

CAO may occur in settings other than the above, and over the last decade a variety of clinicopathologic syndromes have been defined.

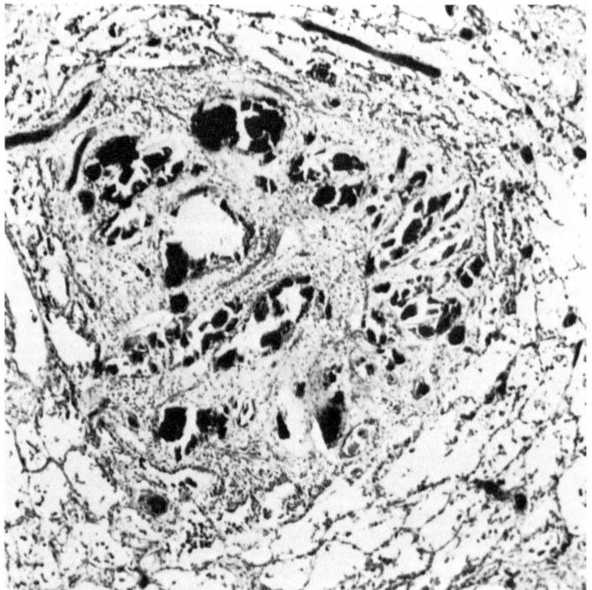

Figure 12–8 Obliterative bronchiolitis due to measles 6 months after the acute infection.

Irritants and Viral Infections

A large number of irritant gases, if respired at the appropriate concentrations, may produce severe bronchiolitis, with acute ulceration and inflammation, followed by occlusion of the airways by loose granulation tissue, and finally by complete stenosis and obliteration. The best known agents are nitrogen dioxide (Horvath et al, 1978), sulfur dioxide (Woodford et al, 1979), and ammonia (Close et al, 1980). Other important causes are viral infections, perhaps the most important one of which currently is adenovirus (Becroft, 1971). Mycoplasma pneumoniae should also be recognized as a frequent cause (Edwards et al, 1983). Measles is now an uncommon cause but is still seen (Fig. 12–8). The course of events is similar to that involving the toxic gases. Extensive bronchiectasis may result because of bronchiolar obliteration. In only rare instances is a lung biopsy performed and then usually because of clinically unusual airflow obstruction, often in a young person. The airway lesions are, of course, not specific and the diagnosis depends on past history. In nearly all instances the information is apparent, obviating the need for biopsy.

Rheumatoid Bronchiolitis

First described by Geddes and colleagues in 1977, rheumatoid bronchiolitis is now a well-recognized condition. Five of their six patients had classic rheumatoid arthritis; the sixth had positive antinuclear antibody and developed rapidly progressive dyspnea and airflow obstruction. All were nonsmoking women, and death occurred 5 to 18 months after the onset. Radiologically the lungs were characterized by gross overinflation but without radiologic evidence of the peripheral arterial insufficiency, as is seen in emphysema. The diffusing capacity and volume-pressure curves were normal. Morphologically, occlusion of scattered small bronchi and bronchioles was seen due to the presence of loose connective tissue in the lumina (Fig. 12–9). One of the authors (WT) has seen a case in which all gradations from rheumatoid-like granulomas in the walls of airways to fibrous obliteration were present. From a practical point of view, the lesions are spotty within the airways, often in bronchi, and may not be apparent in a biopsy specimen. It has now become apparent that chronic airflow obstruction is more common in rheumatoid arthritis than was previously recognized (Geddes et al, 1979), but even in patients with more severe CAO the course has not been as severe as in the original cases. Because of the widespread clinical recognition of rheumatoid bronchiolitis, biopsy is hardly encountered today.

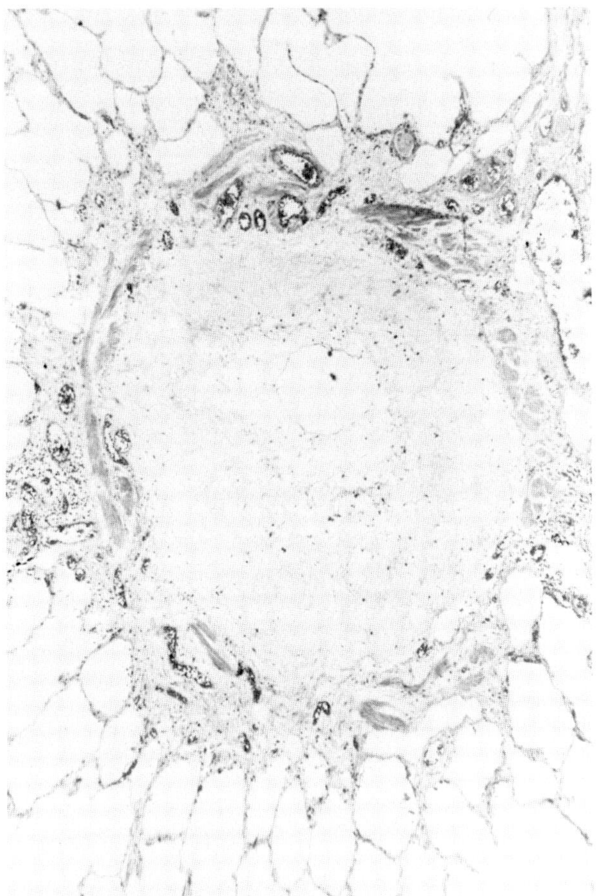

Figure 12–9 Rheumatoid bronchiolitis with occlusion of the lumen with loose fibrous tissue.

Diffuse Panbronchiolitis

This curious condition appears confined or almost confined to Japanese in Japan, where it is quite common; 1,238 cases were recorded in the Japanese panbronchiolitis registry between 1977 and 1980 (Homma et al, 1983). Males are more commonly affected than females, and the age range is 20 to 60 years. The presenting complaints are chronic productive cough and dyspnea, and three of four patients have sinusitis. Radiologically there is variable hyperinflation and multiple scattered fine opacities less than 2 mm in diameter, more profuse in the lower zones. Functionally there is chronic airflow obstruction that is progressive, terminating in respiratory failure. Morphologically the lesion is distinctive. There is severe chronic inflammation of respiratory bronchioles with a mural infiltrate of lymphocytes, plasma cells, and histiocytes (Fig. 12–10). Polymorphonuclear leukocytes and eosinophils in airway lumina, airway walls, and airspaces may be

present. As the lesions progress, there is extension to involve distal bronchioles. The walls of the airways become fibrotic and thickened. The more proximal bronchioles dilate and become irregular in shape. An as-yet unemphasized feature of diffuse panbronchiolitis is the accumulation of a large number of macrophages with abundant clear cytoplasm (presumably lipid or mucus) in the walls and lumina of bronchioles and in adjacent airspaces (see Fig. 12–2). The lesions are widespread but are worse in the lower lobes than the upper lobes. One of the authors (WT) has seen nine cases in consultation and is convinced that this is a specific entity. The Japanese have speculated that the condition occurs in the United States and is unrecognized. They have suggested that some of the cases of "obstructive disease of the small airways" reported by Macklem and colleagues (1971) and some cases of "bronchiolitis obliterans" reported by Gosink and colleagues (1973) were examples of diffuse panbronchiolitis. However, a subsequent review of Macklem's cases has not shown lesions similar to diffuse panbronchiolitis.

Many of the clinical features resemble bronchiectasis as seen in North America, but the condition does not date back to childhood respiratory infection. Morphologically, dilatation occurs in more proximal airways (bronchi) in bronchiectasis, and peripheral bronchiolar disease is also more central and more obliterative, involving distal bronchi and proximal bronchioles. Lymphoid follicles in airway walls are not a feature of diffuse panbronchiolitis.

Graft-versus-Host Disease

Bronchiolitis has become a well recognized complication of graft-versus-host disease (GVHD) in patients treated with bone marrow transplantation since the case reported by Roca and coworkers in 1982. It has been estimated that it occurs in about 4 to 10 percent of patients (Krowka et al, 1986; Ralph et al, 1984) following bone marrow transplantation. The clinical appearance is of rapidly progressive airflow obstruction, with radiologic evidence of overinflation, starting 3 months to 2 years after transplantation. Other manifestations of GVHD are usually present, and treatment is of the reaction. Bronchiolitis (Fig. 12–11), necrotizing bronchiolitis, and bronchiolitis obliterans have been described (Roca et al, 1982; Kurzrock et al, 1984), as have interstitial fibrosis, mild interstitial inflammation, and peribronchiolar fibrosis (Johnson et al, 1984).

Lymphocytic bronchitis and bronchiolitis were described at autopsy in patients following bone marrow transplantation, together with bronchial epithelial necrosis and submucosal gland necrosis. These airway lesions were more obvious in patients with

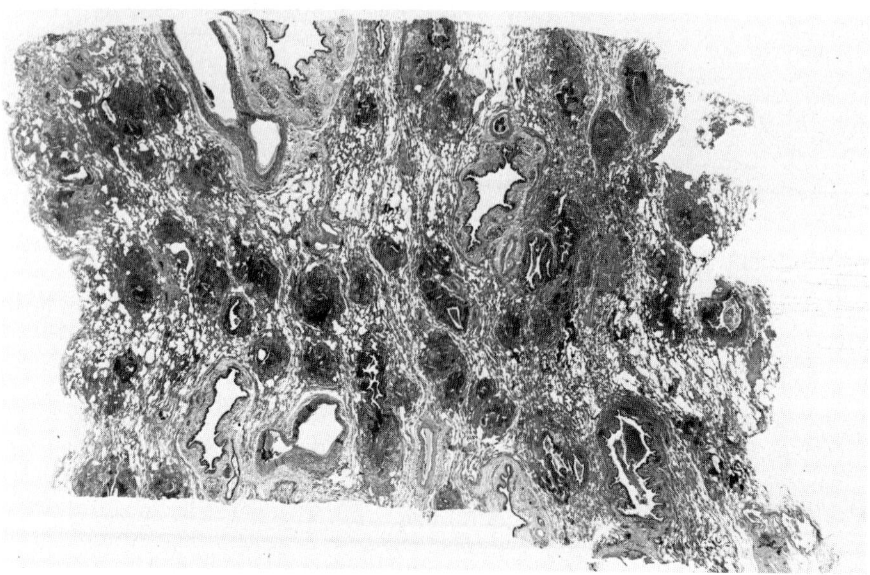

A

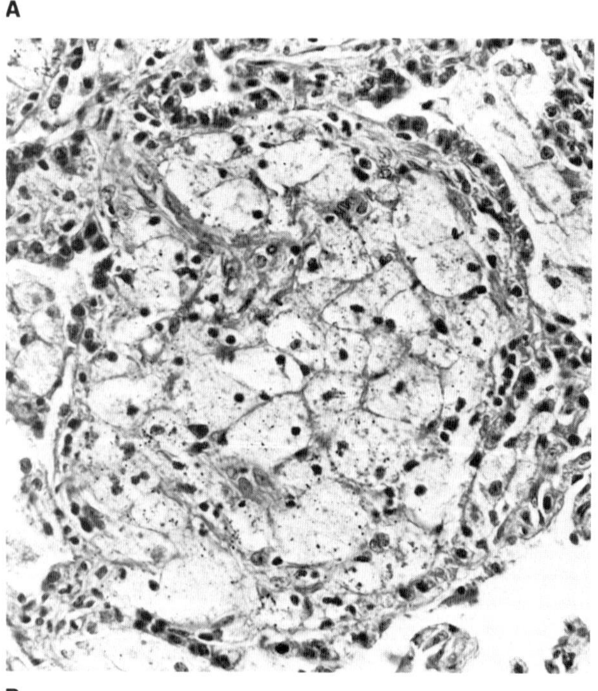

B

Figure 12–10 Diffuse panbronchiolitis. *A*, Scanning view shows bronchiolar distribution of intense inflammation. *B*, Characteristic foamy macrophages.

severe GVHD (Beschorner et al, 1978), but they are not specific.

Heart-Lung Transplantation

Airway disease is now recognized as a serious complication of patients undergoing heart-lung transplantation and was the major cause of death in five of 16 patients surviving beyond the postoperative period (Burke et al, 1984). The patients had recurrent bronchopulmonary infections and developed dyspnea and airflow obstruction 6 months to 2 years after transplantation. Morphologically there was widespread bronchiolitis, bronchiolitis obliterans, and mucous plugging (Fig. 12–12). Extensive bronchiectasis was present in two of the five cases.

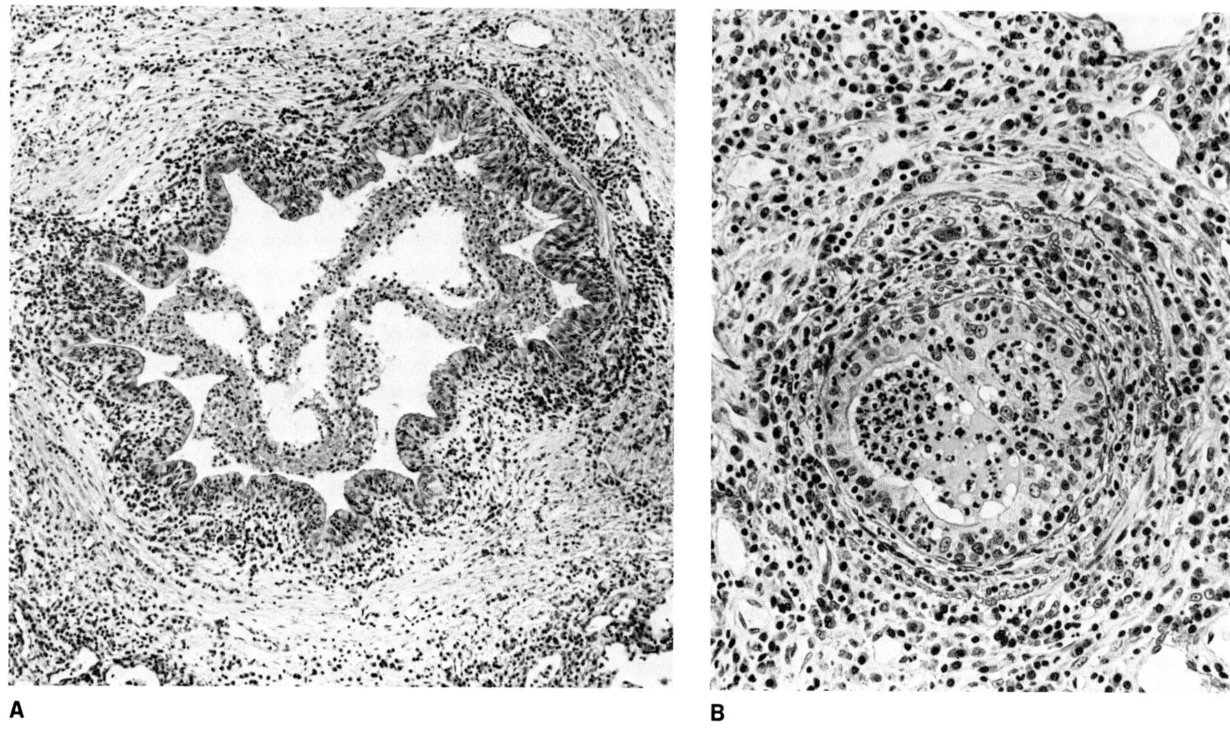

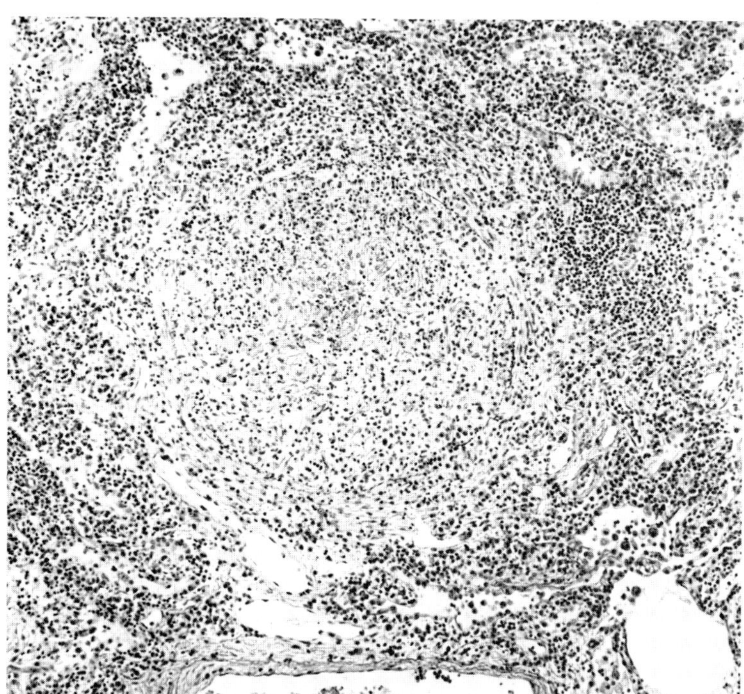

Figure 12–11 Graft-versus-host disease. Mild (*A*), moderate (*B*), and total occlusion of the lumen (*C*).

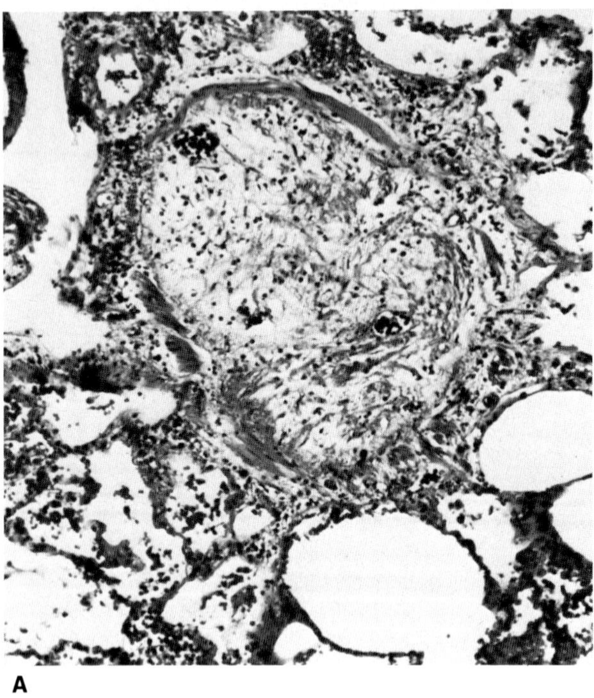

A

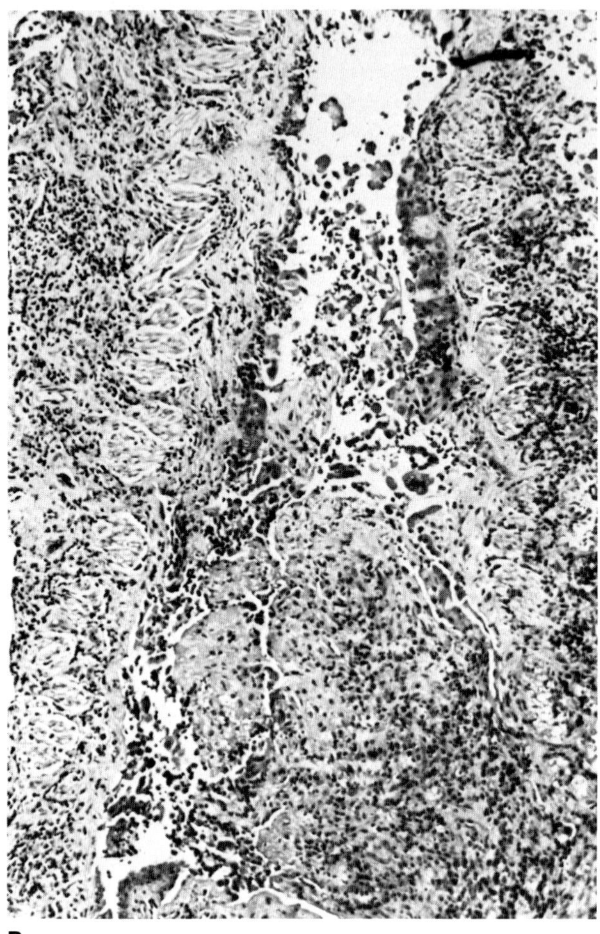

B

Figure 12–12 Heart-lung transplantation. *A,* Obliterative bronchiolitis. *B,* Severe bronchiolitis with ulceration. (Courtesy of Dr. M. Billingham.)

Pleural scars, patchy interstitial fibrosis, and accelerated arterial and venous arteriosclerosis also occurred (Yousem et al, 1985a).

Skeens and colleagues (1989) described the radiologic findings in 11 patients with bronchiolitis obliterans following heart-lung transplantation. CT scans were done in two patients. In all patients the chest radiographs showed parenchymal abnormalities consisting of reticulonodular, nodular, or airspace opacities. Radiographic evidence of central bronchiectasis was present in nine of the 11 patients. Chest CT scans in two patients confirmed the radiographic findings of bronchiectasis by showing dilated airways adjacent to pulmonary arteries.

The cause is unknown, but there is no shortage of possibilities, including repeated bronchopulmonary infection, bronchial artery ligation, mucociliary defect, cyclosporine and other drugs, and aspiration due to loss of the cough reflex. The general view favors rejection (Yousem et al, 1990). This lesion does not seem to occur as much in unilateral lung transplant patients.

Follicular Bronchitis/Bronchiolitis

In a review of a large series of surgical lung biopsies, 19 biopsies were encountered that showed lymphoid follicles with coalescent germinal centers adjacent to small bronchi and/or bronchioles (Fig. 12-13) in the absence of evidence of bronchiectasis or CAO (Yousem et al, 1985b).

The patients were classified into three groups. Seven patients had evidence of auto-immune disease —i.e., six of the seven patients had rheumatoid arthritis and the seventh had unclassifiable collagen-vascular disease. Four patients had immunodeficiency of varying sorts. Eight were classified as hypersensitivity, as seven of the eight with adequate information had peripheral eosinophilia. Other than this there was no common thread.

The age range was wide (1.5 to 77 years), and two thirds of the patients were females. The most common symptom was progressive dyspnea or dyspnea on exertion, which occurred in 15. Bilateral interstitial infiltrates, reticular or nodular, were seen

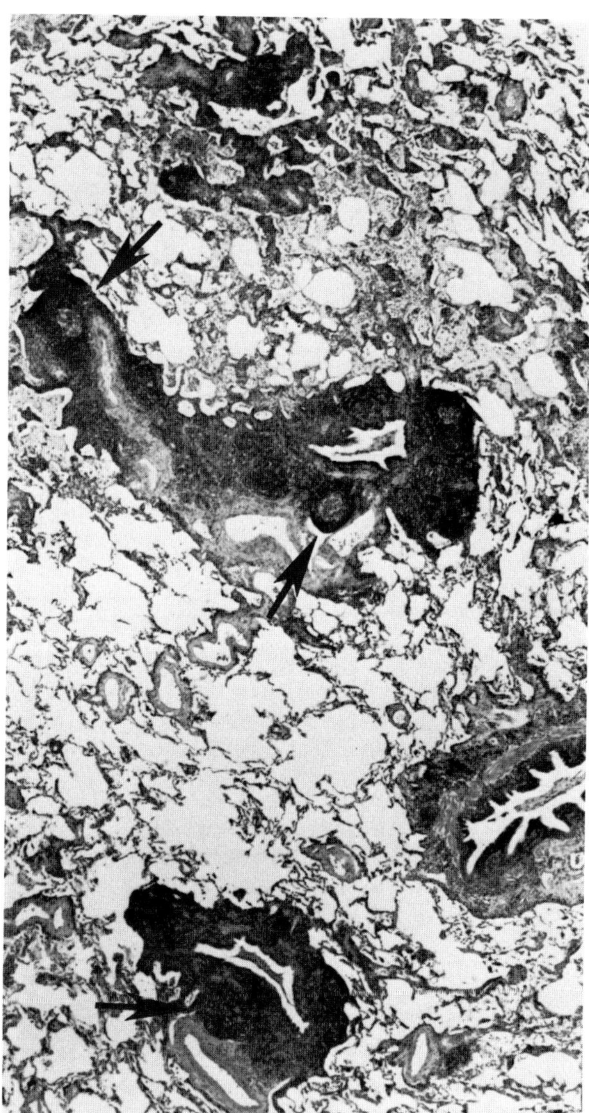

Figure 12–13   Follicular bronchitis/bronchiolitis. Note formation of the germinal center (*arrows*).

radiographically. In general, patients under the age of 30 years had progressive disease.

Respiratory Bronchiolitis

Respiratory bronchiolitis, the presence of greenish-brown pigmented macrophages in the lumen, walls, and adjacent airspaces of respiratory bronchioles (Fig. 12–14), has been a recognized result of cigarette smoking for a number of years (Niewoehner et al, 1974). It has been thought to be the predecessor of centrilobular emphysema since it occurs in the same region within the acinus (respira-

tory bronchioles) and the same region within the lungs (upper zones). It has also been shown to be associated with thickening of the walls of respiratory bronchioles and thought to be a cause of mild chronic airflow obstruction in smokers (Wright et al, 1987). Most recently, Myers and coworkers (1987) have pointed out that respiratory bronchiolitis may be a cause of infiltrative lung disease. These authors reported six young patients (mean age, 36 years), all heavy smokers; five presented with cough and dyspnea (one was asymptomatic), four had mild restrictive lung disease and diminished diffusing capacity, and all had abnormal chest radiographs. Five had diffuse fine reticulonodular densities. Evidence of airflow obstruction was minimal. All had the features of respiratory bronchiolitis, as described above, on lung biopsy. Peribronchiolar inflammation extended into adjacent alveolar septa and was associated with patchy type-II cell metaplasia. At times this is a very striking finding (see Fig. 12–14). Aggregates of macrophages were also seen in more peripheral airspaces. Mild localized interstitial fibrosis was observed. In the NIH interstitial lung disease trial, 18 further examples were found in approximately 200 biopsies for interstitial lung disease. One main differential diagnosis is with desquamative interstitial pneumonitis (DIP), but respiratory bronchiolitis differs in the almost selective aggregation of the macrophages in and around respiratory bronchioles. Diffuse pulmonary hemorrhage can be distinguished by the fine granularity of the pigment in the macrophages, which also stains strongly for iron. Classic "smokers' inclusions" of kaolinite are seen ultrastructurally.

Mineral Dust Airways Disease

A distinctive lesion has been observed in the airways of workers exposed to mineral dust, and this has been referred to as mineral dust airways disease (Churg and Wright, 1983; Churg et al, 1985). A similar appearance has been noted in asbestos workers (Wright and Churg, 1984). The lesion consists of dense fibrosis and heavy pigmentation of respiratory bronchioles (Fig. 12–15). The more proximal bronchioles also had extensive fibrosis; the lesions were widespread in the airways. The researchers found the lesions in about one of four workers exposed to dust and in less than 1 percent of those not exposed. The patients with mineral dust airways disease showed expiratory flow obstruction, generally mild, with abnormalities of the single-breath nitrogen test. Although the data are to some extent controversial, there is evidence that airflow obstruction does occur in mineral-dust–exposed workers (Churg et al, 1985). Churg and colleagues (1985) pointed out that since

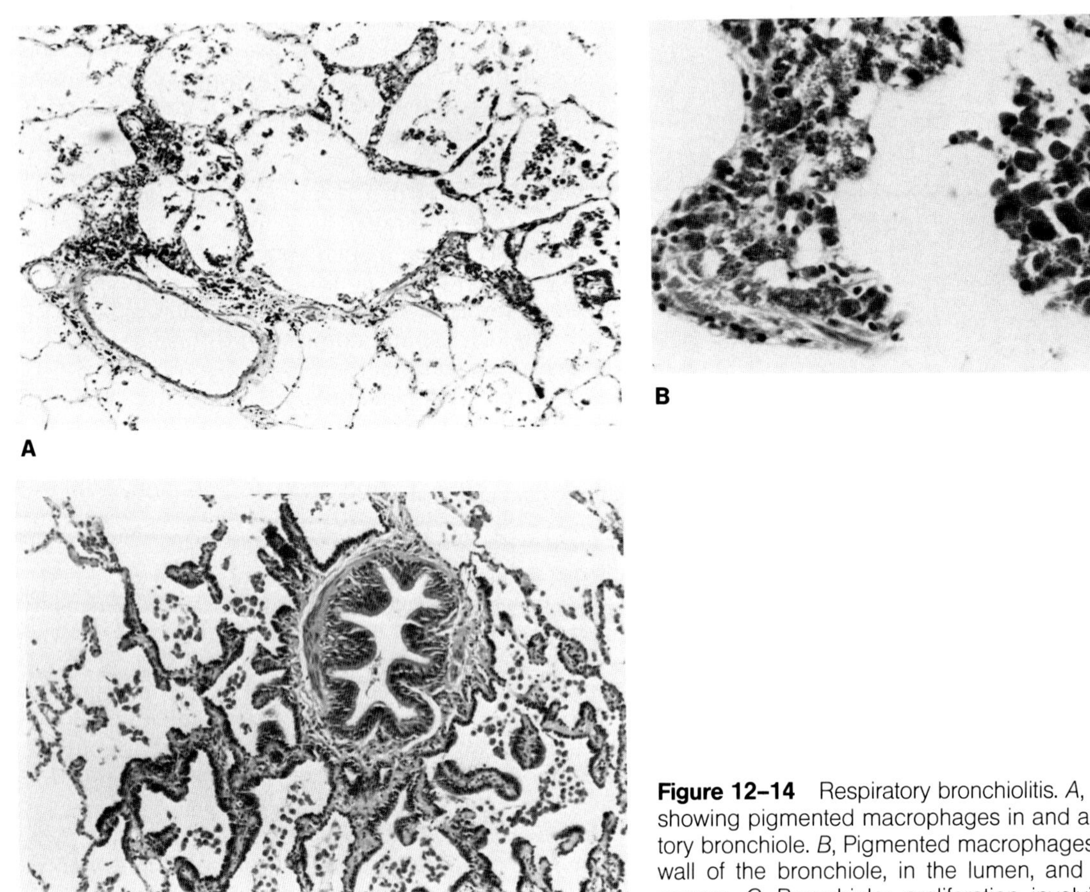

Figure 12–14   Respiratory bronchiolitis. *A*, Low-power view showing pigmented macrophages in and around a respiratory bronchiole. *B*, Pigmented macrophages are seen in the wall of the bronchiole, in the lumen, and in adjacent airspaces. *C*, Bronchiolar proliferation involving the walls of adjacent airspaces.

only a minority of workers developed mineral dust airways disease, a survey of workers as a whole might not detect airflow obstruction in them.

Tryptophan Bronchiolitis

The syndromes of eosinophilia-myalgia, fasciitis, and scleroderma with ingestion of tryptophan is of very recent interest (Silver et al, 1990; Hertzman et al, 1990). Tryptophan is used as a "health food" that formerly could be bought over the counter but it now has been withdrawn. One of the authors (WT) has seen a case that was immediately diagnosed by Dr. Tom Colby, who had previously seen two cases. The tryptophan background of the case referred to was unknown at the time of diagnosis, but subsequent investigation revealed a history of tryptophan ingestion. The histologic features include severe chronic bronchiolitis with occasional follicle formation, a mild chronic interstitial infiltrate with eosinophilia, and a perivasculitis and vasculitis of small

arteries, veins, and alveolar capillaries (Fig. 12–16) (Tazelaar et al, 1990).

Cryptogenic Bronchiolitis

Some idea of the frequency of unexplained chronic airflow obstruction can be obtained from the interesting study by Turton and colleagues (1981), who examined the records of 2,094 patients who had an FEV_1 of less than 60 percent of predicted value from the pulmonary function laboratory. They excluded any patients with asthma, chronic bronchitis, emphysema, current smokers and former smokers, and patients with specific lung disease, such as lung cancer. Ten patients remained: nine were female and one was male, with an age range of 27 to 60 years. Five had rheumatoid arthritis and presumably had rheumatoid bronchiolitis; the others had airflow obstruction of unknown cause, thought to be due to bronchiolitis of unknown cause. The most likely cause is probably a viral infection,

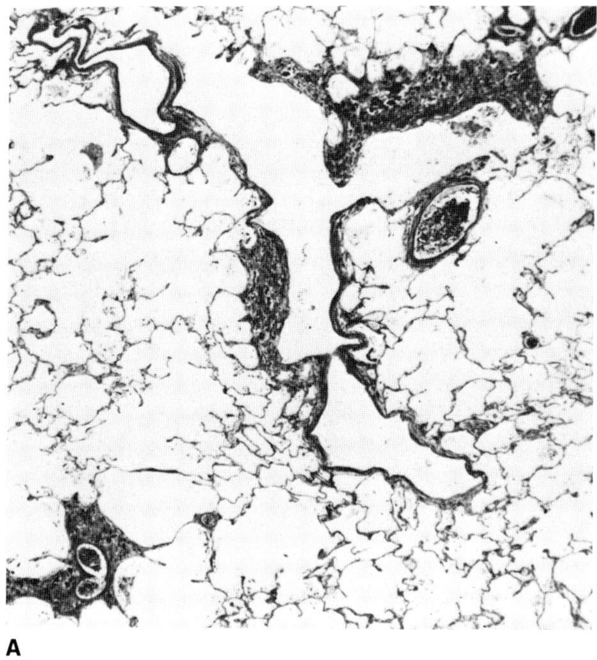

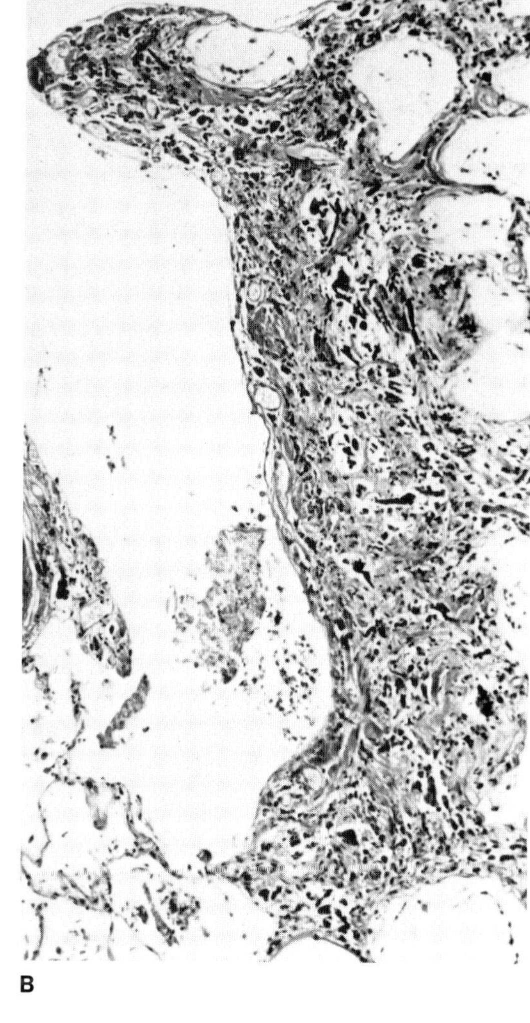

Figure 12–15   Mineral dust–associated airway disease. *A,* Extensive fibrosis of a respiratory bronchiole is seen. *B,* Marked pigmentation and thickening of the wall is present. (Courtesy of Dr. A. Churg.)

unrecognized at the time. The pathology is, of course, not known.

The chest radiograph in bronchiolitis obliterans is often normal. In some patients, mild hyperinflation or subtle peripheral attenuation of the vascular markings may be seen (McLoud et al, 1986; Breatnach and Kerr, 1982). Sweatman and coworkers (1990) described the CT findings in 15 patients with cryptogenic bronchiolitis obliterans. The chest radiography was normal in five patients and showed mild hyperinflation and decreased vascular markings in the remaining 10 patients. In 13 of 15 patients (87 percent) CT showed widespread changes consisting of patchy irregular areas of high and low density. These changes were accentuated in expiration.

PRIMARY SPONTANEOUS PNEUMOTHORAX IN YOUNG ADULTS

Pneumothorax, the presence of air in the pleural space, may be traumatic, iatrogenic, or spontaneous. Spontaneous pneumothorax either may complicate known underlying disease such as extensive emphysema or cavitatory lung infections or tumors (secondary pneumothorax), or the lungs may have been thought to have been previously normal (primary pneumothorax). About 70 percent of spontaneous pneumothoraces are primary (Killem and Gobbel, 1968). Primary spontaneous pneumothorax usually occurs in young adult males. Spontaneous pneumothorax is quite a common condition,

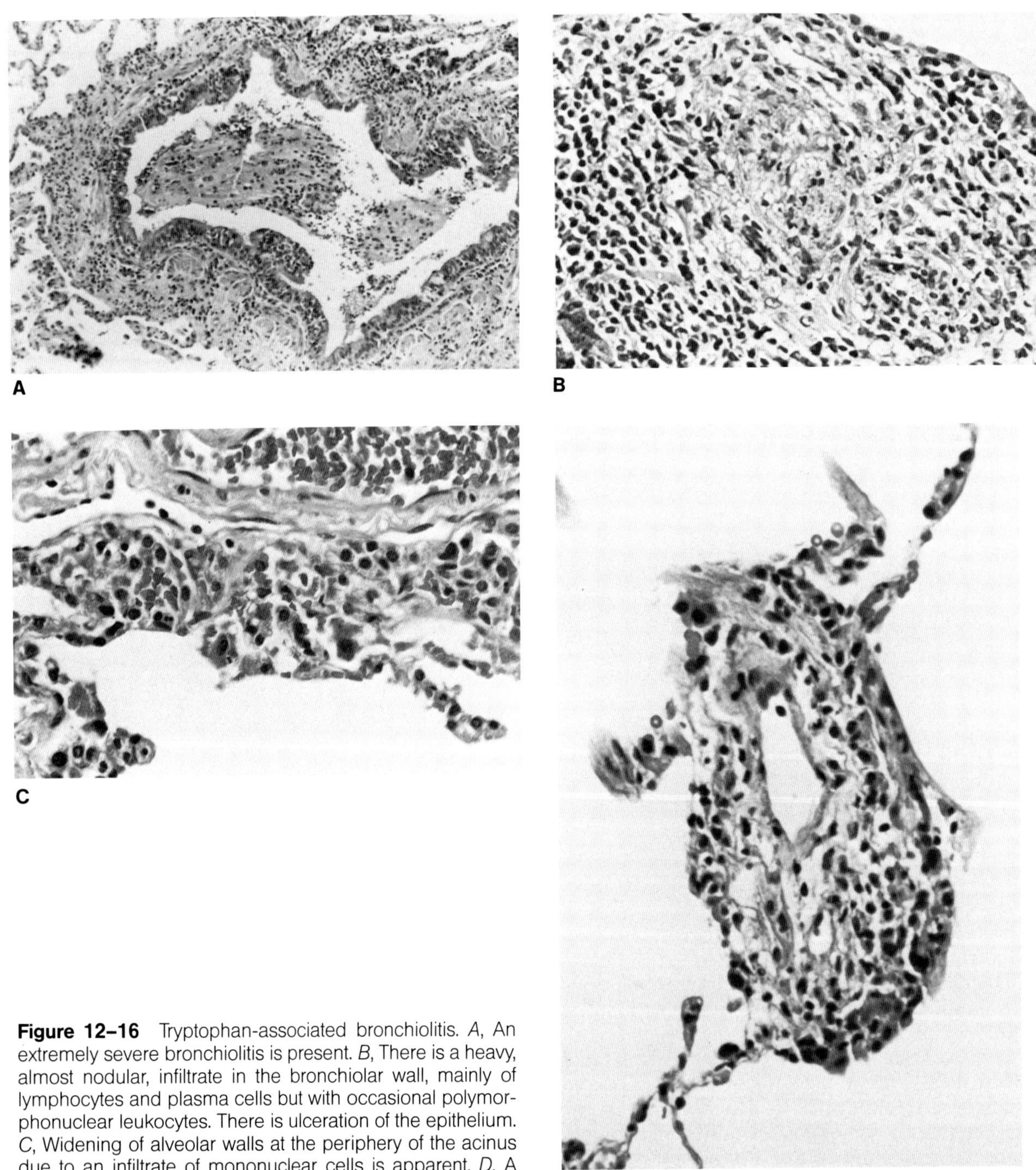

Figure 12–16   Tryptophan-associated bronchiolitis. *A*, An extremely severe bronchiolitis is present. *B*, There is a heavy, almost nodular, infiltrate in the bronchiolar wall, mainly of lymphocytes and plasma cells but with occasional polymorphonuclear leukocytes. There is ulceration of the epithelium. *C*, Widening of alveolar walls at the periphery of the acinus due to an infiltrate of mononuclear cells is apparent. *D*, A heavy inflammatory infiltrate surrounds a small vein.

affecting about one in 400 of the population at some time. Typically, a tall, young man, while exercising vigorously, experiences sudden pain in the chest and then dyspnea. A pneumothorax is discovered clinically and confirmed radiologically. In approximately 20 percent of cases the condition recurs, and wedge bullectomy may be required.

The cause of spontaneous pneumothorax is classically thought to be due to rupture of distal acinar (paraseptal) emphysema into the pleura to form blebs, and rupture through the pleura into the pleural space (Thurlbeck, 1976). (Blebs have a precise definition as collections of air *in* the *pleura* (Ciba Symposium 1959); the term is, however, often used loosely.) Alternatively, the foci of distal acinar emphysema (DAE) may rupture directly, such that the walls of the lesion are emphysematous bullae rather than pleura (Lichter and Glynne, 1971).

The responsible bullae are almost always found in either the apex of the upper lobe or the tip of the superior segment. The underlying tissue shows varying degrees of fibrosis and airspace enlargement and an infiltrate of chronic inflammatory cells (Fig. 12–17). Small arteries show marked thickening of their walls. Because of the obvious fibrosis, the lesions are probably better referred to as airspace enlargement with fibrosis rather than DAE, according to the definitions described above. The scarring and airspace enlargement are presumably sequelae to inflammation. The apex of the lung is subjected to the most negative intrapleural pressure and is greatest in tall patients; this becomes even more negative with exercise. This force presumably precipitates the episode of spontaneous pneumothorax.

The pleura usually shows subacute inflammation, characterized by an infiltrate of lymphocytes and eosinophils and cuboidal metaplasia of the mesothelial cells. The tissue eosinophilia, together with the plump mesothelial cells, may superficially mimic the appearance of eosinophilic granuloma (Askin et al, 1977). Because the latter manifests as a spontaneous pneumothorax in some 20 percent of patients and also often involves younger male patients, it is important to recognize eosinophilic pleuritis, which is a common nonspecific pleural reaction.

CENTRAL AIRWAY LESIONS

Both chronic bronchitis and asthma are important common conditions that may produce diagnostic lesions on bronchial biopsy. However, the diagnosis of neither condition should be made at biopsy since they are clinically defined and recognized. It is inappropriate to discuss these lesions here, and the reader is referred elsewhere (Thurlbeck, 1976). One lesion of the central airways may be important at biopsy. It is now apparent that ultrastructural alterations of the cilia may be associated with abnormal ciliary motility and result in chronic airway inflammation or bronchiectasis and diffuse lung disease (McDowell et al, 1976).

Immotile Cilia Syndrome (Ciliary Dyskinesia Syndrome) (Kuhn, 1988)

Kartagener's Syndrome

Electron-microscopic studies have shown that the fine structure of all cilia, regardless of species or

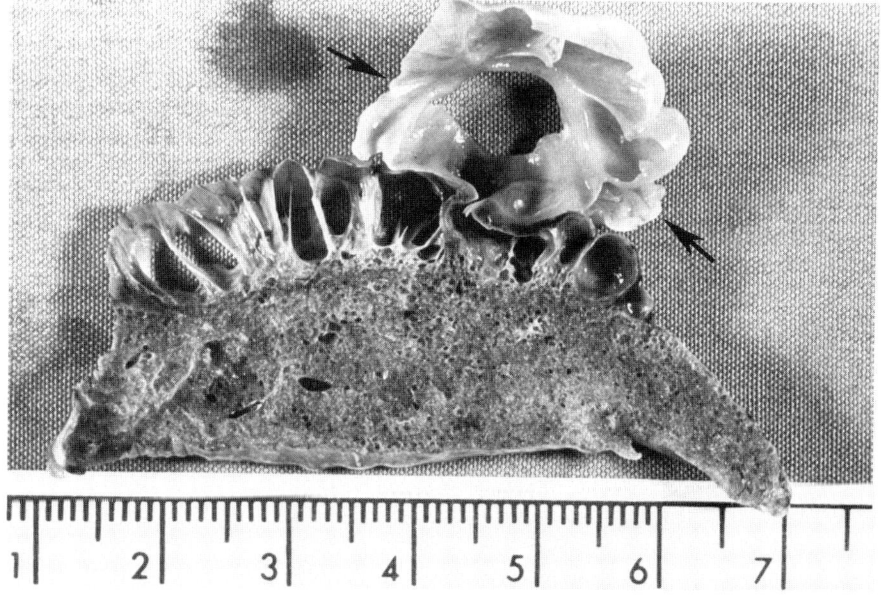

Figure 12–17 Wedge bullectomy for spontaneous pneumothorax in a young man. Much of the lesion involves the distal part of the acinus but is fibrotic. An apparent bleb (*arrow*) is also seen.

organ, is the same. The axoneme of the cilia consists of an outer ring of nine paired microtubules (doublets) and two centrally situated single microtubules. This arrangement is often referred to as the "9 + 2 configuration." The doublets are connected to each other by single strands known as nexin links. The central tubules are surrounded by a sheath and connected to each doublet by radial spoke links. The A tubules, or the clockwise-positioned tubule of the doublets, have two hooked sidearms of dynein, an ATPase protein. These are referred to as dynein arms and are thought to link adjacent doublets and to induce a sliding movement between them, analogous to the cross bridges that cause sliding between actin and myosin in muscle.

A number of syndromes now appear to be associated with defects in the detailed structure of the tubules or their interconnections, with consequent ineffective or absent beating of respiratory cilia. The best known is dynein arm deficiency, and the abnormalities were first encountered in studies of infertile men who had immotile spermatozoa (which have an identical 9 + 2 structure in their tails). Kartagener's syndrome of bronchiectasis, sinusitis, and situs inversus has been well recognized for years, and affected men are generally sterile (Kartagener and Stucki, 1962). The syndrome occurs in only approximately 20 percent of patients with situs inversus. The condition is familial, but the precise genetic abnormality is uncertain. It is now known that absence of the dynein arms of the doublets is associated with this syndrome (Eliasson et al, 1977). There is loss of mucociliary clearance of the airways, and this predisposes to airway infection and the development of bronchiectasis, which is morphologically identical with the usual "postinfective" bronchiectasis. Why dynein arm deficiency should lead to situs inversus is unclear, but bronchiectasis and sinusitis without situs inversus have been well documented in relatives of patients with Kartagener's syndrome. At this time, it is appropriate to refer to patients with the complete triad, together with dynein arm deficiency, as having Kartagener's syndrome, and patients without situs inversus as having dynein arm deficiency. In addition, it has long been known that bronchiectasis is unusually common in Polynesians, specifically Maoris in New Zealand and Samoan Islanders. It has been shown that dynein arm deficiency is characteristic of these patients, although situs inversus is quite uncommon in them (Waite et al, 1978).

Other Causes

Since then, many other abnormalities of the axoneme have been shown to be associated with the immotile cilia syndrome. In general, the clinical features are similar to those of Kartagener's syndrome because of defective or absent ciliary beat. These include absence of the radial spoke between the central tubules and outer doublets (Sturgess et al, 1979), selective absence of the spoke heads, or selective absence of inner and outer dynein arms (Afzalius and Eliasson, 1979). Complex abnormalities have also been reported. These include combined absence of the inner dynein arm and spoke head (Schneeberger et al, 1980), absence of the entire axoneme (Buccetti et al, 1980; Fonzi et al, 1982) and microtubular transposition in which the two central microtubules are absent and one of the peripheral doublets crosses to the center of the lower third of the axoneme to take a central position (Sturgess et al, 1980). Secondary ciliary changes may be seen ultrastructurally in affected patients. Normally, the plane of the central singlet tubules are parallel and the basal feet project from the basal bodies in the same direction. In the immotile ciliary syndrome, orderly orientation may be lost (Veerman et al, 1980). Some patients have cilia with supernumerary microtubules. When the primary defect involves radial spokes, there is loss of the regular spacing of the peripheral doublets from the central pair.

A variety of nonspecific abnormalities may be seen in the cilia of human tracheobronchial epithelium, primarily as a result of cigarette smoking. Mucociliary clearance is often impaired in such patients so they may be thought of as having acquired, rather than congenital, airway ciliary dysfunction. Morphologically the proportion of abnormal cilia is much smaller in patients with acquired dysfunction than in patients with primary ciliary dyskinesia (Rossman et al, 1984). Some abnormal cilia are found in normal patients and more are found in those with bronchial disease. The abnormalities include compound cilia, abnormalities of microtubules, especially the central pair, and minor loss of dynein arms.

Screening can be carried out by light microscopic examination of the motility of living ciliated cells. Nasal biopsy not infrequently fails to provide ciliated cells, but an adequate sample for light microscopy and electron microscopy can be obtained from the inferior turbinate with a curette or bronchial brush (Rutland and Cole, 1980). Adding 0.1 percent tannic acid to the fixative for electron microscopy improves the visualization of the axoneme. A sufficient number of properly oriented cilia should be examined to determine that a consistent abnormality is seen in the great majority, if not all, of the cilia.

REFERENCES

Afzelius BA, Eliasson R. Flagellar mutants in man: on the heterogeneity of the immotile cilia syndrome. J Ultrastruct Res 1979; 69:43–52.

American Thoracic Society. Chronic bronchitis, asthma and pulmonary emphysema: a statement by the committee on diagnostic standards for non-tuberculosis respiratory disease. Am Rev Respir Dis 1962; 85: 762–768.

Askin FB, McCann BG, Kuhn C. Reactive eosinophilic pleuritis. Arch Pathol Lab Med 1977; 101:187–191.

Becroft DMO. Bronchiolitis obliterans, bronchiectasis and other sequelae of adenovirus type 21 infection in young children. J Clin Pathol 1971; 24:72–82.

Berend N, Woolcock AJ, Marlin GE. Correlation between the function and structure of the lung in smokers. Am Rev Respir Dis 1979; 119:695–705.

Bergin CJ, Müller NL, Nichols DM, et al. The diagnosis of emphysema: a computed tomographic-pathologic correlation. Am Rev Respir Dis 1986; 133:541–546.

Beschorner WE, Saral R, Hutchins GM, et al. Lymphocytic bronchitis associated with graft-versus-host disease in recipients of bone marrow transplants. N Engl J Med 1978; 299:1030-1036.

Breatnach E, Kerr I. The radiology of cryptogenic obliterative bronchiolitis. Clin Radiol 1982; 33:657–661.

Buccetti B, Burrini AG, Pallini V. Spermatozoa and cilia lacking axoneme in an infertile male. Andrologia 1980; 12:525–532.

Burke CM, Theodore J, Dawkins KD, et al. Post-transplant obliterative bronchiolitis and other late sequelae in human heart-lung transplantation. Chest 1984; 86: 824–829.

Carr DH, Pride NB. Computed tomography in pre-operative assessment of bullous emphysema. Clin Radiol 1984; 35:43–45.

Case Records of the Massachusetts General Hospital, 32-1990. N Engl J Med 1990; 323:398–406.

Churg A, Wright JL. Small-airway lesions in patients exposed to nonasbestos mineral dusts. Hum Pathol 1983; 14:688–693.

Churg A, Wright JL, Wiggs B, et al. Small airways disease and mineral dust exposure: prevalence, structure, and function. Am Rev Respir Dis 1985; 131:139–143.

Ciba Guest Symposium Report. Terminology, definitions and classification of chronic pulmonary emphysema and related conditions. Thorax 1959; 14:286–299.

Close LG, Catlin FI, Cohn AM. Acute and chronic effects of ammonia burns of the respiratory tract. Arch Otolaryngol 1980; 106:151–158.

Cooney TP, Thurlbeck WM. Pulmonary hypoplasia in Down's syndrome. N Engl J Med 1982; 307:1170-1173.

Cooney TP, Wentworth PJ, Thurlbeck WM. A diminished radial count is only found post-natally in Down's syndrome. Pediatr Pulmonol 1988; 5:204–209.

Edge J, Simon G, Reid L. Peri-acinar (paraseptal) emphysema: its clinical, radiologic and physiologic features. Br J Dis Chest 1966; 60:10–18.

Edwards C, Penny M, Newman J. Mycoplasma pneumonia, Stevens-Johnson syndrome and chronic obliterative bronchiolitis. Thorax 1983; 38:867–869.

Eliasson R, Mossberg B, Camner P, Afzelius B. The immotile cilia syndrome: a congenital ciliary abnormality as an etiologic factor in chronic airway infections and male sterility. N Engl J Med 1977; 297:1–6.

Fonzi L, Lungarella G, Palatresi R. Lack of kinocilia in the nasal mucosa in the immotile cilia syndrome. Eur J Respir Dis 1982; 63:158–163.

Foster WL, Pratt PC, Roggli VL, et al. Centrilobular emphysema: CT-pathologic correlation. Radiology 1986; 159:27–32.

Gaensler EA, Jederlinic PJ, FitzGerald MX. Patient work-up for bullectomy. J Thorac Imag 1986; 1:75–93.

Geddes DM, Corrin B, Brewerton DA, et al. Progressive airway obliteration in adults and its association with rheumatoid disease. Q J Med 1977; 46:427–444.

Geddes DM, Webley M, Emerson PA. Airways obstruction in rheumatoid arthritis. Ann Rheum Dis 1979; 38: 222–225.

Gosink BB, Friedman PJ, Liebow AA. Bronchiolitis obliterans: roentgenologic-pathologic correlation. AJR 1973; 117:816–832.

Heppleston AG. The pathological anatomy of simple pneumoconiosis of coal-workers. J Path Bact 1955; 66: 235–246.

Hertzman PA, Blevens WL, Mayer J, et al. Association of eosinophilia-myalgia syndrome with the ingestion of tryptophan. N Engl J Med 1990; 322:869–873.

Hislop A, Reid L. New pathological findings of childhood: polyalveolar lobe. Thorax 1970; 25:682–690.

Hogg JC, Macklem PT, Thurlbeck WM. Site and nature of airway obstruction in chronic obstructive lung disease. N Engl J Med 1968; 278:1355–1360.

Homma H, Yamanaka A, Tanimota S, et al. Diffuse panbronchiolitis: a disease of the transitional zone of the lung. Chest 1983; 83:63–69.

Horvath EP, DoPico GA, Barbee RA, Dickie HA. Nitrogen dioxide-induced pulmonary disease. J Occup Med 1978; 20:103–110.

Hruban RH, Meziane MA, Zerhouni EA, et al. High resolution computed tomography of inflation-fixed lungs: pathologic-radiologic correlation of centrilobular emphysema. Am Rev Respir Dis 1987; 136: 935–940.

Idell S, Cohen AB. Alpha-1–antitrypsin deficiency. Clin Chest Med 1983; 4:359–375.

Janoff A. Elastases and emphysema: current assessment of the proteinase-antiproteinase hypothesis. Am Rev Respir Dis 1985; 132:417–433.

Johnson FL, Stokes DC, Ruggiero M, et al. Chronic obstructive airway disease after bone marrow transplantation. J Pediatr 1984; 105:370-376.

Kappos AD, Rodarte JR, Lai-Fook SJ. Frequency dependence and partitioning of respiratory impedence in dogs. J Appl Physiol 1981; 51:621–629.

Kartagener M, Stucki P. Bronchiectasis with situs inversus. Arch Pediatr 1962; 79:193–207.

Killem DA, Gobbel WG. Spontaneous pneumothorax. Boston: Little, Brown and Company, 1968.

Kinsella M, Müller NL, Staples C, et al. Hyperinflation in asthma and emphysema: assessment by pulmonary function testing and computed tomography. Chest 1988; 94:286–289.

Krowka MJ, Rosenow EC III, Hoagland HC. Pulmonary complications of bone marrow transplantation. Chest 1986; 87:237–246.

Kuhn C III. Immotile cilia syndrome. In: Thurlbeck WM, (ed). Pathology of the lung. New York: Thieme, 1988: 566–567.

Kurzrock R, Zander A, Kanojia M, et al. Obstructive lung disease after allogenic bone marrow transplantation. Transplantation 1984; 37:156–160.

Kuwano K, Matsuba K, Ikeda T, et al. The diagnosis of mild emphysema: correlation of computed tomography and pathology scores. Am Rev Respir Dis 1990; 141:169–178.

Laurenzi GA, Turino GM, Fishman AP. Bullous disease of the lung. Am J Med 1962; 32:361–378.

Lichter I, Glynne JF. Spontaneous pneumothorax in young subjects: a clinical and pathological study. Thorax 1971; 26:409–417.

McDowell EM, Barrett LA, Harris CC, Trump BF. Abnormal cilia in human bronchial epithelium. Arch Pathol Lab Med 1976; 100:429–436.

McLoud TC, Epler GR, Colby TV, et al. Bronchiolitis obliterans. Radiology 1986; 159:1–8.

Macklem PT, Thurlbeck WM, Fraser RG. Chronic obstructive lung disease of the small airways. Ann Intern Med 1971; 74:167–177.

Martelli NA, Goldman E, Roncoroni AJ. Lower zone emphysema in young patients without $alpha_1$-antitrypsin deficiency. Thorax 1974; 29:234–244.

Marti-Bonmati L, Ruiz Perales F, Catala F, et al. CT findings in Sawyer-James syndrome. Radiology 1989; 172:447–480.

Miller RR, Müller NL, Vedal S, et al. Limitations of computed tomography in the assessment of emphysema. Am Rev Respir Dis 1989; 139:980-983.

Morgan MDL, Strickland B. Computed tomography in the assessment of bullous lung disease. Br J Dis Chest 1984; 78:10–25.

Murata K, Khan A, Herman PG. Pulmonary parenchymal disease: evaluation with high-resolution CT. Radiology 1989; 170:629–635.

Myers JL, Veal CF, Shin MS, Katzenstein A-L A. Respiratory bronchiolitis causing interstitial lung disease: a clinicopathologic study of six cases. Am Rev Respir Dis 1987; 135:880-884.

Nagai A, West WW, Thurlbeck WM. The National Institutes of Health Intermittent Positive Pressure Breathing trial: correlation between morphologic findings, and evidence of expiratory airflow obstruction. Am Rev Respir Dis 1985; 132:946–953.

Niewoehner DE, Kleinerman J, Rice DB. Pathologic changes in the peripheral airways of young cigarette smokers. N Engl J Med 1974; 291:755–758.

Ralph DD, Springmeyer SC, Sullivan KM, et al. Rapidly progressive air-flow obstruction in marrow transplant recipients. Am Rev Respir Dis 1984; 129:641–644.

Reid L. The pathology of emphysema. Chicago: Year Book, 1967.

Roca J, Granena A, Rodriguez-Roison R, et al. Fatal airway disease in an adult with chronic graft-versus-host disease. Thorax 1982; 37:77–78.

Rossman CM, Lee RMKW, Forrest JB, Newhouse MT. Nasal ciliary ultrastructure and function in patients with primary ciliary dyskinesia compared with that in normal subjects and in subjects with various respiratory diseases. Am Rev Respir Dis 1984; 129:161–167.

Rutland J, Cole PJ. Non-invasive sampling of nasal cilia for measurement of beat frequency and study of ultrastructure. Lancet 1980; 2:564–565.

Schneeberger EE, McCormack J, Issenberg HJ, et al. Heterogeneity of ciliary morphology in the immotile-cilia syndrome in man. J Ultrastruct Res 1980; 73: 34–43.

Silver RM, Heyes MP, Matze JC, et al. Scleroderma, fasciitis, and eosinophilia associated with the ingestion of tryptophan. N Engl J Med 1990; 322: 874–881.

Skeens JL, Fuhrman CR, Yousem SA. Bronchiolitis obliterans in heart-lung transplantation patients: radiologic findings in 11 patients. AJR 1989; 153:253–256.

Snider GL, Kleinerman J, Thurlbeck WM, Bengali ZN. The definition of emphysema: report of a National Heart, Lung and Blood Institute, Division of Lung Diseases Workshop. Am Rev Respir Dis 1985; 132: 182–185.

Snider GL, Lucey EC, Faris B, et al. Cadmium chloride-induced airspace enlargement with interstitial fibrosis is not associated with destruction of elastin: implications for the pathogenesis of human emphysema. Am Rev Respir Dis 1988; 137:912–917.

Sturgess JM, Chao J, Turner JAP. Transposition of ciliary microtubules: another cause of impaired ciliary motility. N Engl J Med 1980; 303:318–322.

Sturgess JM, Chao J, Wong J, et al. Cilia with defective radial spokes: A cause of human respiratory disease. N Engl J Med 1979; 300:53–56.

Sweatman MC, Millar AB, Strickland B, Turner-Warwick M. Computed tomography in adult obliterative bronchiolitis. Clin Radiol 1990; 41:116–119.

Tazelaar HD, Myers JL, Drage CW, et al. Pulmonary disease associated with L-tryptophan induced eosinophilic myalgia syndrome. Chest 1990; 97:1032–1036.

Thurlbeck WM. Chronic airflow obstruction in lung disease. Philadelphia: WB Saunders, 1976.

Thurlbeck WM. Chronic airflow obstruction. In: Petty TL, ed. Correlation of structure and function in chronic obstructive pulmonary disease. 2nd ed. New York: Marcel Dekker, 1985:129.

Thurlbeck WM. Chronic airflow obstruction. In: Thurlbeck WM, ed. Pathology of the lung. New York: Thieme, 1988.

Thurlbeck WM. Pathology of chronic airflow obstruction. In: Cherniack NS, ed. Chronic obstructive pulmonary disease. Philadelphia. WB Saunders 1990.

Thurlbeck WM, Dunnill MS, Hartung W, et al. A comparison of three methods of measuring emphysema. Hum Pathol 1970; 1:215–226.

Thurlbeck WM, Simon G. Radiographic appearance of the chest in emphysema. AJR 1978; 130: 429–440.

Turton CW, Williams G, Green M. Cryptogenic obliterative bronchiolitis in adults. Thorax 1981; 36:805–810.

Van Brabandt H, Cauberghs M, Verbeken E, et al. Partitioning of pulmonary impedence in excised human and canine lungs: functional-structural relationships. J Appl Physiol 1983; 55:1733–1742.

Veerman AJP, Van Delden L, Feenstra L, Leene W. The immotile cilia syndrome, phase contrast microscopy, scanning and transmission microscopy. Pediatrics 1980; 65:698–702.

Waite D, Steele R, Ross I, et al. Cilia and sperm tail abnormalities in Polynesian bronchiectasis. Lancet 1978; 2:132–133.

Webb WR, Stein MG, Finkbeiner WE, et al. Normal and diseased isolated lungs: high-resolution CT. Radiology 1988; 166:81–87.

Woodford DM, Coutu RE, Gaensler EA. Obstructive lung disease from acute sulphur-dioxide exposure. Respiration 1979; 38:238–245.

World Health Organization Report. Chronic cor pulmonale: report of an expert committee. Circulation 1963; 27:594–615.

Wright JL, Churg A. Morphology of small-airway lesions in patients with asbestos exposure. Hum Pathol 1984; 15:68–74.

Wright JL, Cosio M, Wiggs B, Hogg JC. A morphologic grading system for membranous and respiratory bronchioles. Arch Pathol Lab Med 1985; 109:163–165.

Wright JL, Wiggs BJ, Paré PD, Hogg JC. Ranking the severity of emphysema on whole lung slices: concordance of upper lobe, lower lobe, and entire lung ranks. Am Rev Respir Dis 1986; 133:930-931.

Wright JL, Hobson J, Wiggs BR, et al. Effect of cigarette smoking on structure of the small airways. Lung 1987; 165:91–100.

Yousem SA, Burke CM, Billingham ME. Pathologic pulmonary alterations in long-term heart-lung transplantation. Hum Pathol 1985a; 16:911–923.

Yousem SA, Colby TV, Carrington CB. Follicular bronchitis/bronchiolitis. Hum Pathol 1985b; 16:700-706.

Yousem SA, Ray L, Paradis IL, et al. Potential role of dendritic cells in bronchiolitis obliterans in heart-lung transplantation. Ann Thorac Surg 1990; 49:424–428.

CHAPTER 13

PULMONARY VASCULAR DISEASE

PULMONARY ARTERIAL HYPERTENSION

Pulmonary hypertension can be divided according to the anatomic site: precapillary, capillary, and postcapillary. Precapillary hypertension may be caused by either increased flow or increased resistance; usually the alveolar walls are normal. This mechanism underlies the pulmonary hypertension of various forms of congenital heart disease (Edwards and Edwards, 1978), recurrent pulmonary emboli, and primary pulmonary hypertension. Capillary hypertension is caused by destruction of alveoli, distortion of the alveolar capillary bed, or chronic hypoxia. Various diffuse lung diseases, including emphysema, interstitial fibrosis, and pneumoconiosis, may give rise to capillary hypertension. The basic change is medial hypertrophy of small muscular arteries—a change that is commonly seen in lung biopsies and lung resections but is rarely the primary abnormality and will not be specifically addressed in this chapter. [Further discussion is available elsewhere (Edwards and Edwards, 1978; Heath and Smith, 1988).] Postcapillary hypertension is associated with passive congestion of alveolar walls. This mechanism operates in cases of severe mitral valve disease and veno-occlusive disease.

Precapillary Pulmonary Hypertension

When cardiac surgery became common, attention was drawn to the morphologic changes in the pulmonary arterial tree in patients with congenital heart disease, and lung biopsy was recommended for prognostic purposes (Reid, 1979). Heath and Edwards (1958) defined six grades of structural changes in pulmonary arteries. *Grade 1* is seen in patients with congenital heart disease and pulmonary hypertension from birth and represents retention of the fetal pulmonary vessel morphology. The media of small arteries are thickened to up to 25 percent of the vessel diameter, but no intimal fibrosis is present (Fig. 13-1). *Grade 2* is seen in vessels less than 300 μm in diameter and is characterized by intimal proliferation. In *grade 3*, the proliferative intimal changes extend into the medium-sized vessels of from 300 to 500 μm in diameter and become concentric and fibrotic (Fig 13-2). In this grade, the limit of medial hypertrophy is reached with a medial thickness of up to 30 percent of wall diameter. Although hypertrophy is the rule, it is now that dilatation is first noted, with thinning of the media near an area of occlusion. Dilatation lesions are the hallmark of *grades 4 to 6* (Heath and Smith, 1988). There are two main types of dilatation lesions: plexiform and vein-like branches. The plexiform lesion is composed of a small muscular artery, a portion of which is greatly distended. Within the distended part, complicated fine vascular sinuses develop. In the early stages of the plexiform lesion, there is considerable endothelial cell proliferation, resembling a vascular plexus (Fig. 13-3). In time, the walls of the sinuses become fibrotic. The lesions may resemble organized thrombi; in fact, thrombotic material is quite often present in plexiform lesions.

Vein-like branches are thin-walled vessels with almost no muscle, arising from an obstructed artery. These greatly dilated channels cluster around the parent vessel, giving the appearance of having herniated out from the vessel at several points (Fig. 13-4). In addition to dilatation lesions, *grade 5* displays

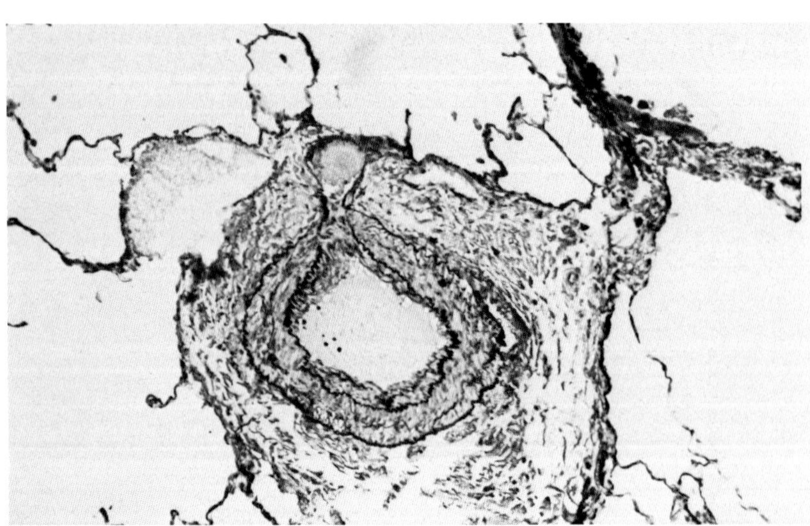

Figure 13-1 Grade-1 vasculopathy in a patient with congenital heart disease, characterized by medial thickening of the muscular artery.

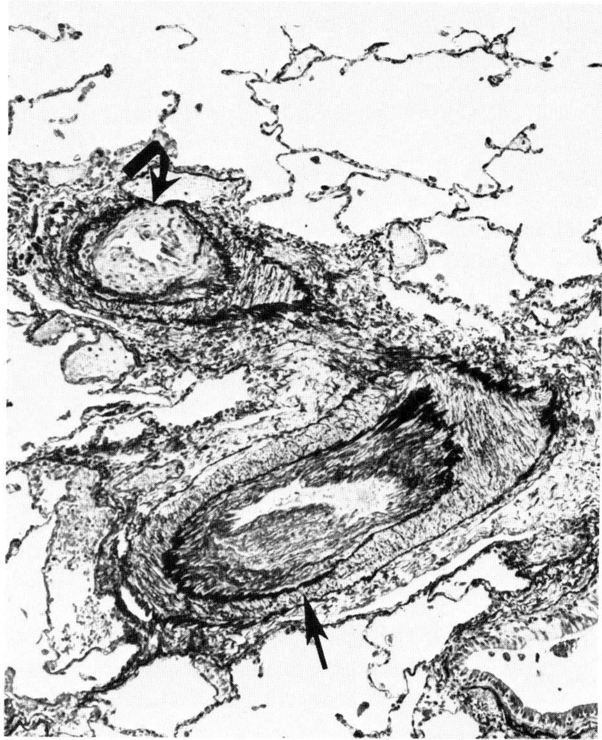

Figure 13–2 Grade-3 vasculopathy with intimal fibrosis (*straight arrow*) and intimal cellular proliferation (*curved arrow*).

hemosiderosis. *Grade 6* lesions are uncommon and are characterized by necrotizing arteritis.

Attention has focused on assessment of reversibility of pulmonary vasculopathy in patients with congenital heart disease by lung biopsy (Edwards and Edwards, 1978). Reid and colleagues (1979) have shown that peripheral extension of muscle—that is, extension of muscle into small arteries previously free of muscle—was characteristic of high-flow states. Workers from Reid's laboratory have suggested a different grading system in children less than 2 years of age (Rabinovitch et al, 1980). Diameter and thickness of arterial walls, peripheral extension of muscle, and the alveolar/arterial ratio were assessed, and three grades of disease were proposed. In *grade A*, there is peripheral extension of vascular smooth muscle into the acinus. This is the earliest stage and is associated with increased pulmonary blood flow but not with pulmonary hypertension. *Grade B* is characterized by increased medial thickness, thus corresponding to Heath and Edwards' grade 1. More severe degrees of grade B are usually associated with pulmonary hypertension. There also may be an associated decrease in size of the intra-acinar pulmonary arteries. In *grade C*, in addition to the changes of grades A and B, there is a reduction in the number of small peripheral arteries. This grade is associated with marked pulmonary hypertension and is usually accompanied by grade 3 changes of Heath and Edwards. The lesions in the A,B,C grading system

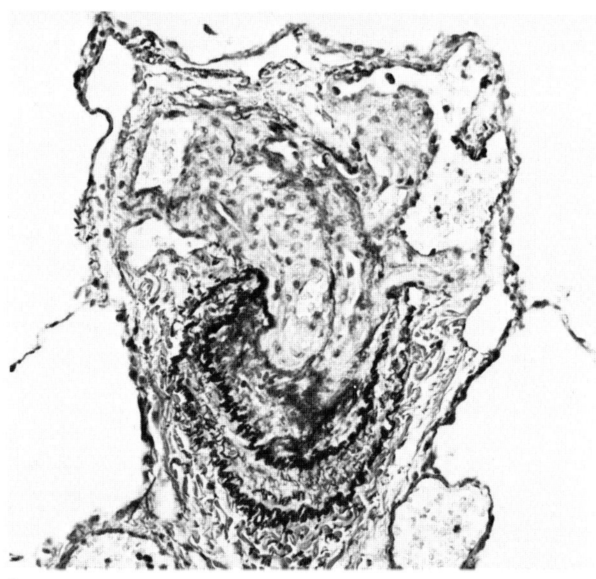

A

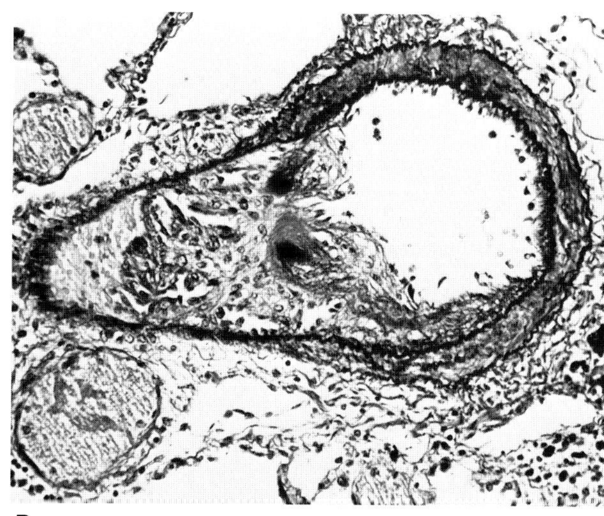

B

Figure 13–3 Grade-4 vasculopathy with plexiform lesions. *A*, Cellular lesion with obvious disruption of elastin. *B*, More fibrotic lesion simulating thrombus.

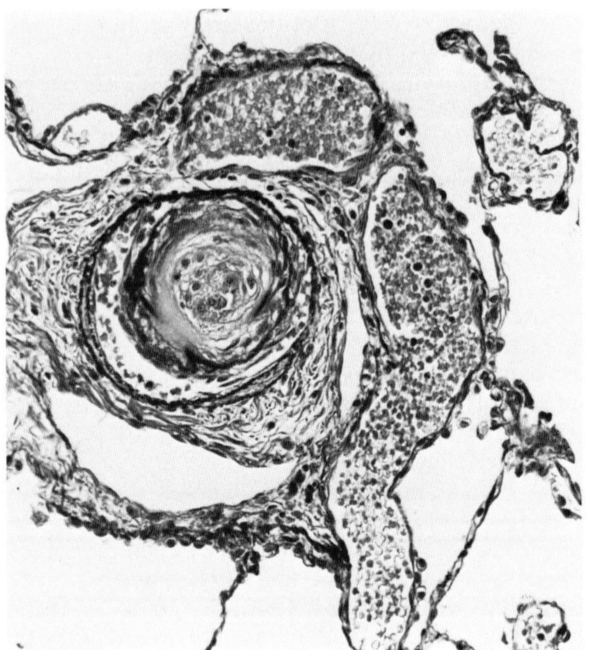

Figure 13–4   Grade-4 vasculopathy: vein-like "herniation" forming vascular cluster around parent artery. Note concentric intimal sclerosis of artery.

are uniform through the lung, except for the lingula (Haworth and Reid, 1978). This system of grading has not been widely accepted, and it also appears that grade-C changes have little predictive value and may be reversible (Langston and Holder, 1987). In general, the Heath-Edwards system may still be the best estimate of reversibility. Medial hypertrophy regresses readily, as do cellular intimal proliferation and the early stages of concentric laminar intimal fibrosis. However, severe intimal laminar fibrosis does not reverse, and dilatation lesions and fibrinoid necrosis are ominous findings (Wagenvoort, 1987).

Radiologically, conditions associated with left-to-right shunt and increased pulmonary blood flow (atrial septal defect, ventricular septal defect, patent ductus arteriosus) are characterized by an increase in caliber of pulmonary arteries throughout the lungs. As pulmonary arterial hypertension develops, the central arteries become larger and they taper rapidly as they extend to the periphery of the lung (Rees, 1968). In patients with longstanding pulmonary hypertension and Eisenmenger physiology, the central pulmonary arteries may become quite large and may have calcification in their walls due to atherosclerosis (Fig. 13–5).

It should be noted that it is often difficult to recognize radiologically the presence of pulmonary

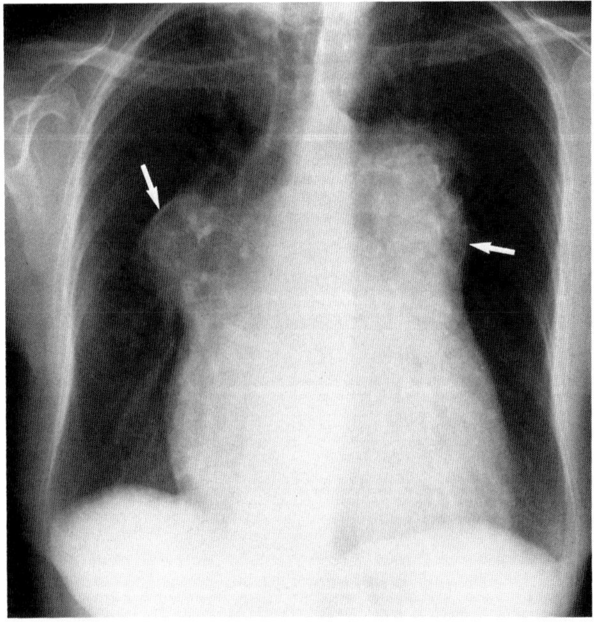

A

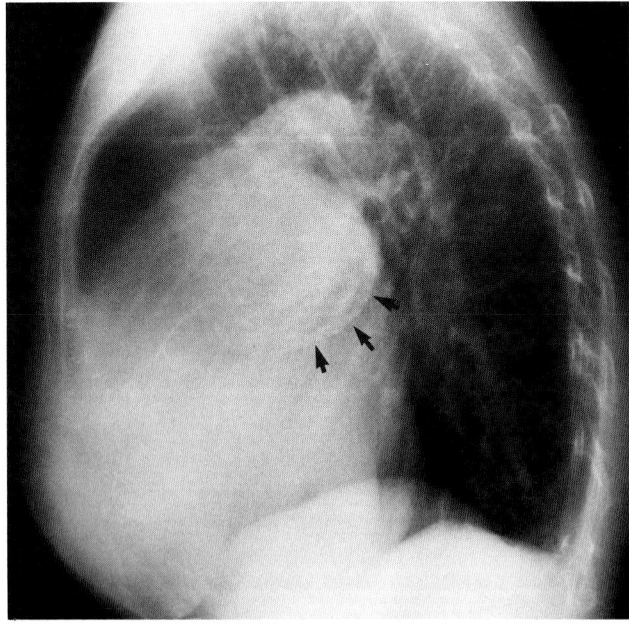

B

Figure 13–5   A 57-year-old woman with severe pulmonary arterial hypertension due to an atrial septal defect. Posteroanterior (*A*) and lateral (*B*) chest radiographs show markedly enlarged central pulmonary arteries that taper rapidly. Calcification can be seen on the pulmonary artery walls (*arrows*), indicating systemic pulmonary arterial pressures.

arterial hypertension in patients with left-to-right shunt. Enlarged central pulmonary arteries in these patients may reflect only increased flow rather than increased pressure, and tapering of peripheral vessels may not be present until the patients have severe pulmonary arterial hypertension (Doyle et al, 1957).

The clinical features of primary pulmonary hypertension (PPH; plexogenic pulmonary arteriopathy) are well documented (Shepherd et al, 1957; Edwards and Edwards, 1978). There is a marked female predominance, except in childhood, when the sex incidence is equal. Patients are young, with the usual age at presentation in the 20s and 30s. Death usually occurs within 2 or 3 years. Cardiac catheterization shows pulmonary hypertension in the face of a normal wedge pressure. Dyspnea is usual and is associated with an angina-like pain and signs of congestive heart failure. Hemoptysis, syncope, and palpitations are less frequent. The electrocardiogram shows evidence of right ventricular hypertrophy. Enlargement of the central pulmonary artery branches that taper rapidly is seen radiologically (Fig. 13–6). The latter is confirmed on angiography with demonstration of vascular "pruning." The histologic changes of primary pulmonary hypertension are the same as those described above for congenital heart disease (Edwards and Edwards, 1978).

By definition, primary pulmonary hypertension is of unknown etiology. Many factors may play a part in this disease, and many diagnoses must be excluded. The Wagenvoorts (1970) studied 156 patients with the diagnosis of primary hypertension and were able to exclude 46 cases on the basis of other histologically recognizable diagnoses. Drugs, including aminorex (Kay et al, 1971a) and Crotalaria (Kay et al, 1971b), have been identified either epidemiologically or by experimental evidence as causing pulmonary hypertension. Genetic factors may play a major role in PPH (Thompson and McRae, 1970; Loyd et al, 1984). Inglesby and coworkers (1973) found abnormally elevated antiplasmin levels in seven of ten members in a four-generation kindred and suggested that the pulmonary hypertension was related to inability to lyse undocumented microthrombi.

Blockage to pulmonary blood flow at the precapillary level can be due to multiple recurrent pulmonary emboli (MRPE). The clinical signs and symptoms depend on the size, number, and location of the emboli; the time interval between embolic episodes; whether vessel occlusion is complete or partial; and on the presence or absence of cardiopulmonary disease. Failure to locate a venous source of emboli does not exclude MRPE. Symptoms may

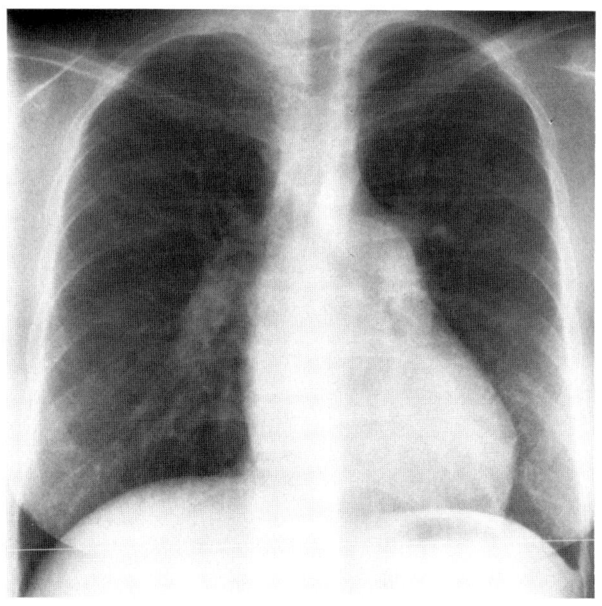

A

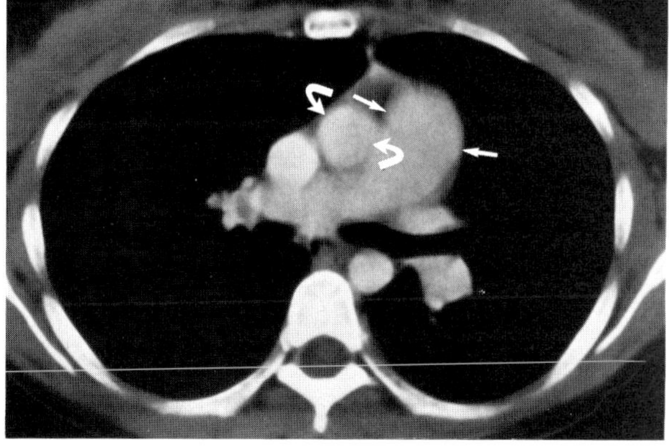

B

Figure 13–6 A 22-year-old woman with primary pulmonary hypertension (PA pressure, 80/40 mm Hg). *A*, Chest radiograph shows enlarged central pulmonary arteries that taper rapidly. *B*, CT scan shows to a better advantage the enlarged main pulmonary artery (*straight arrows*). Compare the diameter of the enlarged pulmonary artery with the normal ascending aorta (*curved arrows*).

range from absent to cardiac arrhythmias, hypotension, and sudden death. Pulmonary hypertension is not sustained until at least 50 to 70 percent of the pulmonary vascular bed is occluded. Obstruction to flow in thromboembolic disease involves muscular arteries rather than the elastic arteries. Although widespread, the lesions are focal in nature and are of varying ages (Edwards and Edwards, 1978). Thus, there may be early thrombi, organized and recanalized vessels, or fibrous bands and intimal plaques marking the site of an embolic episode.

The radiologic findings of pulmonary embolism include pulmonary consolidation, atelectasis, pleural effusion, or elevated hemidiaphragm (Alderson and Martin, 1987). In some cases, pleural-based truncated cone-shaped areas of consolidation ("Hampton hump") and regional areas of hyperlucency due to oligemia (Westermark sign) may be present (Fig. 13–7). The chest radiograph, however, has limited sensitivity and specificity in the diagnosis of acute pulmonary embolism (Greenspan et al, 1982). In acute pulmonary embolism, the diagnosis is usually made by ventilation-perfusion scintigraphy or pulmonary angiography. The combination of multiple segmental perfusion defects and normal ventilation on scintigraphy in areas that are radiographically clear is highly suggestive of pulmonary embolism. However, while scintigraphy is a sensitive method for detection of a localized or diffuse area of decreased pulmonary blood flow, it is nonspecific (Alderson

and Martin, 1987). A definitive diagnosis requires pulmonary angiography. Because angiography is an invasive procedure, it is usually not performed when the pulmonary nuclear medicine scan is highly suggestive of pulmonary embolism. Angiography is indicated, however, when there is a strong clinical suspicion of pulmonary embolism and a low probability or indeterminate ventilation-perfusion scan and in patients with a high probability scan and a contraindication to anticoagulation. Definitive diagnosis of pulmonary embolism on angiography requires the demonstration of intraluminal filling defects or vessel occlusion (Fig. 13–8). Large central emboli may be detected by magnetic resonance imaging (MRI) or computed tomography (CT) (Fig. 13–9).

The majority of patients with pulmonary arterial hypertension from unresolved or recurrent pulmonary embolism have cardiomegaly with right ventricular dilatation and prominent central pulmonary arteries (Woodruff et al, 1985). Localized areas

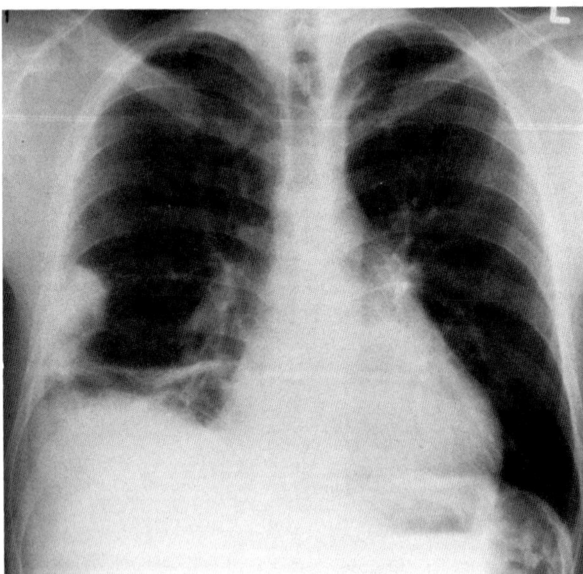

Figure 13–7   A 25-year-old man with pulmonary embolism. Chest radiography shows a pleural-based opacity in the right lower lung zone (Hampton hump) and plate-like atelectasis. The pulmonary angiogram confirmed the diagnosis of pulmonary embolism.

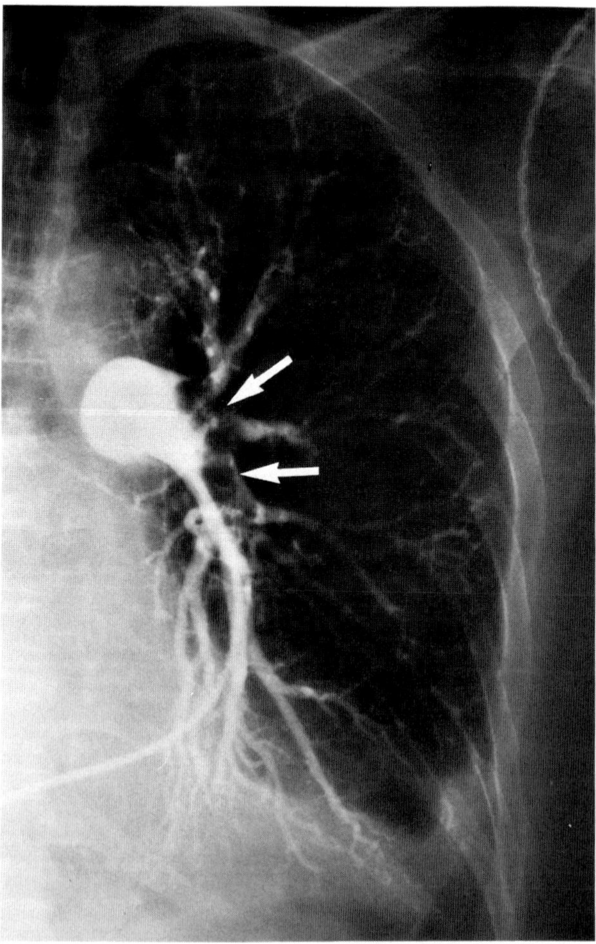

Figure 13–8   Selective left pulmonary angiogram shows large intraluminal filling defect (*arrows*) due to pulmonary embolism.

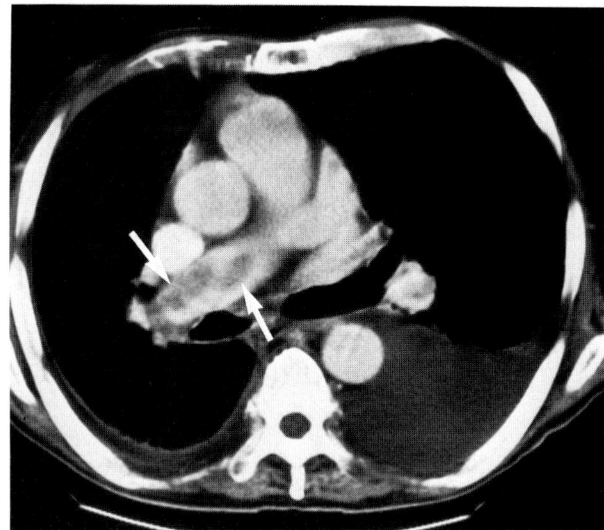

Figure 13–9 A 10-mm collimation CT scan in a 65-year-old man shows a large embolus in the right pulmonary artery (*arrows*). The patient also has bilateral pleural effusions.

of increased lucency due to decreased vascularity (mosaic oligemia) can be seen on the radiograph in 60 percent of cases. The areas of diminished vascularity were shown by pulmonary angiography to correspond to areas with emboli (Woodruff et al, 1985). Other findings such as atelectasis or pleural effusion, often present in patients with acute embolism, are seen in only 20 percent of patients with pulmonary arterial hypertension from recurrent thromboembolism. Definitive diagnosis of pulmonary hypertension due to MRPE traditionally has required the use of pulmonary angiography. Recently CT has been shown to be helpful in the assessment of these patients (Kereiakes et al, 1983). CT with intravenous bolus of contrast material allows differentiation of chronic organized thrombus from vessel walls and delineation of the proximal extent of thrombus. It therefore can be helpful in selecting patients for thromboarterectomy (Kereiakes et al, 1983). CT is well tolerated in patients with severe pulmonary hypertension, in whom the morbidity and mortality of pulmonary angiography are considerably increased.

The distinction between MRPE and PPH is still difficult in some cases. In both conditions, there is thickening of the media of the pulmonary arteries and thrombi are often seen in the vessels. In PPH, there is a decrease in the number of arteries less than 40 μm in dimension, whereas this does not occur in MRPE (Reid, 1979). Concentric laminar intimal fibrosis is characteristic of PPH (Wagenvoort, 1987); however, eccentric intimal fibrosis is not specific for MRPE. Organizing thromboemboli and intravas-

cular fibrous septa (webs) are more in keeping with MRPE. However, organized thrombi can closely resemble fibrotic plexiform lesions in many cases (Bjornsson and Edwards, 1985). Medial disruption as demonstrated by elastin stains are more typical of plexiform lesions than of organized thrombi. The general recommendation is that the diagnosis of MRPE should be made only when thromboembolic occlusive lesions are found which do not resemble plexiform lesions and when classic plexiform and vein-like dilatation lesions are not present (Edwards and Edwards, 1978; Bjornsson and Edwards, 1985). Borderline cases are probably best classified as PPH.

Postcapillary Pulmonary Hypertension

Pulmonary veno-occlusive disease (VOD) typically affects individuals in the first or second decade of life. The clinical presentation is very similar to that of primary pulmonary hypertension, with progressive dyspnea, pulmonary hypertension, and cor pulmonale. Radiographically, VOD is characterized by enlarged central pulmonary arteries with thickened interlobular septa (Kerley B lines) and a normal left atrium (Rubin, 1989). The venous pressure, as assessed by the pulmonary wedge pressure, is sometimes normal but this is quite variable. Histologically the parenchymal abnormalities are often more obvious than the venous changes. Hemosiderosis with alveolar wall thickening and alveolar capillary engorgement are seen. There may be patchy interstitial inflammation and fibrosis, simulating fibrosing alveolitis (Case Records, 1983). Elastin fibers from vessels and from alveolar walls undergo fraying and encrustation with iron and calcium, inciting a foreign-body granulomatous reaction. The diagnostic features are found in veins of various sizes and consist of luminal occlusion by myxoid fibrous tissue (Fig. 13–10). The occlusive lesions may be total or partial; in the latter case, the appearance may be like a recanalized thrombus or eccentric intimal fibrosis. Medial hypertrophy ("arterialization") of veins may be seen. In general, the lesions appear to be old rather than fibrinous and cellular. The variability in venous morphology possibly explains the variability in pulmonary wedge pressures as noted above. Similarly severe degrees of intimal fibrosis are found in the pulmonary arteries in approximately half of patients (Wagenvoort et al, 1985) although plexiform dilatation lesions are not a feature of VOD. It is not clear whether the arterial lesions are secondary to venous obstruction or whether they represent an independent lesion in the disease complex. The vascular changes may be subtle and overshadowed by the other abnormalities; elastin stains are quite useful in these difficult cases.

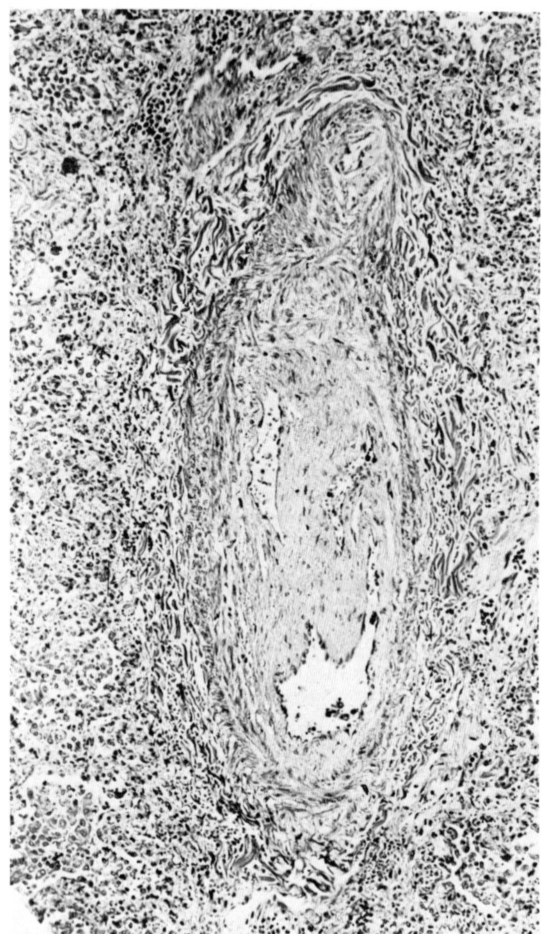

Figure 13–10   Veno-occlusive disease: fibrotic luminal occlusion with appearance of organized thrombus.

The etiology of VOD is unknown, although several associations have been noted (Wagenvoort et al, 1985), including viral infections (Carrington and Liebow, 1970), other infections, autoimmunity, familial predisposition, and toxins. The latter association is believed to be important in cases of VOD in patients treated with cytotoxic drugs (Lombard et al, 1987). It is the general view that VOD is a syndrome with different etiologies, rather than a specific disease with a specific cause.

FOREIGN BODY EMBOLI

On occasion, one may find foreign-body granulomas in pulmonary arteries due to contamination of catheters or intravenous fluid solutions, but these are typically incidental findings (Heath and Smith, 1988). In instances of intravenous drug abuse, contamination of drugs by talc or other foreign material may lead to massive perivascular foreign-body reaction and clinical pulmonary hypertension (Tomashefski and Hirsch, 1980). In florid cases, the lungs are grossly gritty and nodular (Fig. 13–11). Angiothrombosis and foreign-body granulomas with birefringent material are the characteristic histologic findings. Plexiform lesions are not found.

Figure 13–11   Diffuse nodular foreign body (talc) granulomas in a drug addict. *A,* Scanning view shows diffuse fine nodularity. *B,* Each nodule consists of foreign body reaction.

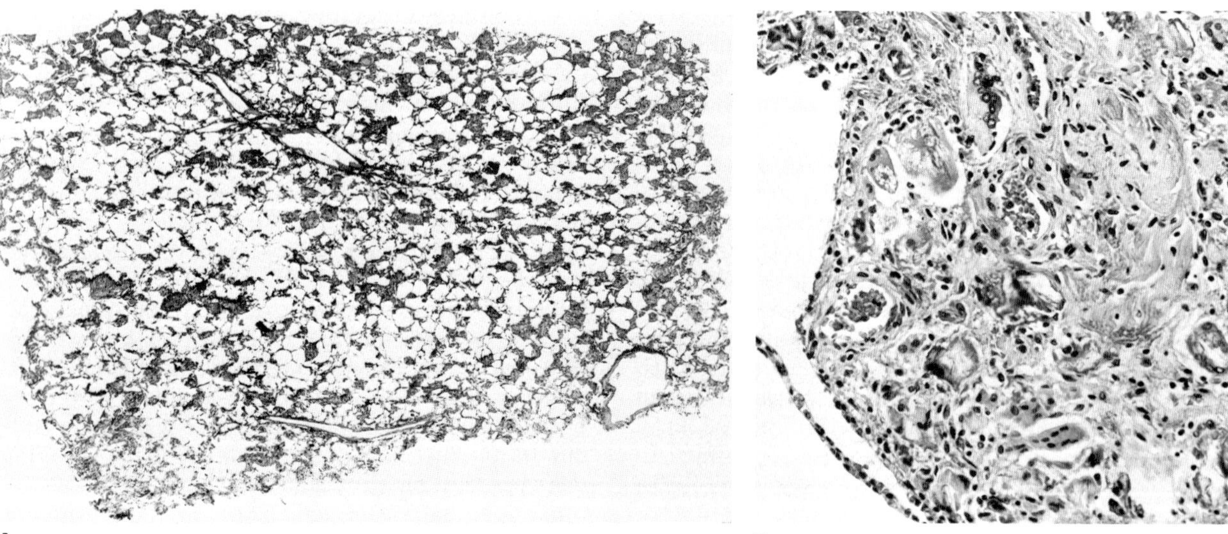

A

B

OTHER EMBOLIC LESIONS

Fat, air, amniotic fluid, and trophoblast emboli are all well-described phenomena, much more likely to be seen at autopsy than at lung biopsy.

Bone marrow emboli are associated with skeletal trauma, and particularly with chest trauma including surgery (Heath and Smith, 1988). We have seen several cases of bone marrow emboli in open lung biopsies, presumably due to the relatively minor trauma from the rib spreader. These emboli had no apparent postoperative clinical significance.

Brain emboli are occasionally seen in patients with severe head injury (Fig. 13–12) (Torry, 1987). The implication of such an event in the setting of lung transplantation is uncertain.

Tumor emboli are a common pathogenetic factor in the development of metastatic disease. Rarely, massive tumor emboli can result in bilateral radio-

logic lesions, pulmonary hypertension, and cor pulmonale (Fildes et al, 1988; Benditt and Celli, 1990).

Leukemic cell thrombi can result in respiratory distress and bilateral infiltrates (Tryka et al, 1982; Myers et al, 1983). Such patients usually have nonlymphocytic leukemia with leukocyte counts in excess of 100,000 per cubic millimeter, and the crisis occurs within hours to a few days of initiation of chemotherapy. The diagnostic feature pathologically is the presence of plugs of degenerating leukemic cells in small arteries, veins, and capillaries. Edema, infarcts, and diffuse alveolar damage may also be present.

REFERENCES

Alderson PO, Martin EC. Pulmonary embolism: diagnosis with multiple imaging modalities. Radiology 1987; 164:297–312.

Benditt JO, Celli B. Bilateral pleural-based densities in a patient with hip pain. Chest 1990; 97:467–468.

Bjornsson J, Edwards WD. Primary pulmonary hypertension: a histopathologic study of 80 cases. Mayo Clin Proc 1985; 60:16–25.

Carrington CB, Liebow AA. Pulmonary veno-occlusive disease. Hum Pathol 1970; 1:322–324.

Case Records of the Massachusetts General Hospital, 14–1983. N Engl J Med 1983; 308:823–834.

Doyle AE, Goodwin JF, Harrison CV, Steiner RE. Pulmonary vascular patterns in pulmonary hypertension. Br Heart J 1957; 19:353–365.

Edwards WD, Edwards JE. Recent advances in the pathology of the pulmonary vasculature. In: Thurlbeck WM, Abell MR, eds. The lung: structure, function and disease. Baltimore: Williams & Wilkins, 1978.

Fildes J, Narvaez GP, Baig KA, et al. Pulmonary tumor embolization after peritoneovenous shunting for malignant ascites. Cancer 1988; 61:1973–1976.

Greenspan RH, Ravin CE, Polansky SM, McCloud TC. Accuracy of the chest radiograph in diagnosis of pulmonary embolism. Invest Radiol 1982; 17:539–543.

Haworth SG, Reid L. A morphometric study of regional variation of lung structure in infants with pulmonary hypertension and congenital cardiac defect: a justification of lung biopsy. Br Heart J 1978; 40:825–831.

Heath D, Edwards JE. The pathology of hyperactive pulmonary vascular disease: a description of six grades of structural changes in the pulmonary arteries with special reference to congenital cardiac septal defects. Circulation 1958; 18:533–547.

Heath D, Smith P. Disorders of the vascular system. In: Thurlbeck WM ed. Pathology of the lung. New York: Thieme, 1988.

Inglesby TV, Singer JW, Gordon DS. Abnormal fibrinolysis in familial pulmonary hypertension. Am J Med 1973; 55:5–14.

Kay JM, Heath D, Smith P, et al. Fulvine and the pulmonary circulation. Thorax 1971b; 26:249–261.

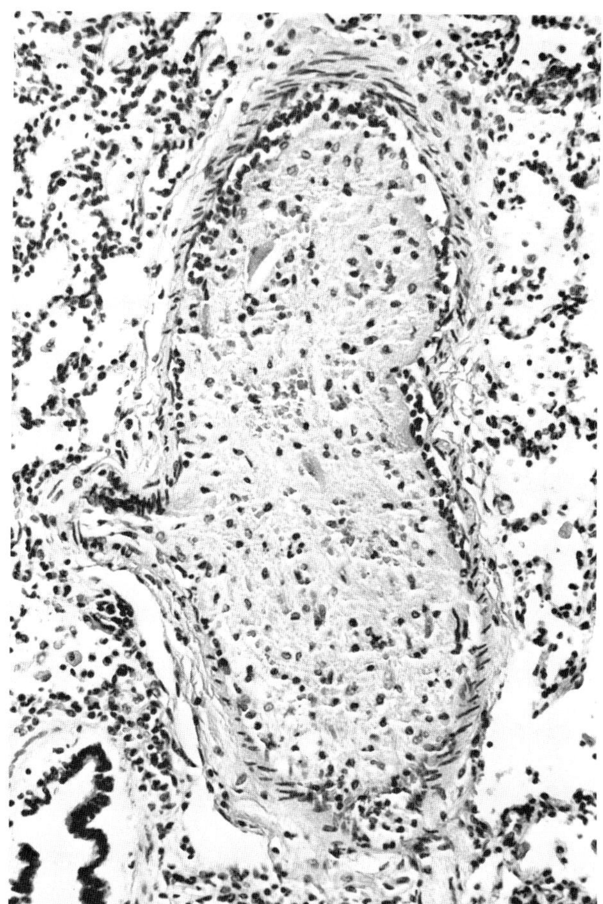

Figure 13–12 Brain embolus in a child dying after severe head trauma.

Kay JM, Smith P, Heath D. Aminorex and the pulmonary circulation. Thorax 1971a; 26:262–270.

Kerciakes DJ, Herfkens RJ, Brundage BH, et al. Computerized tomography in chronic thromboembolic pulmonary hypertension. Am Heart J 1983; 106:1432–1436.

Langston C, Holder P. Pulmonary vascular changes in infants and children. In: Will JA, Dawson CA, Weir EK, Buckner CK, eds. The pulmonary circulation in health and disease. Orlando, FL: Academic Press, 1987:57.

Lombard CM, Churg A, Winokur S. Pulmonary veno-occlusive disease following therapy for malignant neoplasms. Chest 1987; 92:871–876.

Loyd JE, Primm RK, Newman JH. Familial primary pulmonary hypertension: clinical patterns. Am Rev Respir Dis 1984; 129:194–197.

Myers TJ, Cole SR, Klatsky AU, Hild DH. Respiratory failure due to pulmonary leukostasis following chemotherapy of acute nonlymphocytic leukemia. Cancer 1983; 51:1808–1813.

Rabinovitch M, Haworth SG, Vance Z, et al. Early pulmonary vascular changes in congenital heart disease studied in biopsy tissue. Hum Pathol 1980; 11:499–509.

Rees S. The chest radiograph in pulmonary hypertension with central shunt. Br J Radiol 1968; 41:172–179.

Reid LM. The pulmonary circulation: remodeling in growth and disease. Am Rev Respir Dis 1979; 119:531–546.

Rubin LJ. Approach to the diagnosis and treatment of pulmonary hypertension. Chest 1989; 96:659–664.

Shepherd JT, Edwards JE, Burchell HB, et al. Clinical, physiologic and pathologic considerations in patients with idiopathic pulmonary hypertension. Br Heart J 1957; 19:70-82.

Thompson P, McRae C. Familial pulmonary hypertension: evidence of autosomal dominant inheritance. Br Heart J 1970; 32:758–760.

Tomashefski JF, Hirsch CS. The pulmonary vascular lesions of intravenous drug abuse. Hum Pathol 1980; 11:133–145.

Torry JM. Massive brain tissue and fat pulmonary embolism following severe head injury. Med Sci Law 1987; 27:128–131.

Tryka AF, Godleski JJ, Fanta CH. Leukemic cell lysis pneumopathy. Cancer 1982; 50:2763–2770.

Wagenvoort CA. The pathology of human pulmonary hypertension: pattern recognition and specificity. In: Will JA, Dawson CA, Weir EK, Buckner CK, eds. The pulmonary circulation in health and disease. Orlando, FL: Academic Press, 1987:15.

Wagenvoort CA, Wagenvoort N. Primary pulmonary hypertension: a pathologic study of the lung vessels in 156 clinically diagnosed cases. Circulation 1970; 42:1163–1184.

Wagenvoort CA, Wagenvoort N, Takahashi T. Pulmonary veno-occlusive disease: involvement of pulmonary arteries and review of the literature. Hum Pathol 1985; 16:1033–1041.

Woodruff WW, Hoeck BE, Chitwood Jr WR, et al. Radiographic findings in pulmonary hypertension from unresolved embolism. AJR 1985; 144:681–686.

Index

G

Gallium-67 scanning, in diffuse lung disease, 35–36
Gas exchange, measurements of, 10
Generation, airway, cross section of, *2*
Goblet cells, 2, *3*
Goodpasture's syndrome. *See* Antiglomerular basement
    membrane disease (AGBMD)
Graft-versus-host disease
    bronchiolitis and, 213–214, *215*
    in immunocompromised hosts, 87, *87–88*
Granuloma
    eosinophilic, *42*
    foreign-body, in pulmonary arteries, 234, *234*
    in respiratory bronchioles, *41*
    round, in coccidiomycosis, *42*
Granulomatosis, 169–188
    bronchocentric, 182–186, *184, 185*
        in allergic bronchopulmonary aspergillosis, *58*
        description, 182–183
    lymphomatoid, 162, 177–182
        clinical features, 177–178
        histologic findings, 180, *180–181*
        and lymphoma, distinguishing features, 178
        and necrotizing sarcoidal granulomatosis, distinguishing
            features, 182
        prognosis, 182
        radiologic findings, 178, *179*
    necrotizing sarcoidal, 176–177
        characteristics, 176
        clinical findings, 176
        description, 117–118
        diagnosis, 177
        and lymphomatoid granulomatosis, distinguishing features,
            182
        radiologic findings, 176–177, *176–177*
        and sarcoidosis, distinguishing features, 177
    Wegener's. *See* Wegener's granulomatosis

H

Hamartoma, leiomyomatous, and benign metastasizing
    leiomyoma, comparison, 167
Heart-lung transplantation, and chronic airway obstruction, 214,
    216, *216*
Hemorrhage
    in diffuse lung disease, 26
    diffuse pulmonary, 93–100
        angiosarcomas and, *97*
        causes, 95, *95*, 97–98
        and collagen vascular disease, 96
        description, 94
        in immunocompromised hosts, 89, 98–99
        and mixed collagen vascular disease, *94*
        in nonimmunocompromised hosts, 95–98
        in SLE, 142
Hemosiderosis, idiopathic pulmonary, in
    nonimmunocompromised hosts, 96–97, *97*
Herpes simplex virus (HSV), in immunocompromised hosts, 71,
    71–72
Herpes varicella-zoster, in immunocompromised hosts, 71–72
Histiocytosis X, 120, *121*
Histoplasma capsulatum, and pulmonary disease, 81–82, *82*
Histoplasmosis, in immunocompromised hosts, 81–82, *82*
Hodgkin's disease, lung involvement in, 161, *162*
Hyperplasia, lymphoid, with germinal centers, in rheumatoid
    arthritis, 142, *143*

Hypertension, pulmonary
    arterial, 228–234
    postcapillary, 233–234, *234*
    precapillary, 228–233
    primary, *43*
        causes, 231
        clinical features, 231, *231*
        and multiple recurrent pulmonary emboli, distinguishing
            features, 233
        symptoms, 231–232
    in rheumatoid arthritis, 142
    types, 228

I

Idiopathic pulmonary fibrosis, description, 26
Immotile cilia syndrome, 221–222
Immunocompromised hosts
    acute infiltrative lung disease in, 65–91
        differential diagnosis, 66–71, 66t
    bacterial infections in, 75–77
    diffuse pulmonary hemorrhage in, 89, 98–99
    drug reactions in, 85–86
    fungal infections in, 77–81
    graft-versus-host disease in, 87, *87–88*
    lung biopsy in, 36–37, 66–71
    mycobacterial infections in, 77
    protozoal infections in, 82–85
    pulmonary alveolar proteinosis in, 89
    radiation pneumonitis in, 86–87
    tumors in, 89
    viral infections in, 71–75
Infections
    bacterial, in immunocompromised hosts, 75–77
    fungal, in immunocompromised hosts, 77–81
    in immunocompromised hosts, 66, 75–85
    of the lung
        bacterial, 49–53
        fungal, 55–58, *57–58*
        viral, 53–55, 53t, *54, 55*
    and lung disease, 23
    mycobacterial, in immunocompromised hosts, 77
    protozoal, in immunocompromised hosts, 82–85
    viral
        in immunocompromised hosts, 71–75
        irritants and, 212
Infiltrative lung disease
    acute
        biopsy, 36–37
        in immunocompromised hosts, 65–91
            differential diagnosis, 66–71, 66t
        in nonimmunocompromised hosts, 45–63
    chronic, 101–138
        biopsy, 37–38, 37t
        causes, 102t
    diffuse
        ARDS in, 23
        biopsy, 33–44
        causes, 19t, 20
        chest radiograph in, 34
        clinical approach, 18–26
        connective tissue disease and, 24–26
        CT in, 34–35
        definition, 14
        diagnosis, tissue sample in, 21t
        differential diagnosis, 19t, 22–26, 26t, 28t
            radiographic patterns in, 25t